TOP TRAILS™

San Francisco Bay Area

MUST-DO HIKES FOR EVERYONE

Written by
David Weintraub and Ben Pease

Series edited by
Joe Walowski

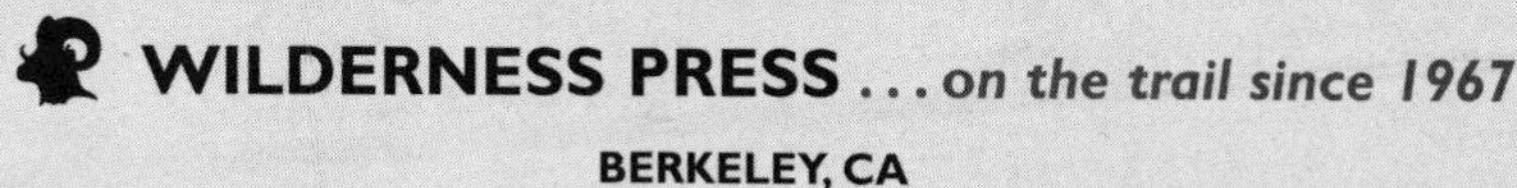

BERKELEY, CA

Top Trails San Francisco Bay Area: Must-Do Hikes for Everyone

1st EDITION 2004
2nd EDITION 2009

Maps: Pease Press and Fineline Maps
Cover design: Frances Baca Design and Andreas Schueller
Interior design: Frances Baca Design
Typesetting and composition: Lapiz Digital

ISBN: 978-0-89997-484-2

Manufactured in the United States of America

Published by: **Wilderness Press**
1345 8th Street
Berkeley, CA 94710
(800) 443-7227; FAX (510) 558-1696
info@wildernesspress.com
www.wildernesspress.com
Visit our Web site for a complete listing of our books and for ordering information.

The Top Trails™ Series

Wilderness Press

When Wilderness Press published *Sierra North* in 1967, no other trail guide like it existed for the Sierra backcountry. The first print run sold out in less than two months, and its success heralded the beginning of Wilderness Press. Since we were founded more than 40 years ago, we have expanded our territories to cover California, Alaska, Hawaii, the US Southwest, the Pacific Northwest, the Midwest, the Southeast, New England, Canada, and Baja California.

Wilderness Press continues to publish comprehensive, accurate, and readable outdoor books. Hikers, backpackers, kayakers, skiers, snowshoers, climbers, cyclists, and trail runners rely on Wilderness Press for accurate outdoor adventure information.

Top Trails

In its Top Trails guides, Wilderness Press has paid special attention to organization so that you can find the perfect hike each and every time. Whether you're looking for a steep trail to test yourself on or a walk in the park, a romantic waterfall or a city view, Top Trails will lead you there.

Each Top Trails guide contains trails for everyone. The trails selected provide a sampling of the best that the region has to offer. These are the "must-do" hikes, walks, runs, and bike rides, with every feature of the area represented.

Every book in the Top Trails series offers:

- The Wilderness Press commitment to accuracy and reliability
- Ratings and rankings for each trail
- Distances and approximate times
- Easy-to-follow trail notes
- Maps and permit information

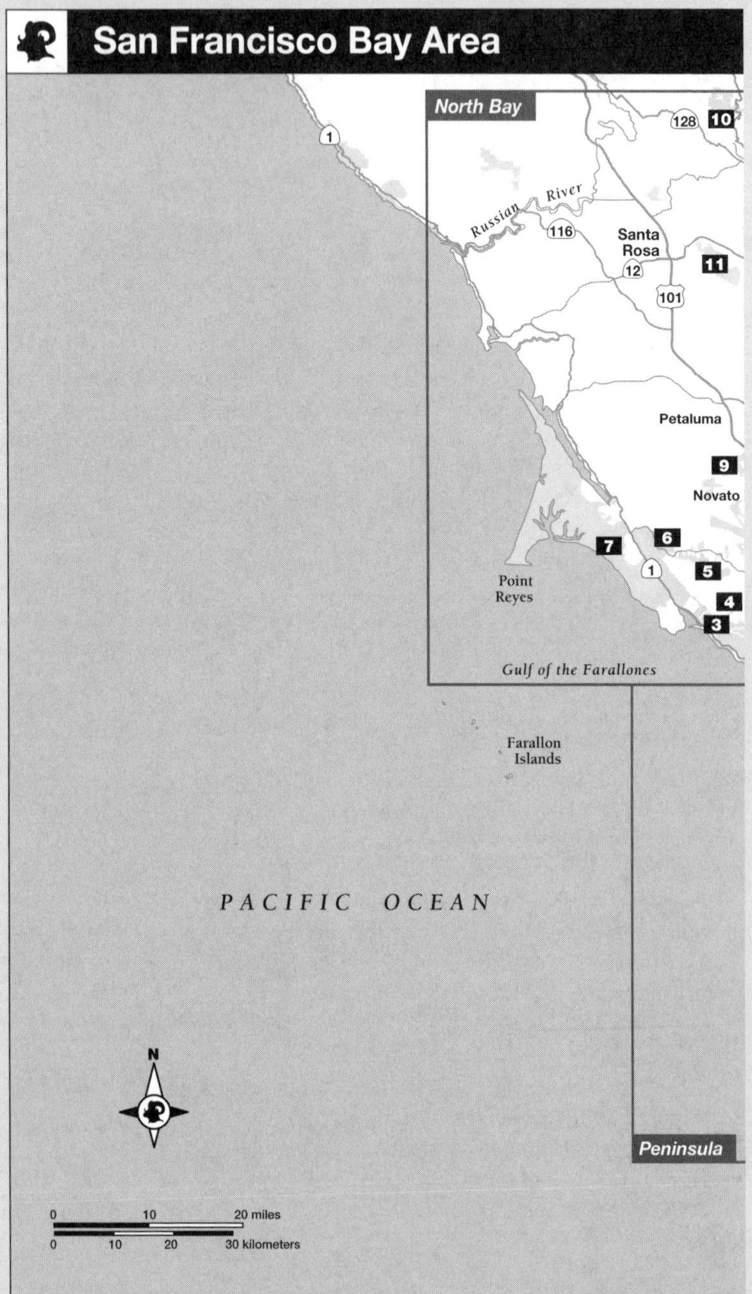
San Francisco Bay Area
North Bay
1
128
10
Russian River
116
Santa Rosa
12
11
101
Petaluma
9
Novato
6
7
1
5
Point Reyes
4
3
Gulf of the Farallones
Farallon Islands
PACIFIC OCEAN
N
Peninsula
0 10 20 miles
0 10 20 30 kilometers

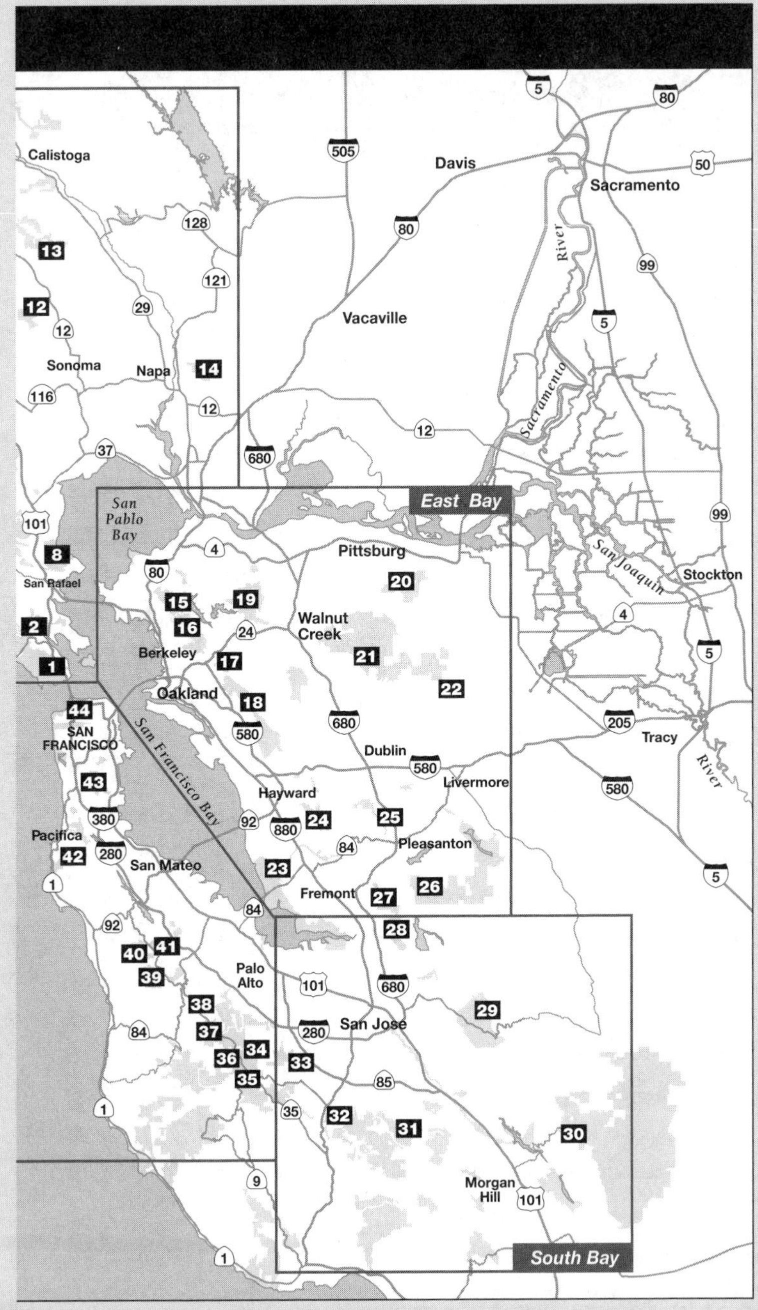
Calistoga
Sonoma
Napa
San Rafael
Davis
Sacramento
Vacaville
Sacramento River
San Pablo Bay
East Bay
Pittsburg
Stockton
San Joaquin River
Walnut Creek
Berkeley
Oakland
SAN FRANCISCO
San Francisco Bay
Tracy
Dublin
Livermore
Hayward
Pacifica
Pleasanton
San Mateo
Fremont
Palo Alto
San José
Morgan Hill
South Bay
1
2
8
12
13
14
15
16
17
18
19
20
21
22
23
24
25
26
27
28
29
30
31
32
33
34
35
36
37
38
39
40
41
42
43
44

San Francisco Bay Area Trails

TRAIL NUMBER & NAME	Page	Difficulty –12345+	Length in Miles	Type	Hiking	Running	Biking	Child Friendly
1. NORTH BAY								
1 Marin Headlands: Gerbode Valley	27	3	5.4	↺	✓	✓	✓	
2 Muir Woods Nat'l. Monument: Dipsea Trail	33	3	4.0	↺	✓			
3 Mount Tamalpais: High Marsh Loop	39	4	5.8	↺	✓	✓		
4 Mount Tamalpais: Middle Peak	47	3	5.1	↺	✓	✓		
5 Pine Mountain	53	3	4.7	↗	✓	✓	✓	
6 Samuel P. Taylor State Park	57	4	6.5	↺	✓	✓		
7 Point Reyes National Seashore: Sky Trail	61	5	10.5	↺	✓	✓		
8 China Camp State Park	67	4	8.4	↺	✓	✓	✓	
9 Mt. Burdell Open Space Preserve	73	4	5.6	↺	✓	✓	✓ [1]	✓
10 Mount St. Helena	79	5	10.6	↗	✓	✓	✓ [1]	
11 Annadel State Park: Lake Ilsanjo	85	4	8.8	↺	✓	✓	✓	
12 Jack London State Historic Park	91	3	2.9	↺	✓	✓		✓
13 Sugarloaf Ridge State Park	97	5	6.7	↺	✓	✓		
14 Skyline Wilderness Park	101	4	6.0	↗	✓	✓		
2. EAST BAY								
15 Wildcat Canyon Regional Park	117	4	7.0	↺	✓	✓	✓	
16 Tilden Regional Park: Wildcat Peak	123	3	3.3	↺	✓	✓		✓
17 Sibley Volcanic Regional Preserve	129	2	1.8	↺	✓	✓		✓
18 Redwood Regional Park: East Ridge	135	3	6.0	↺	✓	✓		
19 Briones Regional Park: Briones Crest	141	4	6.8	↺	✓	✓	✓	
20 Black Diamond Mines Regional Preserve	147	4	7.6	↺	✓	✓	✓ [1]	
21 Mount Diablo State Park: Grand Loop	155	5	6.5	↺	✓	✓	✓ [1]	
22 Morgan Territory Regional Preserve	163	4	5.9	↺	✓	✓	✓ [1]	
23 Coyote Hills Regional Park: Red Hill	169	2	1.0	↺	✓	✓	✓ [1]	✓
24 Dry Creek Pioneer Regional Park	173	4	5.7	↺	✓	✓	✓ [1]	
25 Pleasanton Ridge Regional Park	179	5	12.3	↺	✓	✓	✓	
26 Sunol Regional Wilderness	185	4	5.9	↺	✓	✓	✓ [1]	
27 Mission Peak Regional Preserve	191	5	6.3	↗	✓	✓	✓	

Dogs Allowed	Permit	Fee	River/Stream	Waterfall	Lake	Canyon	Mountain	Summit	Autumn Color	Wildflowers	Birds	Wildlife	Historic	Geologic Interest	Great Views	Photo Opportunity	Secluded	Cool & Shady	Camping	Steep
USES & ACCESS			**TERRAIN**						**FLORA & FAUNA**				**OTHER**							
								●		●	●				●	●			●	
			●			●					●		●					●		
●			●	●		●	●				●						●	●		
●		●	●			●	●				●				●			●		
●							●	●			●				●	●	●			
			●			●	●			●	●				●		●			
			●						●	●	●				●			●	●	
		●									●				●			●	●	
●					●		●			●	●				●	●				
							●	●			●		●	●	●		●			●
					●				●		●	●					●	●		
		●			●					●	●		●		●		●	●		
		●					●	●		●	●				●				●	
		●					●			●	●				●		●			
●			●			●		●		●	●	●			●	●				
			●			●	●	●			●				●					
●											●			●	●					
●		●	●								●				●					
●		●			●			●		●	●				●	●				
●		●					●			●	●		●	●			●		●	
		●					●	●		●	●		●		●	●	●		●	
●						●			●		●				●		●			
●		●			●			●		●	●				●	●				
●		●			●			●			●	●			●		●			
●			●			●		●		●	●				●	●	●			
●	●					●		●		●	●				●		●			
●							●				●				●					●

San Francisco Bay Area Trails

USES & ACCESS
- Hiking
- Running
- Biking
- Child Friendly
- Dogs Allowed
- $ Fee
- Permit Required

TYPE
- Loop
- Out & Back
- Point to Point

DIFFICULTY
–12345+
less — more

TERRAIN
- River or Stream
- Waterfall
- Lake or Shore
- Canyon
- Mountain
- Summit

FLORA & FAUNA
- Autumn Colors
- Wildflowers
- Birds
- Wildlife

OTHER
- Historic
- Geologic Interest
- Great Views
- Photo Opportunity
- Secluded
- Cool & Shady
- Camping
- Steep

[1] *Bicyclists use described alternate trails or trailheads*

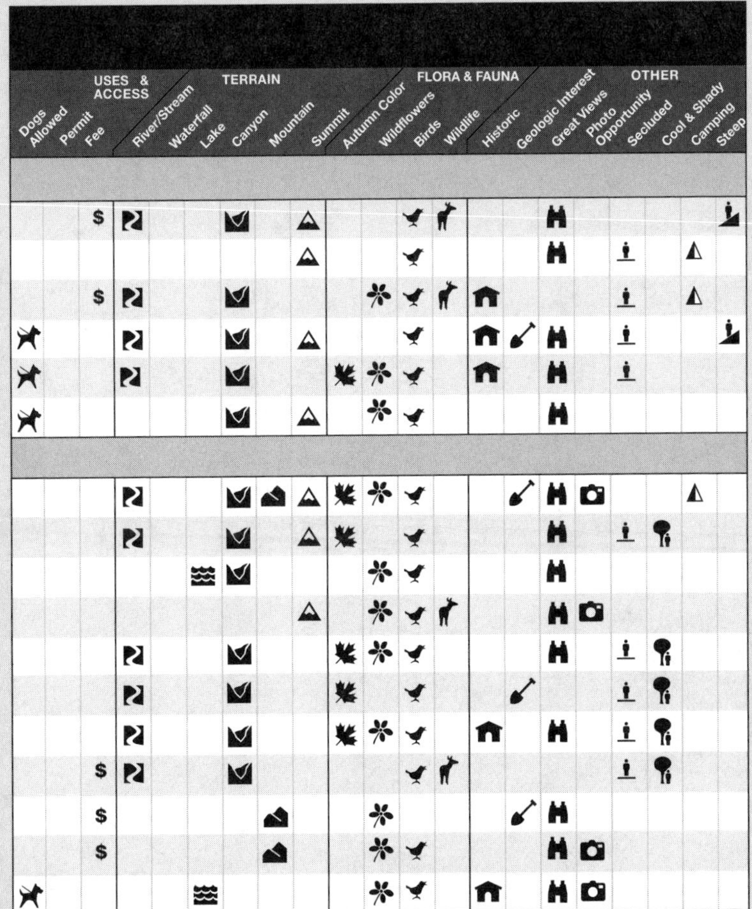
USES & ACCESS
Dogs Allowed
Permit
Fee
TERRAIN
River/Stream
Waterfall
Lake
Canyon
Mountain
Summit
FLORA & FAUNA
Autumn Color
Wildflowers
Birds
Wildlife
OTHER
Historic
Geologic Interest
Great Views
Photo Opportunity
Secluded
Cool & Shady
Camping
Steep
$
$
$
$
$
$

Contents

Using Top Trails™

Organization of Top Trails

Top Trails is designed so you can find the perfect trail and make every outing a success and a pleasure. With this guide you'll find it's a snap to find the right trail, whether you're planning a major hike or just a sociable stroll with friends.

The Region

At the very front of this guide, the **San Francisco Bay Area regional map** (pages iv–v) provides a geographic overview of the San Francisco Bay Area, and shows the areas covered by each chapter. The adjacent **Bay Area Trails table** (pages vi-ix) lists every trail covered in this guide along with attributes for each trail. A quick reading of the regional map and the trails table gives you a quick overview of the entire region covered by the guide.

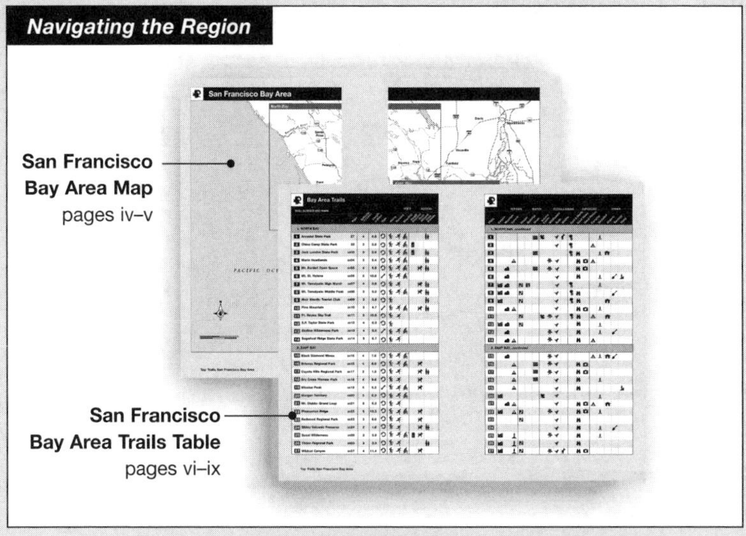

The Areas

The region covered in each guide is divided into areas, with each chapter corresponding to one area in the region. Each area chapter starts with information to help you choose and enjoy a trail every time out. Use the table of contents or the regional map to identify an area of interest, then turn to the area chapter to find the following information:

- An overview of the area's parks and trails
- An area map showing trail locations
- A trail feature table providing trail-by-trail details
- Trail summaries highlighting each trail's special features

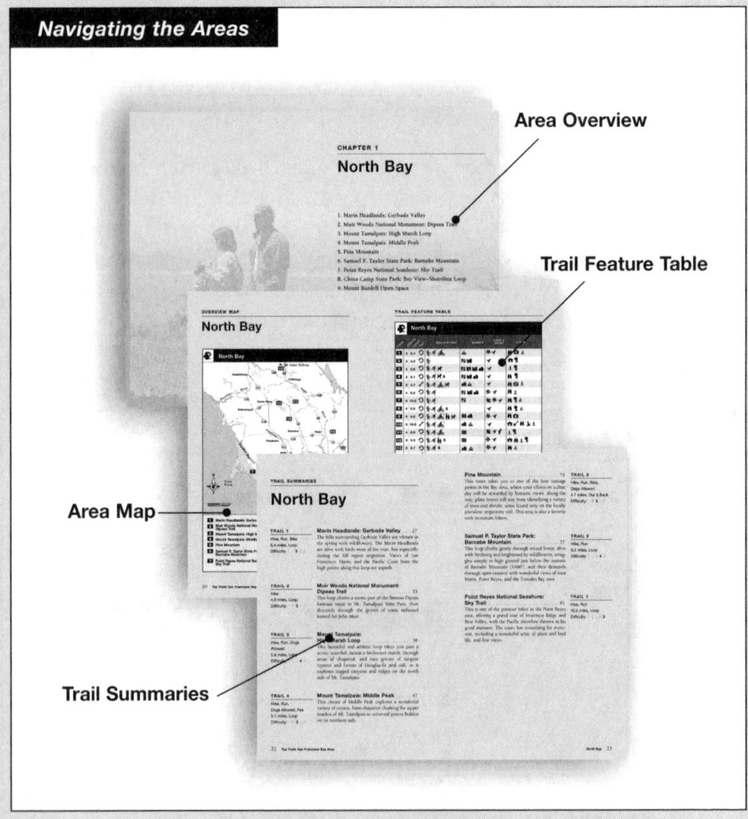

The Trails

The basic building block of the Top Trails guide is the trail entry. Each one is arranged to make finding and following the trail as simple as possible, with all pertinent information presented in this easy-to-follow format:

- A detailed trail map
- Trail descriptors covering difficulty, length, and other essential data
- A written trail description
- Trail milestones providing easy-to-follow, turn-by-turn trail directions

Some trail descriptions offer additional information:

- An elevation profile
- Trail options
- Trail highlights

In the margins of the Trail Entries, keep your eyes open for graphic icons that signal features mentioned in the text.

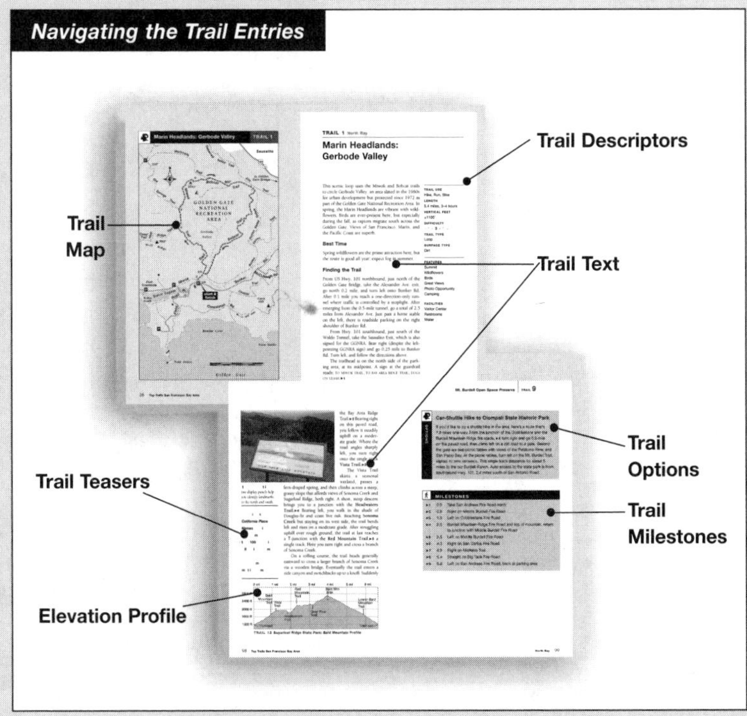

Choosing a Trail

Top Trails provides several different ways of choosing a trail, using easy-to-read tables and maps.

Location

If you know in general where you want to go, Top Trails makes it easy to find the right trail in the right place. Each chapter begins with a large-scale map showing the starting point of every trail in that area.

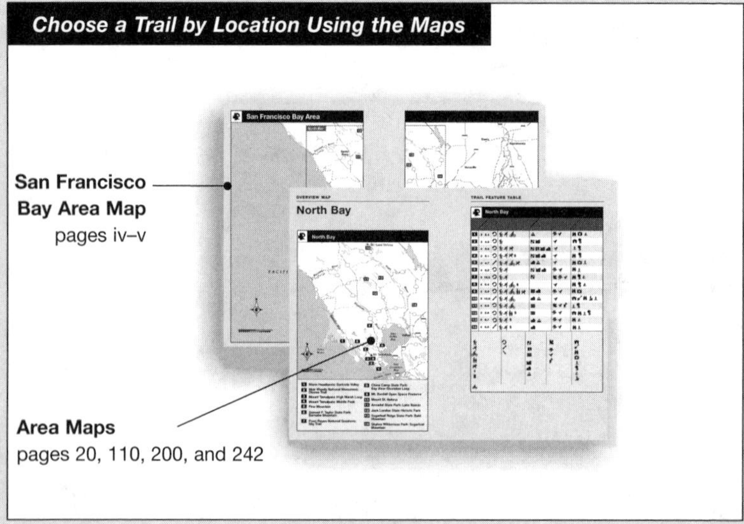

Features

This guide describes the top trails of the San Francisco Bay Area. Each trail has been chosen because it offers one or more features that make it interesting. Using the trail descriptors, summaries, and tables, you can quickly examine all the trails to find out what features they offer, or seek a particular feature among the list of trails. Included here is information about park fees. Some parks charge fees seasonally or only when the park's entrance kiosk is attended; others have self-registration stations. Where dogs are allowed, there may be an additional fee.

Best Time

Time of year and current conditions can be important factors in selecting the best trail. For example, an exposed grassland trail may be a riot of color in early spring, but an oven-baked taste of hell in midsummer. Other trails may be cool and shady all year. Where relevant, Top Trails identifies the best and worst conditions for the trails you plan to visit.

Difficulty

Each trail has an overall difficulty on a scale of 1 to 5, which takes into consideration length, elevation change, exposure, trail quality, and more to create one (admittedly subjective) rating.

The difficulty ratings assume you are an able-bodied adult in reasonably good shape using the trail for hiking. The ratings also assume normal weather conditions—clear and dry.

Readers should make an honest assessment of their own abilities and adjust time estimates accordingly. Also rain, snow, heat, mud, and poor visibility can all affect the pace on even the easiest of trails.

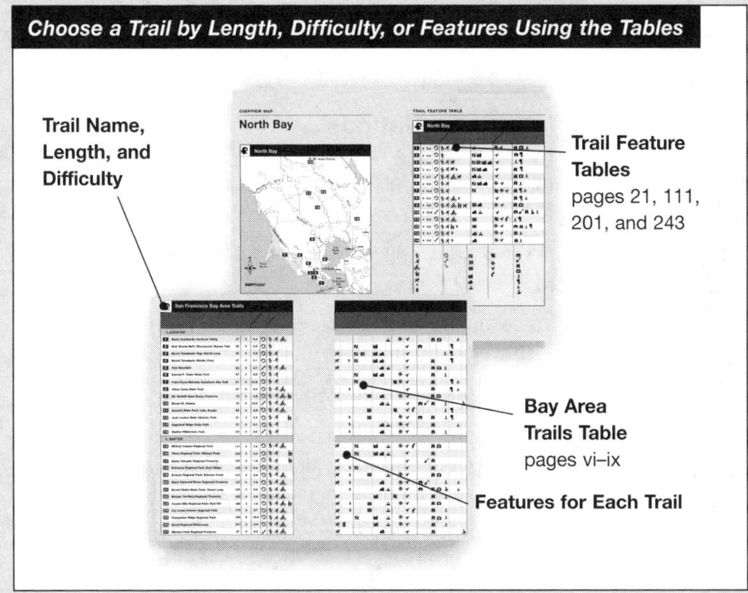

Vertical Feet

Elevation change is often underestimated by hikers and bikers when gauging the difficulty of a trail. Vertical feet accounts for all elevation change, not simply the difference between the highest and lowest points, so that rolling terrain with lots of up and down is not ignored.

For routes that begin and end at the same spot—i.e., loop or out and back—the vertical gain exactly matches the vertical descent. With a point-to-point route the vertical gain and loss will most likely differ, and both figures are provided in the text.

The more strenuous routes have an **elevation profile,** an easy means for visualizing the topography of a route. These profiles graphically depict the elevation throughout the length of the trail.

Surface Type

Each trail entry provides information about the surface of the trail. This is useful in determining what type of footwear or bicycle is appropriate. Surface type should also be considered when checking the weather—on a rainy day a dirt surface can be a muddy slog; an asphalt surface might be a better choice (although asphalt can be slick when wet).

Top Trails Difficulty Ratings

1 A short trail, generally level, which can be completed in 1 hour or less.

2 A route of 1 to 3 miles, with some up and down, which can be completed in 1 to 2 hours.

3 A longer route, up to 5 miles, with uphill and/or downhill sections.

4 A long or steep route, perhaps more than 5 miles, or climbs of more than 1000 vertical feet.

5 The most severe route, both long and steep, more than 5 miles long, with climbs of more than 1000 vertical feet.

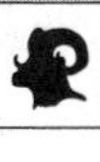

Map Legend

Trail	Stream
Trail Option	Seasonal Stream
Other Trails	Body of Water
Freeway	Dam
Major Road	Marsh/Swamp
Minor Road	Park/Preserve
Tunnel	Boundary
Bridge	Milestones 1 2 3 4
Trailhead Parking P	North Arrow N
Picnic Area	Start/Finish start & finish
Camping	
Gate	
Building	
Point of Interest	
Peak	

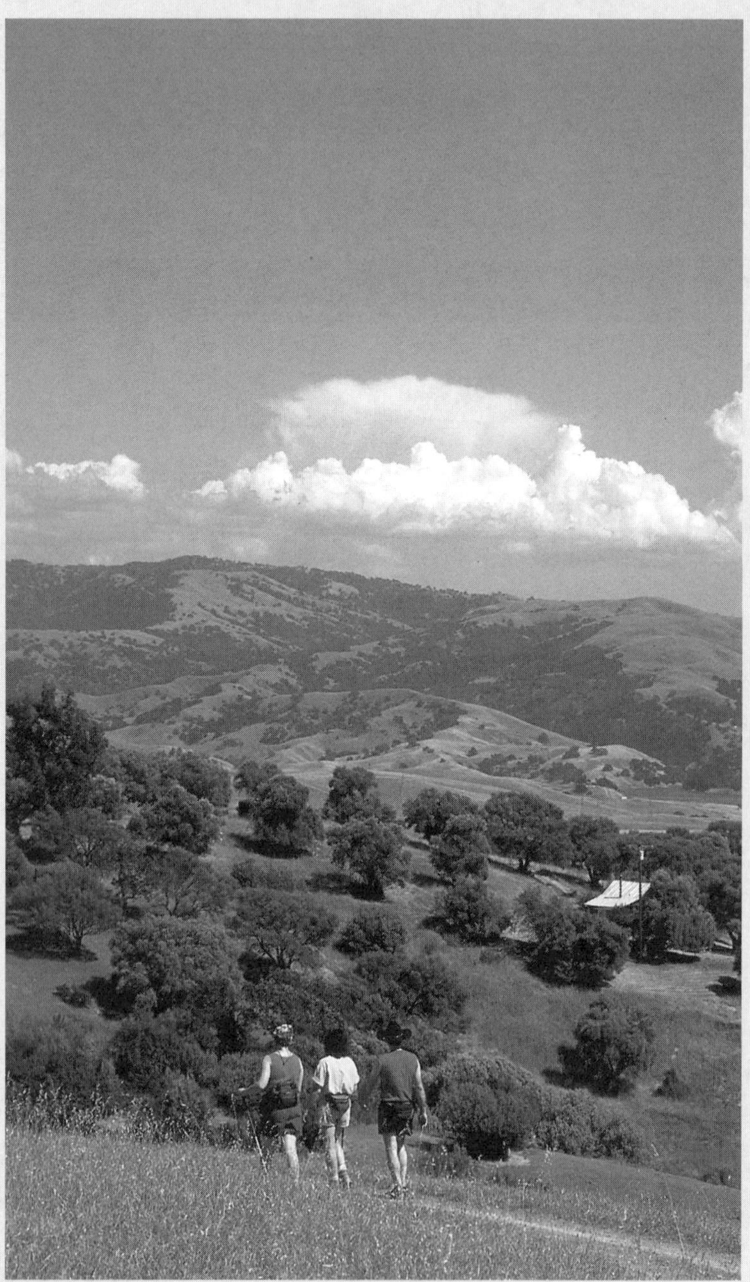

Pleasanton Ridge *(Trail 25)*

Introduction to the San Francisco Bay Area

The Bay Area is usually divided into four regions—**North Bay, East Bay, South Bay**, and **Peninsula**—and this guide follows that scheme, making a roughly clockwise circuit of the Bay, starting at the Golden Gate. The North Bay includes Marin, Napa, and Sonoma counties; the East Bay consists of Alameda and Contra Costa counties; the South Bay takes in most of Santa Clara County; and the Peninsula covers San Francisco, San Mateo, and the northwestern part of Santa Clara County. Within the Bay Area are bustling urban areas such as San Francisco, Oakland, San Jose, and Silicon Valley, along with tranquil forests, mountains, beaches, marshes, and farmlands.

The parks and open spaces here are administered by an alphabet soup of local, state, and federal agencies, including California State Parks (CSP); East Bay Regional Park District (EBRPD); Golden Gate National Recreation Area (GGNRA); Midpeninsula Regional Open Space District (MROSD); Santa Clara County Parks and Recreation; San Mateo County Parks; Marin Municipal Water District (MMWD); and Marin County Open Space District (MCOSD).

Geography

The San Francisco Bay Area is distinguished by its rolling hills, grassy valleys, and rugged mountain ranges, all encircling a great body of water, San Francisco and San Pablo bays, and bordering an even greater body of water, the Pacific Ocean.

The Bay Area lies within a geological province called the **Coast Ranges,** a complex system of ridges and valleys that stretches from Arcata to the north to near Santa Barbara in the south, and inland to the edge of the Central Valley. Several important subranges run through our area, including the **Sonoma, Mayacamas,** and **Vaca mountains** in the North Bay; the **Diablo Range** in the East Bay and South Bay; and the **Santa Cruz Mountains** on the Peninsula and in the South Bay. The tallest peak in the North Bay (and in this guide) is **Mt. St. Helena** (4339'). Other prominent Bay Area summits include **Mt. Hamilton** (4213'), **Mt. Diablo** (3849'), **Loma Prieta** (3806'), **Mt. Tamalpais** (2571'), and **Sonoma Mountain** (2295').

A lead player in the shaping of the Bay Area is the **San Andreas Fault**, which splits the Santa Cruz Mountains, passes under water seaward of the Golden Gate, and then slices through Point Reyes National Seashore. The **Calaveras Fault**, running along the Oakland hills and past Mission Peak, is a major offshoot of the San Andreas.

Movement along these faults, as the Pacific Plate bumps and grinds its way northwest against the North American Plate, is what rattles our teacups and collapses our freeways. Evidence of this movement can be found at the tip of Point Reyes and on Montara Mountain, where granite from the so-called Salinian Block, formed 25 million years ago near the southern end of the Sierra Nevada, has slowly shifted northward along the San Andreas Fault. Greenish serpentine rock, found near faults, creates a challenging growing environment favoring rare native shrubs and wildflowers.

Much of the rock underlying the Bay Area is sedimentary or metamorphic (sandstone, schist, and shales), but there are some delightfully unusual areas, such as the volcanic soils of Mt. St. Helena, Skyline Wilderness Park, and Sibley Volcanic Regional Preserve; granite on Montara Mountain; and the dark, red Franciscan chert of the Marin Headlands. The East Bay's Black Diamond Mines Regional Preserve was a major coal mining area more than a century ago, and mercury was mined near Almaden Quicksilver County Park as recently as the 1970s.

Flora

Bay Area parks have an incredible diversity of plant life. California has more than 5000 native plant species and an estimated 1000 introduced species. Of the native plants, about 30 percent occur nowhere else—these are called endemics. Among the most common endemics are many types of manzanita *(Arctostaphylos)* and monkeyflower *(Mimulus)*. The state has some of the oldest species, in terms of evolution, and also some of the youngest. For example, coast redwoods date back to the dinosaurs, whereas certain species of tarweed *(Madia)* have evolved within the past several thousand years.

The Bay Area's dry interior hills, untouched by summer fog, are characterized by the **oak woodland community**, which is found at elevations between 300 and 3500 feet. Common trees and shrubs found in this generally open woodland, sometimes called a **savanna**, include various oaks, California buckeye, gray pine, California bay, buckbrush, toyon, coffeeberry, snowberry, and poison oak. Especially with oaks, slope aspect and elevation determine which species occur where. Excluding hybrids, there are six common oaks in the Bay Area—valley oak, black oak, blue oak, canyon oak, interior live oak, and coast live oak. Examples of this community can be found at Sugarloaf Ridge State Park, Black Diamond Mines Regional Preserve, and Henry W. Coe State Park.

Members of the **riparian woodland** are usually found beside rivers and creeks. Among the most common are bigleaf maple, white alder, red alder, California bay, various willows, California rose, poison oak, California wild grape, elk clover, and giant chain fern. Point Reyes National Seashore and Monte Bello Open Space Preserve give you opportunities to enjoy this community.

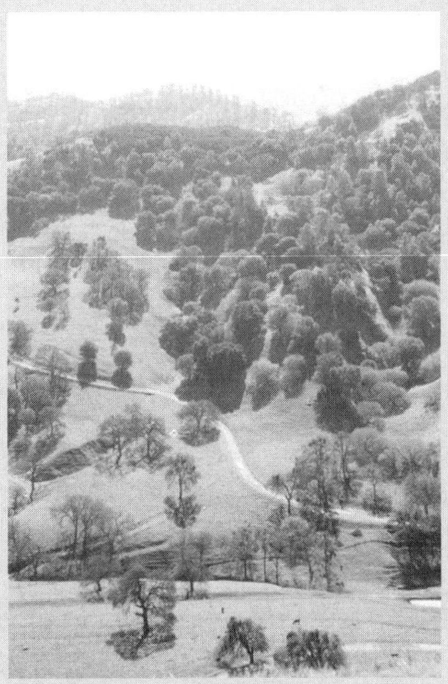

Oak woodland *in Black Diamond Mines Regional Preserve*

Coast redwoods are the world's tallest trees and are among the fastest-growing. Redwood groves once formed an extensive coastal forest that stretched from central California to southern Oregon. Commercially valuable, they were heavily logged. The remaining old-growth coast redwoods in the Bay Area are confined to a few areas, most notably Muir Woods National Monument, in Marin County, and Armstrong Redwoods State Reserve, in northwest Sonoma County. Associated with redwoods are a number of plant species, including tanbark oak, California bay, hazelnut, evergreen huckleberry, wood rose, redwood sorrel, western sword fern, and evergreen violet. You can visit second-growth redwood forests and see a few old-growth giants at Muir Woods National Monument, Redwood Regional Park, and Purisima Creek Redwoods Open Space Preserve.

In many parts of the Bay Area, **Douglas-fir** is the "default" evergreen, easily told by its distinctive cones, which have protruding, three-pointed bracts, sometimes called rat's tails. Douglas-fir and coast redwood are California's two most important commercial trees. Douglas-fir often grows in similar habitats as coast redwood but where soil conditions do not favor redwood growth. Some of the common plants associated with Douglas-fir are the same as those associated with coast redwood, namely California bay, tanbark oak, and western sword fern. Others include blue blossom, coffeeberry, and poison oak. Point Reyes National Seashore, Mt. Tamalpais State Park, and El Corte de Madera Creek Open Space Preserve have beautiful Douglas-fir forests.

A **mixed evergreen forest** contains a mixture of evergreen trees, including California bay, canyon oak, coast live oak, and madrone. The understory to this forest often contains shrubs such as toyon, blue elderberry, hazelnut,

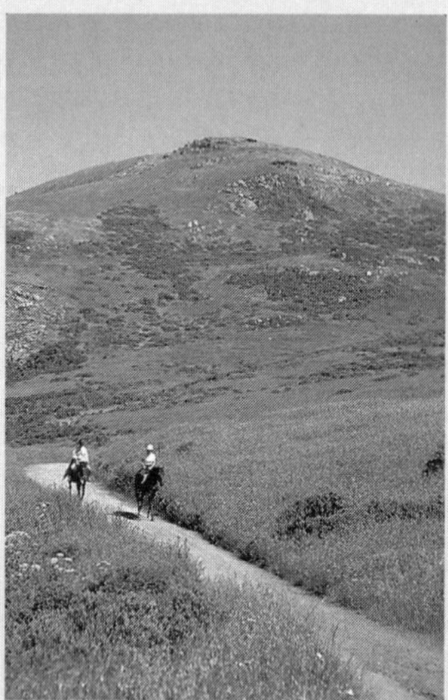

Grassland *and coastal scrub in the Marin Headlands host a wide variety of native wildflowers.*

buckbrush, snowberry, thimbleberry, creambush, and poison oak. Carpeting the forest floor may be an assortment of wildflowers, including milk maids, fairy bells, mission bells, hound's tongue, and western heart's-ease. Take a stroll through a mixed evergreen forest at China Camp State Park, Dry Creek Pioneer Regional Park, and Sierra Azul Open Space Preserve.

The **chaparral community** is made up of hardy plants that thrive in poor soils under hot, dry conditions. Chaparral is very susceptible to fire, and some of its members, such as various species of manzanita, survive devastating blazes by sprouting new growth from ground-level burls. Despite the harsh environment, chaparral can be beautiful year-round, with certain manzanitas blooming as early as December, and other plants continuing into spring and summer. The word itself comes from a Spanish term for "dwarf" or "scrub oak," but in the Bay Area it is chamise, various manzanitas, and various species of ceanothus that dominate the community. Other chaparral plants include mountain mahogany, yerba santa, toyon, chaparral pea, and poison oak. You can study this fascinating assembly of plants on Mt. Tamalpais, Pine Mountain, Mt. Diablo, and in Sierra Azul Open Space Preserve.

Few if any **grasslands** in the Bay Area retain their native character. Human intervention, in the form of fire suppression, farming, and livestock grazing, along with the invasion of nonnative plants, have significantly altered the landscape. Gone from most areas are the native bunchgrasses, perennial species that once dominated our area. Remaining, thankfully, are native wildflowers, which decorate the grasslands in spring and summer. Among the most common are bluedicks, California poppy, owl's-clover, checkerbloom, lupine, and blue-eyed grass. Look for these at Skyline Wilderness Park, Sunol Wilderness, Joseph D. Grant County Park, and Russian Ridge Open Space Preserve.

Sudden Oak Death

Many Bay Area parks are infested with *Phytophthora ramorum*, a plant pathogen that kills tanbark oak, coast live oak, black oak, and canyon live oak. This pathogen also infects other trees and shrubs, including California bay,

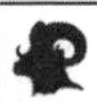

OPTIONS

Help Stop the Spread of Sudden Oak Death

- Avoid parking your vehicle in muddy areas.
- Stay on established trails.
- Avoid walking or riding through damp soil or mud.
- Do not collect any plant material, including leaves, flowers, acorns, wood, and bark.
- Clean soil and mud off shoes, bikes, pets' paws, and vehicles to prevent spreading spores via contaminated soil to new areas.

madrone, rhododendron, bigleaf maple, huckleberry, California buckeye, manzanita, toyon, coast redwood, and Douglas-fir. Its spores may spread via water, soil, and infected plant material. For more information, visit the California Oak Mortality Task Force's Web site: www.suddenoakdeath.org.

Fauna

Besides deer, rabbits, and squirrels, you probably won't see many other land mammals on your hikes in the Bay Area, unless you time your visits near dawn or dusk. These are times when most mammals are active, and then you may be rewarded with a fleeting glimpse of a coyote or a bobcat. Large mammals, such as black bears and mountain lions, are seldom seen. Other more common mammals in our area include foxes, raccoons, skunks, opossums, and chipmunks. Wild pigs are present in Bay Area parks, and in some they have done extensive damage. Never approach wild pigs; they are dangerous. In many East Bay and South Bay parks, you may encounter cows on or near the trail. Though they are often sweet-tempered, give them plenty of space, and never get between cows and their calves.

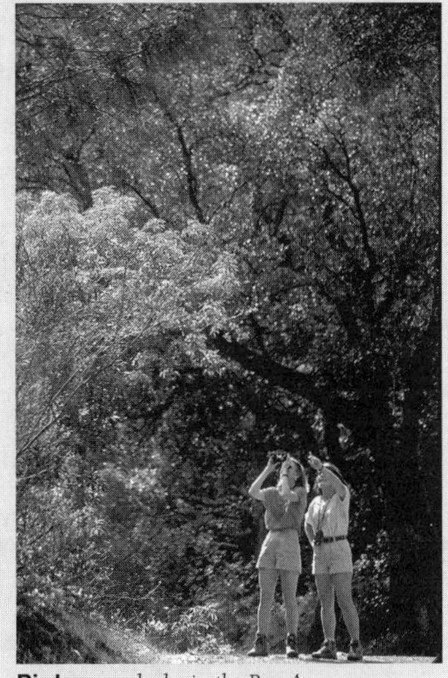

Birders *are lucky in the Bay Area.*

It is not hyperbole to call the Bay Area one of the world's great birding areas. Its location on the western edge of the Pacific Flyway, combined with the presence of so many different habitats, from offshore islands to inland mountains, guarantees both a high species count and an enormous number—in the millions—of individual birds either resident, wintering, or passing through on their migration. Point Reyes National Seashore, perhaps the area with the most variety of birds, has logged an impressive 440 different species, or just under half of all bird species found in North America north of Mexico. The American Ornithologists' Union's (AOU) checklist for birds of the continental US and Canada is the standard reference for common names of birds.

Season, location, weather, and even time of day—these together help determine which birds you are likely to see. Among the most common birds seen from the trail are acorn woodpeckers, western scrub-jays, Steller's jays, spotted towhees, dark-eyed juncos, California quail, and turkey vultures. Raptors such as hawks, falcons, golden eagles, and kites patrol the skies above many Bay Area parks. If you learn to "bird by ear," identifying species by their distinctive notes, calls, and songs, you will quickly expand your list, because many birds are frustratingly hard to spot, especially in dense foliage. Birding with a group also improves your odds of seeing and identifying a large number of species, including rarities.

If a sudden scurrying in the leaves takes you by surprise, it is probably nothing more than a western fence lizard, the Bay Area's most commonly seen reptile. When threatened, these lizards may stand their ground and begin to do "push-ups," which perhaps strike terror into their foes. Also here are the California whiptail, a lizard with a tail as long as its body, the alligator lizard, and the western skink. An animal resembling a lizard but actually an amphibian is the California newt, which spends the summer buried under the forest floor, then emerges with the first rains and migrates to breed in ponds and streams. Briones Regional Park and Monte Bello Open Space Preserve are among good places to witness these migrations. Other amphibians you might see or hear include western toads and Pacific tree frogs.

Gopher snake, California kingsnake, rubber boa, California whipsnake, western rattlesnake, and garter snake are among the snakes present in the Bay Area. Gopher snakes are often mistaken for rattlers, and for a heart-stopping moment you may struggle to recall the differences: A gopher snake has a slim head and a fat body, whereas a rattlesnake has a relatively thin body compared with its large, triangular head. Gopher snakes are common, but rattlers, although present in the Bay Area, are seldom seen.

Seasons

Where else can you find such a perfect climate for outdoor activities? Not too hot in summer, not too cold in winter, and a rain-free season that lasts generally from May through October. The moderating effect of the Pacific Ocean keeps temperatures near the coast in a narrow range year-round. The summer months are characterized by fog at the coast but generally clear and warm conditions elsewhere. The shady canyons of Marin County and the Peninsula are perfect summer places to cool off. If you want to bake on the trail, head away from the Bay.

By the time fall arrives, the hills are brown and seasonal creeks dry. These clear, cool days are perfect just about everywhere, with a modest palette of autumn colors in riparian areas. With the first rains, the change is dramatic: Hillsides turn green and water returns to the creek beds.

Fall and winter storms from the Gulf of Alaska can bring copious rainfall, high winds, and even snow to the tallest Bay Area peaks. In their wakes these storms usually leave a few exceptionally cold but clear days, perfect for bundling up and visiting a vantage point with great views, such as Mt. Tamalpais or even Mt. St. Helena.

As early as December, our manzanitas and currants begin to bloom, decorating chaparral areas with floral displays of white and pink. Other shrubs and the earliest wildflowers begin their show in late winter or early spring. By the time April rolls around, especially after a wet winter, the wildflower display is usually fantastic, so this is the time to head to the grasslands of the East Bay and the Peninsula.

The farther inland you go, the less pronounced is the moderating influence of the ocean. Temperature differences—the average highs and lows for any given location—widen as you leave the coast. Here's an example, using two locations about 65 miles apart: The highest average high temperature for San Francisco is 68.5°F, whereas the same figure for St. Helena in Napa County is 89.2°F. But San Francisco's lowest average minimum, 45.7°F (January), is about 10°F warmer than St. Helena's.

Similarly, rainfall varies as you move around the Bay Area. Each successive range of coastal hills blocks more and more Pacific moisture, creating a rain-shadow effect that intensifies as you move away from the coast and from San Francisco Bay. That is why coast redwoods, which depend on fog-drip to supply moisture during the dry season, grow only in a narrow band near the coast.

Time of day and weather conditions are often as important as time of year when considering a route. A hike that is pleasant in the cool of the morning can be a sweltering ordeal under the noonday sun if there is no shade. An outing can be spoiled (or otherwise transformed) by high winds or a sudden squall. Always check for the most current weather before heading out for the day.

Trail Selection

The goal of this guide is to steer you to the best parks and open spaces in the Bay Area, and also to encourage you to explore on your own. Of course, every book reflects its authors' interests. With so many possible parks, trails, and habitats to choose from, how were the 44 trails in this guide chosen?

Key Features

Taking the series name literally, many of these "top" trails climb high. Outdoor enthusiasts love vantage points with great views but some also climb for sheer enjoyment. So, you will find an assortment of the Bay Area's tallest **peaks**—Mt. St. Helena, Mt. Tamalpais, Mt. Diablo, and Black Mountain—represented here.

If **long-distance routes** sound like fun, check out Annadel State Park, Point Reyes National Seashore, Black Diamond Mines Regional Preserve, Pleasanton Ridge Regional Park, Almaden Quicksilver County Park, and Purisima Creek Redwoods Open Space Preserve. (If short strolls are your preference, many of the trips suggest shorter options.)

If you have a passion for **water,** you'll enjoy exploring Mt. Burdell Open Space Preserve, which has a large vernal pool with rare wildflowers; Redwood Regional Park, where coast redwoods rise majestically above a rushing creek; and Monte Bello Open Space Preserve, where a self-guiding nature trail wanders through the canyon holding Stevens Creek.

If you are interested in **wildflowers** and **native plants**—from tiny flowers to towering redwoods—head for the Marin Headlands, Henry W. Coe State Park, and Russian Ridge Open Space Preserve. Birders may see birds ranging from hawks to hummingbirds just about anywhere in the Bay Area.

Finally, many of the trails in even our remotest parks and preserves touch on the Bay Area's fascinating **human history,** from the earliest Native Americans to today's Silicon Valley entrepreneurs. Many of these trails take you through terrain once trod by Ohlone Indians, Spanish missionaries, Mexican ranchers, Italian winemakers, Portuguese dairymen, Chinese fishermen, and a host of famous and infamous personalities. Without this human history, and generations of environmental activists working to save our hills and shorelines from encroaching development, our experience of the Bay Area's landscape would be much less rich.

Multiple Uses

Many of the trails in the Bay Area are multiuse trails, which means they are shared by hikers, bicyclists, runners, and equestrians—most of these are actually dirt roads. In general, bicycles are not permitted on single-track trails. Exceptions, including Annadel and China Camp state parks and some MROSD preserves, are noted in the text. Whenever possible, if a route described has a segment closed to bikes, the text provides alternate trails that are open. A few trails, designated "hiking only," are closed to both bikes and horses.

Some agencies, such as MROSD, close their multiuse trails to bikes and horses during wet weather, with special gates that allow hikers to pass.

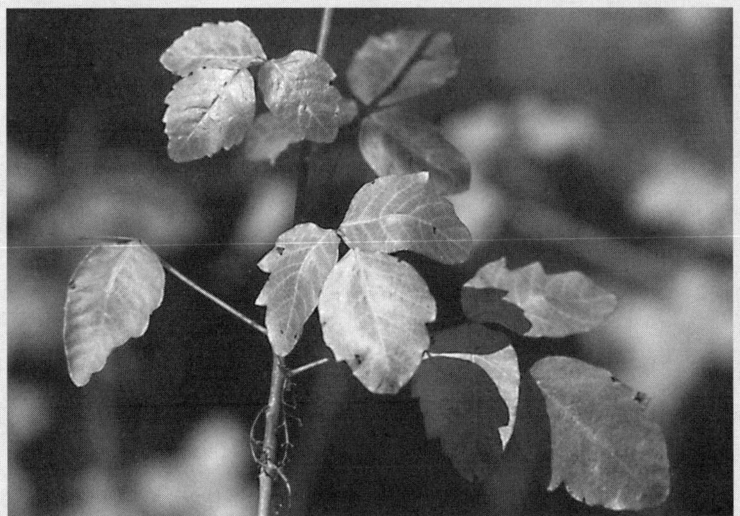

Poison Oak *Learn to recognize the stems and lobed leaves in all seasons.*

Where this is the case, it is noted in the text. Call ahead to the agency in charge of the park or open space you are planning to visit, and have an alternate route selected. Agency phone numbers and their Web site addresses, if any, are listed in Appendix 2 (page 314).

When planning a hike with your dog, check to make sure pets are allowed. Dogs (and other pets) are not allowed on the trails in any Bay Area state park, and there are restrictions at other parks and open spaces as well. Where dogs are allowed, they generally must be on a leash no longer than 6 feet. Some agencies allow dogs off-leash, but the dogs must be under immediate voice command of the person they are with, and must never be allowed to threaten or harm people or wildlife. People with dogs must clean up after their pets and obey all other posted rules and regulations.

Trail Safety

Poison oak produces an itchy rash in people allergic to its oil. Learn to identify poison oak's shiny green foliage—"leaflets three, let it be"—and avoid it. In fall the shrub's leaves turn yellow and red, adding a wonderful touch of color to the woods. In winter, you can identify the plant by its upward-reaching clusters of bare branches. Staying on the trail is the best way to avoid contact with poison oak, and wearing long pants and a long-sleeved shirt helps too. Anything that touches poison oak—clothing or pets, for instance—should be washed in soap and water.

The **tick**, a tiny, almost invisible insect, has been the cause of much woe among hikers and others who spend time outdoors. Western black-legged ticks carry a bacteria that causes **Lyme disease**, which can produce serious symptoms in people who have been bitten. These include flulike aches and pains which, if left untreated, may progress to severe cardiac and neurological disorders. Often the tick bite produces a rash that over time clears from the center, producing a bull's-eye pattern.

You can take several steps to protect against Lyme disease. Wear light-colored clothing, so ticks are easier to spot. Use long-sleeved pants with the legs tucked into your socks (or gaiters over the bottom of your pants and tops of your shoes), and a long-sleeved shirt tucked into your pants. Spray your clothing with an insect repellent containing DEET before hiking. When you return home, shake out and brush all clothing, boots, and packs outdoors. If you find an attached tick, use tweezers to remove it by grasping the tick as close to your skin as possible and steadily pulling it out. Do not squeeze the tick while it is attached, as this may inject the bacterium into your skin. Wash the area and apply antiseptic, then call your doctor.

Although present in the Bay Area, western **rattlesnakes** are shy and seldom seen. Most snake bites are the result of a defensive reaction: A foot or hand has suddenly landed in the snake's territory. A rattlesnake often, but not always, gives a warning when it feels threatened. Stand still until you have located the snake, and then back slowly away. If you are bitten, seek medical attention as quickly and effortlessly as possible, to avoid spreading the venom.

Mountain lions, also called **cougars** or **pumas**, are rarely seen in our area. They hunt at night and feed mostly on deer. If you do encounter a mountain lion, experts advise standing your ground, making loud noises, waving your arms to appear larger, and fighting back if attacked. Above all, never run: You want to avoid being seen as prey by the mountain lion.

Note from the Authors

During the course of several years, we walked every trail included in this guide at least once. In many cases, we returned to favorite areas in different seasons. We try to be accurate and thorough in both our observations and our writing. The natural world, however, is always in a state of flux, and although this is a fine thing in general, it plays havoc with outdoor guides. Your experience on the trail—affected as it is by season, weather, time of day, and acts of God and various federal, state, and local agencies—will very likely be different from ours. We acknowledge this variability by the use of the word "may" in the text, as in "As you tromp along the trail, you may scare up a covey of California quail." We certainly hope you get to see the quail, but like so many other things, the movement of birds is beyond our control.

On the Trail

Every outing should begin with proper preparation. Even the easiest trail can turn up unexpected surprises. People seldom think about getting lost or suffering an injury, but unexpected things can and do happen. A few minutes' worth of simple precautions can make the difference between a marvelous and a miserable outcome—or merely a good story to tell afterward.

Use the Top Trails ratings and descriptions to determine if a particular trail is a good match with your fitness and energy level, given current conditions and time of year.

Have a Plan

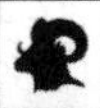

Prepare and Plan

- Know your abilities and your limitations.
- Leave word about your plans.
- Know the area and the route.

Choose Wisely The first step to enjoying any trail is to match the trail to your abilities. It's no use overestimating your experience or fitness—know your abilities and limitations, and use the difficulty rating that accompanies each trail.

Leave Word About Your Plans The most basic of precautions is leaving word of your intentions with family or friends. Many people will hike the backcountry their entire lives without ever relying on this safety net, but establishing this simple habit is free insurance.

It's best to leave specific information—location, trail name, intended time of travel—with a responsible person. If there is a registration process, make use of it. If there is a ranger station or park office, check in.

Review the Route Before embarking on any trail, be sure to read the entire description and study the map. It isn't necessary to memorize every detail, but it is worthwhile to have a clear mental picture of the trail and the general area.

If the trail and terrain are complex, augment the trail guide with a topographic map. Park maps, as well as current weather and trail condition information, are often available from local ranger stations and trailheads.

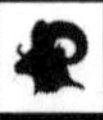

Trail Essentials

- Dress to keep cool but be ready for cold.
- Bring plenty of water and adequate food.

Carry the Essentials

Proper preparation for any type of trail use includes gathering the essential items to carry. Your checklist may vary according to choice of trails and daily conditions.

Clothing When the weather is good, light, comfortable clothing is the obvious choice. It's easy to believe that very little spare clothing is needed, but a prepared hiker has something tucked away for any emergency from a surprise shower to an unexpected overnight in a remote area.

Clothing includes proper footwear, essential for hiking and running trails. As a trail becomes more demanding, you will need footwear that performs. Running shoes are fine for many trails. If you will be carrying substantial weight or encountering sustained rugged terrain, step up to hiking boots and synthetic or wool-blend socks (no cotton) specifically designed for hiking.

In hot, sunny weather, proper clothing includes a hat, sunglasses, long-sleeved shirt, and sunscreen. In cooler weather, particularly when it's wet, carry waterproof outer garments and quick-drying undergarments (avoid cotton). As general rule, whatever the conditions, bring layers that can be combined or removed to provide comfort and protection from the elements in a wide variety of conditions.

Water Never embark on a trail without carrying water. For most outings, you should plan to carry sufficient water to last you and your party for the entire hike. At all times, particularly in warm weather, adequate water is of key importance. Experts recommend at least two quarts of water per day per person, and when hiking in heat a gallon or more may be more appropriate. At the extreme, dehydration can be life threatening. More commonly, inadequate water brings on fatigue and muscle aches.

If it's necessary to make use of trailside water, you should filter or chemically treat it. You should regard all untreated water sources as being contaminated with bacteria, viruses and fertilizers.

There are three methods for treating water: boiling, chemical treatment, and filtering. Boiling is best, but often impractical—it requires a heat source, a pot, and time. Chemical treatments, available in sporting goods and outdoor stores, handle some problems, including the troublesome *Giardia* parasite, but will not combat many human-made chemical pollutants. The preferred method is filtration, which removes *Giardia* and other contaminants and doesn't leave any unpleasant aftertaste.

One final admonishment: Be prepared for surprises. Water sources described in the text or on maps can change course or dry up completely. Never run your water bottle dry in expectation of the next source; fill up when water is available and always keep a little in reserve.

Food Although not as critical as water, food is energy and its importance shouldn't be underestimated. Avoid foods that are hard to digest, such as candy bars and potato chips. Carry high energy, fast-digesting foods, such as nutrition bars, dehydrated fruit, nuts, trail mix, and jerky. Bringing a little extra food is good protection against an outing that turns unexpectedly long, perhaps due to weather or losing your way.

Useful but Less Than Essential

Map and Compass (and the Know-How to Use Them) Many trails don't require much navigation, meaning a map and compass aren't always essential, but can be useful. If the trail is remote or infrequently visited, a map and compass should be considered necessities.

A handheld GPS (Global Positioning System) receiver can also be a useful trail companion, but is really no substitute for a map and compass; knowing your longitude and latitude is not much help without a map.

Cell Phone Most of the Bay Area has some level of cellular coverage. In extreme circumstances, a cell phone can be a lifesaver, but don't depend on it; coverage is unpredictable and batteries fail. And be sure that the occasion warrants the phone call—a blister doesn't justify a call to search and rescue.

Gear Depending on the remoteness and rigor of the trail, there are many additional useful items to consider; pocketknife, flashlight, fire source (waterproof matches, light, or flint), and a first-aid kit.

Every member of your party should carry the appropriate essential items described above; groups often split up or get separated along the trail. Solo hikers should be even more disciplined about preparation, and make a habit of carrying a little more gear than absolutely necessary. Traveling solo is inherently more risky. This isn't meant to discourage solo travel, simply to emphasize the need for extra preparation.

Trail Etiquette

The overriding rule on the trail is "**Leave No Trace.**" Interest in visiting natural areas continues to increase, even as the quantity of unspoiled natural areas continues to shrink. These pressures make it ever more critical that we leave no trace of our visit.

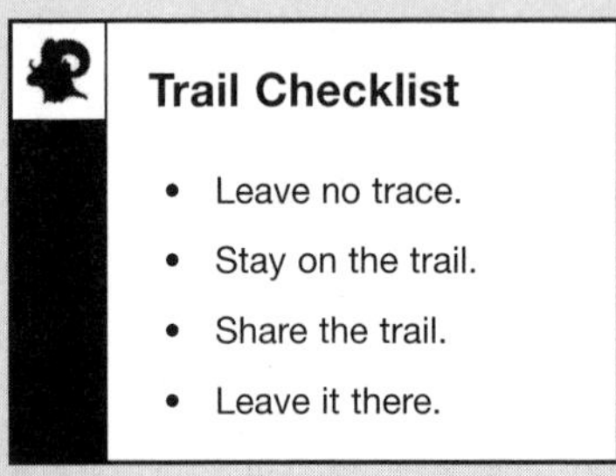

Trail Checklist

- Leave no trace.
- Stay on the trail.
- Share the trail.
- Leave it there.

Never Litter If you carried it in, it's easy enough to carry it out. Leave the trail in the same, if not better, condition than you find it. Try picking up any litter you encounter and packing it out—it's a great feeling! Pack a spare plastic bag to carry litter. Just picking up a few pieces of garbage makes a difference.

Stay on the Trail Paths have been created, sometimes over many years, for many purposes: to protect the surrounding natural areas, to avoid dangers, and to provide the best route. Leaving the trail can cause damage that takes years to undo. Never cut switchbacks. Shortcutting rarely saves energy or time, and it takes a terrible toll on the land, trampling plant life and hastening erosion. Moreover, safety and consideration intersect on the trail. It's hard to get truly lost if you stay on the trail.

Share the Trail The best trails attract many visitors and you should be prepared to share the trail with others. Do your part to minimize impact. Commonly accepted trail etiquette dictates that **bike riders yield to both hikers and equestrians, hikers yield to horseback riders, downhill hikers yield to uphill hikers, and everyone stays to the right.** Not everyone knows these rules of the road, so let common sense and good humor be the final guide.

Leave It There Destruction or removal of plants and animals, or historical, prehistoric, or geological items, is certainly unethical and almost always illegal.

Getting Lost If you become lost on the trail, stay on the trail. Stop and take stock of the situation. In many cases, a few minutes of calm reflection will yield a solution. Consider all the clues available; use the sun to identify directions if you don't have a compass. If you determine that you are indeed lost, stay on the main trail and stay put. You are more likely to encounter other people if you stay in one place.

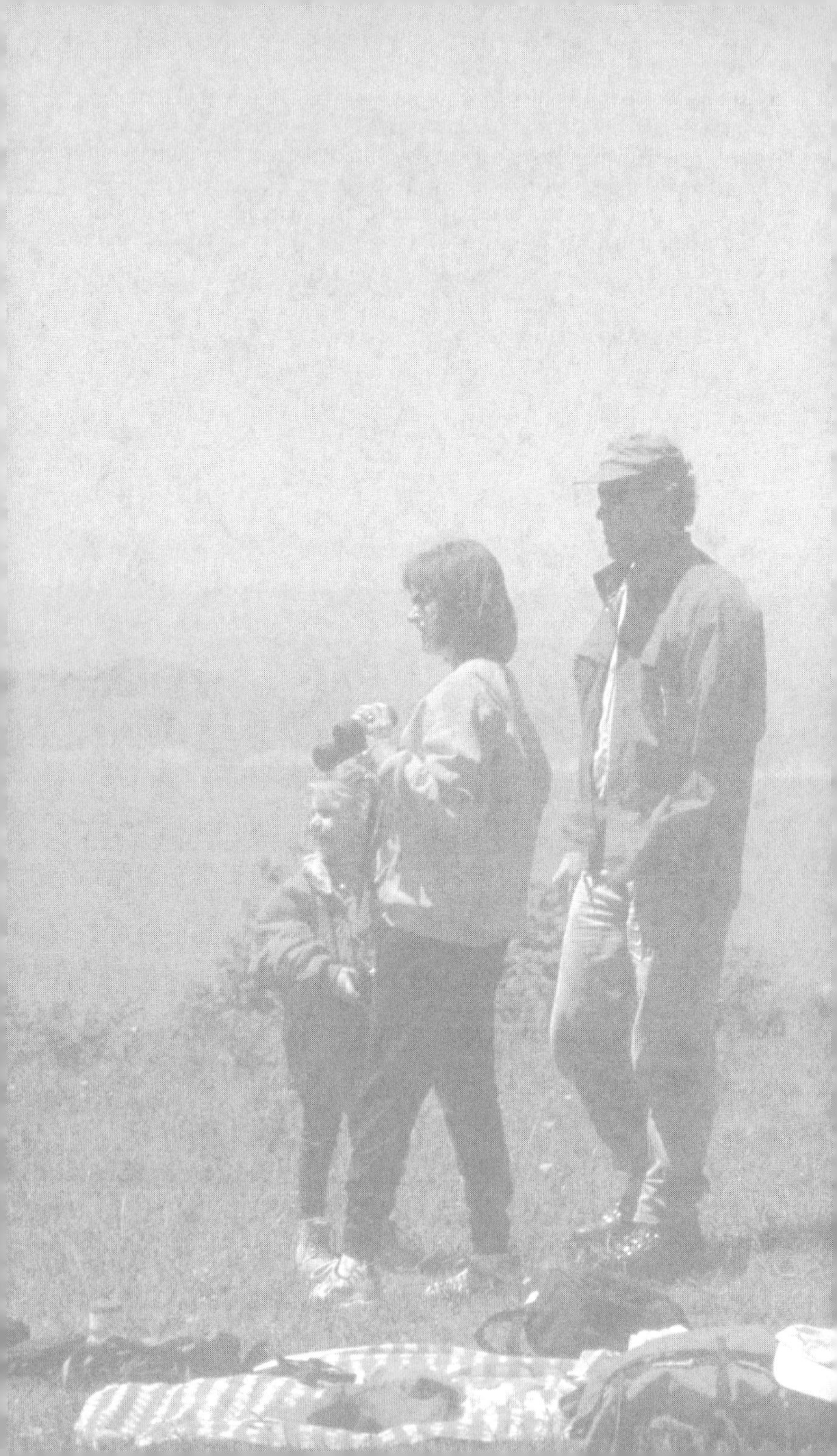

CHAPTER 1

North Bay

1. Marin Headlands: Gerbode Valley
2. Muir Woods National Monument: Dipsea Trail
3. Mount Tamalpais: High Marsh Loop
4. Mount Tamalpais: Middle Peak
5. Pine Mountain
6. Samuel P. Taylor State Park: Barnabe Mountain
7. Point Reyes National Seashore: Sky Trail
8. China Camp State Park: Bay View–Shoreline Loop
9. Mt. Burdell Open Space Preserve
10. Mount St. Helena
11. Annadel State Park: Lake Ilsanjo
12. Jack London State Historic Park
13. Sugarloaf Ridge State Park: Bald Mountain
14. Skyline Wilderness Park: Sugarloaf Mountain

North Bay

For this guide, the North Bay includes all of Marin and Napa counties, and Sonoma County east of US Highway 101.

Marin is the smallest of the North Bay counties, but has the most parks and open spaces—more than 200 square miles in federal, state, and local lands, traversed by hundreds of miles of trails. It includes rugged Pacific shoreline, redwood groves, forested valleys and ridges, open grassland, chaparral, and salt marsh. The jewel in the crown is Mt. Tamalpais, at 2571 feet the highest North Bay peak near the coast. Low on its southern slope lies Muir Woods National Monument, one of the last remaining groves of old-growth coast redwoods. The Marin Municipal Water District (MMWD) watershed surrounding Mt. Tamalpais is also open to respectful recreational use.

The creation of Point Reyes National Seashore in 1969 and the Golden Gate National Recreation Area in 1972 helped protect southern and western Marin from urban sprawl. Conservation easements and strict agricultural zoning protect many of western Marin's cattle and dairy ranches.

Eastern Marin, fronting San Francisco and San Pablo bays, is mostly suburban, but if you look carefully between the towns and cities you'll find more than a dozen Marin County Open Space District (MCOSD) preserves and China Camp State Park, which protect areas of forest, grasslands, and salt marsh. This part of Marin is often 10°F to 20°F warmer than the foggy coastal areas of West Marin, the Marin Headlands, and San Francisco.

Some of Marin's place names, such as Mill Valley and Corte Madera ("a place where wood is cut") are clues to its lumber-producing past. Others, like San Rafael and Sausalito ("little willow grove"), tell of Franciscan missionaries and Mexican ranchos. Still others—Tamalpais and Olompali—are derived from the language of Marin's original inhabitants, the Coast Miwok people.

Sonoma is the largest and most varied of the North Bay counties, stretching from the volcanic highlands of the Mayacmas Mountains and the North Bay's tallest peak, Mt. St. Helena (4339'), to the wave-washed Pacific shore. The focus of this guide is the inland area east of US 101.

Overleaf: *Sky Trail, Point Reyes National Seashore (Trail 7)*

Sonoma has a scattering of public lands, including Annadel, Jack London, and Sugarloaf Ridge state parks, and a growing network of regional parks, some of which also have trails and camping. Voters established the Sonoma County Agricultural Preservation and Open Space District in 1996 to protect the area's varied natural habitat and productive agricultural land from urban development. Though more urban than in years past, the county still supports dairy farming, cattle and sheep ranching, fishing, timber harvesting, and tourism, and has several wine-growing regions.

Napa needs no introduction: Its reputation for world-class wines is well known and well deserved—nearly every tillable acre of land is devoted to growing grapes. Before wine became queen, Napa's economy included large ranchos, fruit and nut orchards, and mines that produced gold, silver, and cinnabar. Today, especially on weekends, the valley seems mainly inhabited by tourists, whose cars move at a snail's pace up and down State Highway 29.

Although Napa has several scenic state parks, it offers the least amount of trails of any North Bay county, and only established its county park district in 2006. The trails that do exist overlook a fascinating patchwork of vineyards. One of the area's finest parks, Skyline Wilderness Park, is operated by a citizen volunteer group for the City of Napa.

See Appendix 2 for agency contact information (page 314) and Appendix 6 for maps (page 321).

North Bay

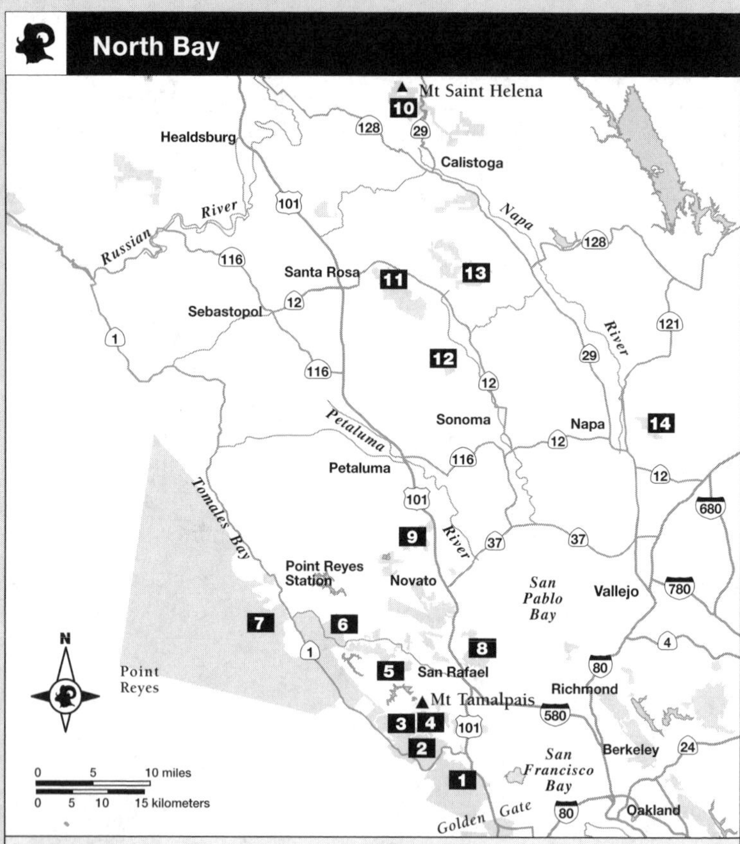

1 Marin Headlands: Gerbode Valley

2 Muir Woods National Monument: Dipsea Trail

3 Mount Tamalpais: High Marsh Loop

4 Mount Tamalpais: Middle Peak

5 Pine Mountain

6 Samuel P. Taylor State Park: Barnabe Mountain

7 Point Reyes National Seashore: Sky Trail

8 China Camp State Park: Bay View–Shoreline Loop

9 Mt. Burdell Open Space Preserve

10 Mount St. Helena

11 Annadel State Park: Lake Ilsanjo

12 Jack London State Historic Park

13 Sugarloaf Ridge State Park: Bald Mountain

14 Skyline Wilderness Park: Sugarloaf Mountain

TRAIL FEATURE TABLE

North Bay

TRAIL	Difficulty	Length	Type	USES & ACCESS	TERRAIN	FLORA & FAUNA	OTHER
1	3	5.4	Loop	Hiking, Running, Biking	Summit	Wildflowers, Birds	Great Views, Photo Opportunity, Camping
2	3	4.0	Loop	Hiking	River or Stream, Canyon	Birds	Historic, Cool & Shady
3	4	5.8	Loop	Hiking, Running, Dogs Allowed	River or Stream, Waterfall, Canyon, Mountain	Birds	Secluded, Cool & Shady
4	3	5.1	Loop	Hiking, Running, Dogs Allowed, Fee	River or Stream, Canyon, Mountain	Birds	Great Views, Cool & Shady
5	3	4.7	Out & Back	Hiking, Running, Biking, Dogs Allowed	Mountain, Summit	Birds	Great Views, Photo Opportunity, Secluded
6	4	6.5	Loop	Hiking, Running	River or Stream, Canyon, Mountain	Wildflowers, Birds	Great Views, Secluded
7	5	10.5	Loop	Hiking, Running	River or Stream	Autumn Colors, Wildflowers, Birds	Great Views, Cool & Shady, Camping
8	4	8.4	Loop	Hiking, Running, Biking, Fee		Birds	Great Views, Cool & Shady, Camping
9	4	5.6	Loop	Hiking, Running, Biking[1], Child Friendly, Dogs Allowed	Lake or Shore, Mountain	Wildflowers, Birds	Great Views, Photo Opportunity
10	5	10.6	Out & Back	Hiking, Running, Biking[1]	Mountain, Summit	Birds	Historic, Geologic Interest, Great Views, Steep, Secluded
11	4	8.8	Loop	Hiking, Running, Biking	Lake or Shore	Autumn Colors, Birds, Wildlife	Secluded, Cool & Shady
12	3	2.9	Loop	Hiking, Running, Child Friendly, Fee	Lake or Shore	Wildflowers, Birds	Historic, Great Views, Secluded, Cool & Shady
13	5	6.7	Loop	Hiking, Running, Fee	Mountain, Summit	Wildflowers, Birds	Great Views, Camping
14	4	6.0	Out & Back	Hiking, Running, Fee	Mountain	Wildflowers, Birds	Great Views, Secluded

USES & ACCESS
- Hiking
- Running
- Biking
- Child Friendly
- Dogs Allowed
- $ Fee
- Permit Required

TYPE
- Loop
- Out & Back
- Point to Point

DIFFICULTY
– 1 2 3 4 5 +
less more

TERRAIN
- River or Stream
- Waterfall
- Lake or Shore
- Canyon
- Mountain
- Summit

FLORA & FAUNA
- Autumn Colors
- Wildflowers
- Birds
- Wildlife

OTHER
- Historic
- Geologic Interest
- Great Views
- Photo Opportunity
- Secluded
- Cool & Shady
- Camping
- Steep

[1] *Bicyclists use described alternate trails or trailheads*

North Bay

TRAIL 1

Hike, Run, Bike
5.4 miles, Loop
Difficulty: 1 2 **3** 4 5

The hills surrounding Gerbode Valley are vibrant in the spring with wildflowers. The Marin Headlands are alive with birds most of the year, but especially during the fall raptor migration. Views of San Francisco, Marin, and the Pacific Coast from the high points along this loop are superb.

TRAIL 2

Hike
4.0 miles, Loop
Difficulty: 1 2 **3** 4 5

This loop climbs a scenic part of the famous Dipsea footrace route in Mt. Tamalpais State Park, then descends through the groves of coast redwood named for John Muir.

TRAIL 3

Hike, Run, Dogs Allowed
5.8 miles, Loop
Difficulty: 1 2 3 **4** 5

This beautiful and athletic loop takes you past a scenic waterfall, beside a freshwater marsh, through areas of chaparral, and into groves of Sargent cypress and forests of Douglas-fir and oak, as it explores rugged canyons and ridges on the north side of Mt. Tamalpais.

TRAIL 4

Hike, Run, Dogs Allowed, Fee
5.1 miles, Loop
Difficulty: 1 2 **3** 4 5

This circuit of Middle Peak explores a wonderful variety of terrain, from chaparral cloaking the upper reaches of Mt. Tamalpais to redwood groves hidden on its northern side.

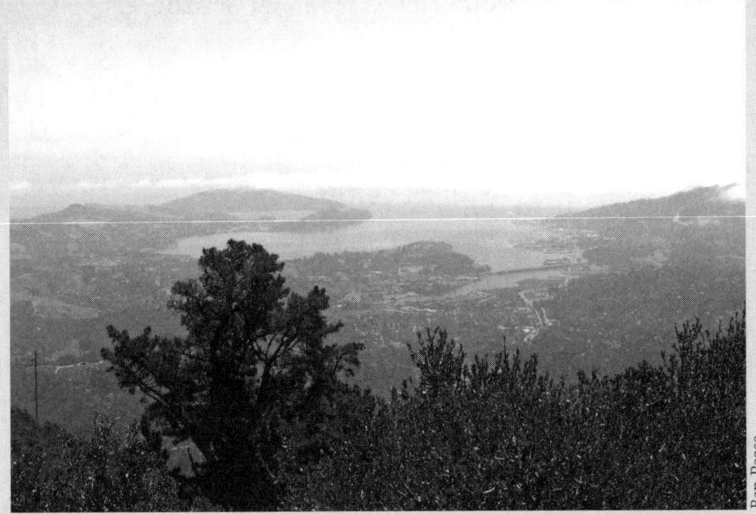
Ben Pease

View *of Richardson Bay from Mt. Tamalpais (Trail 4)*

Pine Mountain 53

TRAIL 5

Hike, Run, Bike, Dogs Allowed
4.7 miles, Out & Back
Difficulty: 1 2 **3** 4 5

This route takes you to one of the best vantage points in the Bay Area, where your efforts on a clear day will be rewarded by fantastic views. Along the way, plant lovers will stay busy identifying a variety of trees and shrubs, some found only on the locally prevalent serpentine soil. This area is also a favorite with mountain bikers.

Samuel P. Taylor State Park: Barnabe Mountain 57

TRAIL 6

Hike, Run
6.5 miles, Loop
Difficulty: 1 2 3 **4** 5

This loop climbs gently through mixed forest, alive with birdsong and brightened by wildflowers, struggles steeply to high ground just below the summit of Barnabe Mountain (1466'), and then descends through open country with wonderful views of west Marin, Point Reyes, and the Tomales Bay area.

Annadel State Park: Lake Ilsanjo 85

Visitors encounter dense forest, oak savanna, and a cattail-lined lake during this tour of the northwestern part of Annadel State Park. The park's single-track trails are popular with hikers, runners, equestrians, and bicyclists.

TRAIL 11

Hike, Run, Bike
8.8 miles, Loop
Difficulty: 1 2 3 **4** 5

Jack London State Historic Park 91

The climb from Jack London's historic Beauty Ranch through beautiful redwood forest to a meadow with great views are a good introduction to this park's growing trail network.

TRAIL 12

Hike, Run,
Child Friendly, Fee
2.9 miles, Loop
Difficulty: 1 2 **3** 4 5

Sugarloaf Ridge State Park: Bald Mountain 97

A superb array of trees, shrubs, and wildflowers, along with some of the best views in the North Bay, are your rewards for tackling the challenging climb to the summit of Bald Mountain.

TRAIL 13

Hike, Run, Fee
6.7 miles, Loop
Difficulty: 1 2 3 4 **5**

Skyline Wilderness Park: Sugarloaf Mountain 101

This route ascends past volcanic outcrops to reach the 1630-foot west peak of Sugarloaf Mountain. Meadows decorated with wildflowers overlook the scenic Napa Valley.

TRAIL 14

Hike, Run, Fee
6.0 miles, Out & Back
Difficulty: 1 2 3 **4** 5

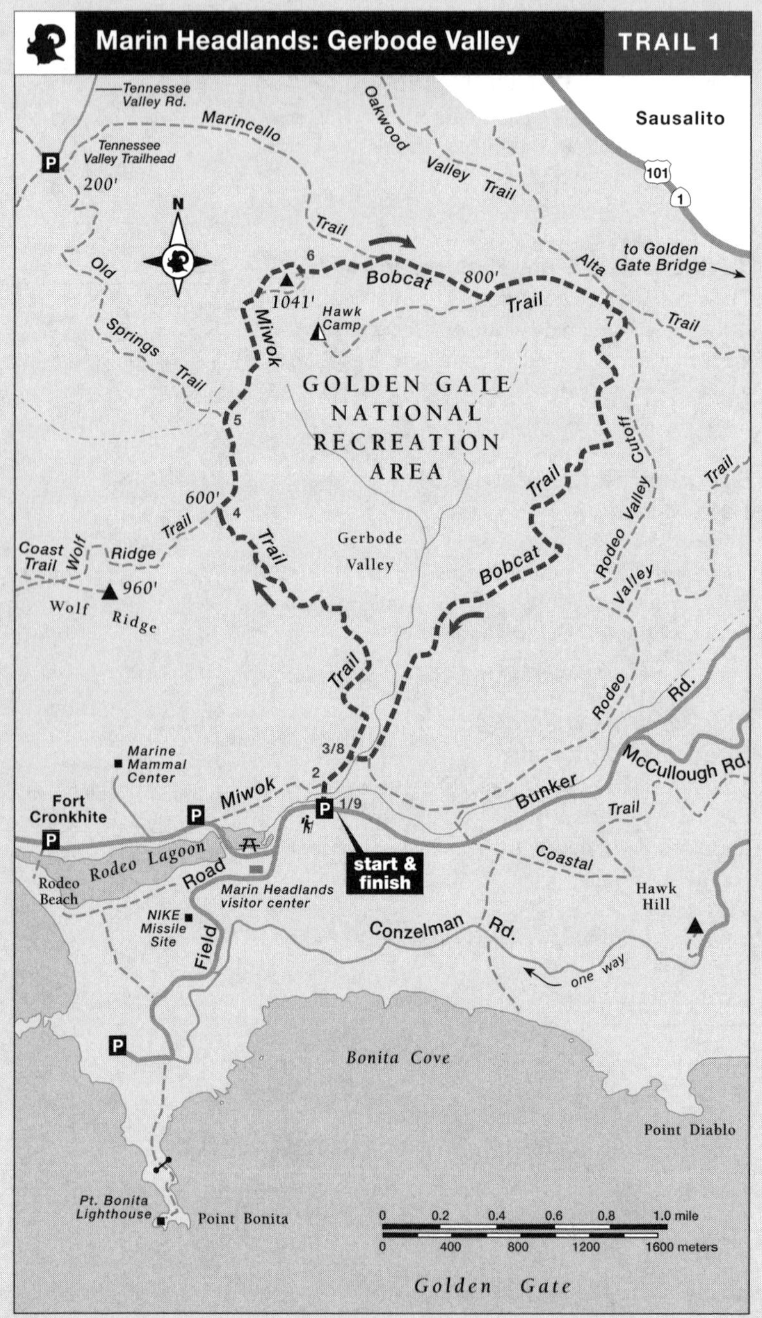
Marin Headlands: Gerbode Valley
TRAIL 1
Tennessee Valley Rd.
Marincello
Tennessee Valley Trailhead
200'
Oakwood Valley Trail
Sausalito
101
1
Trail
Old Springs Trail
6
Bobcat
800'
Trail
Alta Trail
to Golden Gate Bridge
1041'
Hawk Camp
Miwok
7
GOLDEN GATE NATIONAL RECREATION AREA
5
Cutoff
Trail
Rodeo Valley
Trail
600'
4
Trail
Ridge
Wolf
Coast Trail
Gerbode Valley
Bobcat
960'
Wolf Ridge
Valley
Trail
Rodeo
Rd.
3/8
Marine Mammal Center
2
Miwok
McCullough Rd.
Bunker
Fort Cronkhite
1/9
Trail
Rodeo Lagoon
Road
start & finish
Coastal
Rodeo Beach
Marin Headlands visitor center
Hawk Hill
NIKE Missile Site
Field
Conzelman
Rd.
one way
Bonita Cove
Point Diablo
Pt. Bonita Lighthouse
Point Bonita
0 0.2 0.4 0.6 0.8 1.0 mile
0 400 800 1200 1600 meters
Golden Gate

Marin Headlands: Gerbode Valley

This scenic loop uses the Miwok and Bobcat trails to circle Gerbode Valley, an area slated in the 1960s for urban development but protected since 1972 as part of the Golden Gate National Recreation Area. In spring, the Marin Headlands are vibrant with wildflowers. Birds are ever-present here, but especially during the fall, as raptors migrate south across the Golden Gate. Views of San Francisco, Marin, and the Pacific Coast are superb.

TRAIL USE
Hike, Run, Bike

LENGTH
5.4 miles, 3–4 hours

VERTICAL FEET
±1100'

DIFFICULTY
– 1 2 **3** 4 5 +

TRAIL TYPE
Loop

SURFACE TYPE
Dirt

FEATURES
Summit
Wildflowers
Birds
Great Views
Photo Opportunity
Camping

FACILITIES
Visitor Center
Restrooms
Water

Best Time

Spring wildflowers are the prime attraction here, but the route is good all year; expect fog in summer.

Finding the Trail

From US Hwy. 101 northbound, just north of the Golden Gate Bridge, take the Alexander Ave. exit, go north 0.2 mile, and turn left onto Bunker Rd. After 0.1 mile you reach a one-direction-only tunnel where traffic is controlled by a stoplight. After emerging from the 0.5-mile tunnel, go a total of 2.5 miles from Alexander Ave. Just past a horse stable on the left, there is roadside parking on the right shoulder of Bunker Rd.

From Hwy. 101 southbound, just south of the Waldo Tunnel, take the Sausalito Exit, which is also signed for the GGNRA. Bear right (despite the left-pointing GGNRA sign) and go 0.25 mile to Bunker Rd. Turn left, and follow the directions above.

The trailhead is on the north side of the parking area, at its midpoint. A sign at the guardrail reads: TO MIWOK TRAIL, TO BAY AREA RIDGE TRAIL; DOGS ON LEASH.►1

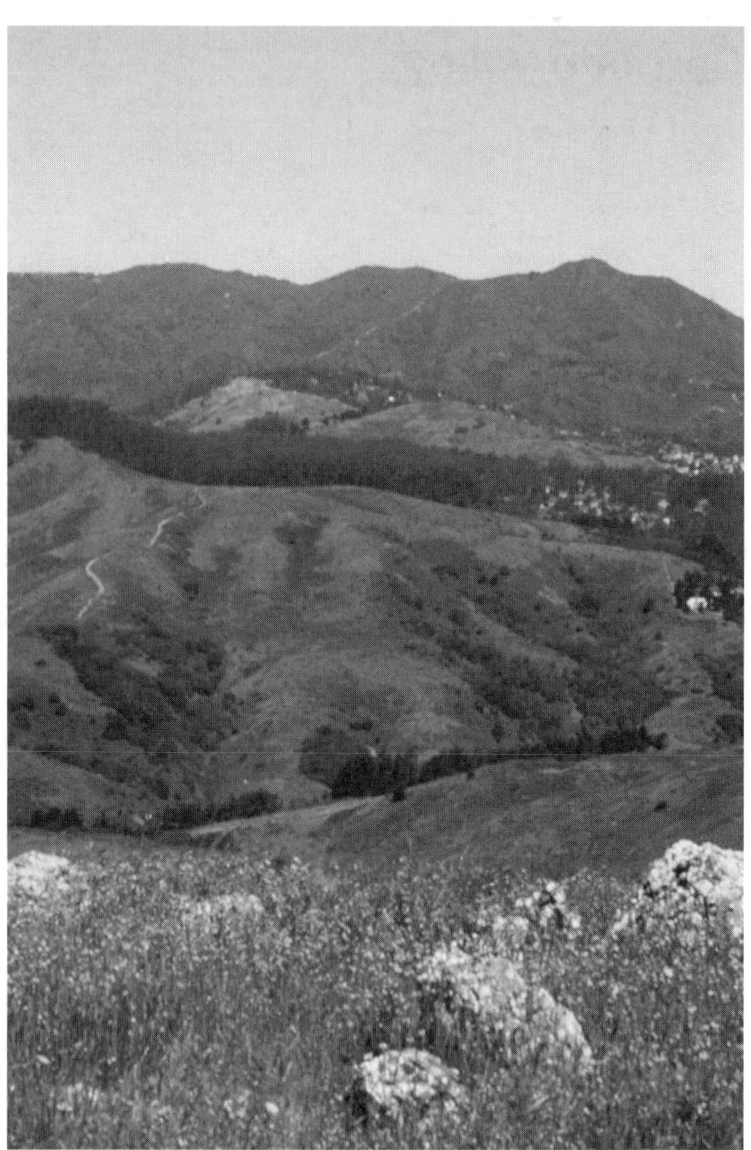

Mt. Tamalpais, *viewed from the Miwok Trail, stretches across the northern horizon.*

Facilities

Just west of the trailhead, the **Marin Headlands visitor center** has interpretive displays, books and maps for sale, helpful rangers, restrooms, and water. Reach it by going 0.2 mile past the first parking area on Bunker Rd.; turn left onto Field Rd. and go 0.1 mile to the parking area on the right.

The Gerbode Valley loop takes you into some of the best wildflower terrain in the North Bay.

Trail Description

Walk north▶**1** on a dirt-and-gravel path to a wood-plank bridge that crosses a willow-shaded creek. In several hundred feet you come to a T-junction▶**2** with the Miwok Trail. You turn right onto this multi-use dirt road, alongside a marsh and willow thicket, right, which are home to red-winged blackbirds and other songbirds. After about 200 yards on this level trail you reach a junction▶**3** were the Bobcat Trail goes right, and your route, the Miwok Trail, continues straight.

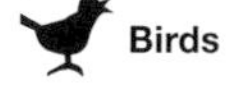

Now the Miwok Trail begins a relentless and unshaded climb toward the east end of Wolf Ridge. The hillside, right, falls steeply to Gerbode Valley. The open, coastal-scrub habitat affords seemingly limitless views, and is some of the best wildflower terrain in the Bay Area. In spring, especially after a wet winter, look for dazzling displays of California poppies, mule ears, paintbrush, Ithuriel's spear, yarrow, blow wives, and blue-eyed grass.

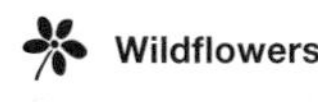

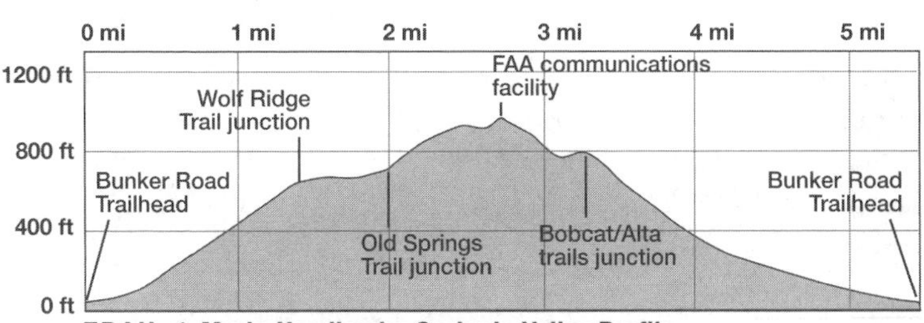

TRAIL 1 Marin Headlands: Gerbode Valley Profile

After a mile or so, you reach a notch at the east end of Wolf Ridge. From this vantage point, you can look northwest to Mt. Tamalpais and west to the Pacific Ocean. A few paces ahead is a junction with the Wolf Ridge Trail,►**4** left, which is hiking-only, with dogs allowed. (From here on, your route is closed to dogs.)

Make a short side trip on the Old Springs Trail►5 to visit lush, spring-fed meadows with sedges and wildflowers.

Bend right on the Miwok Trail and amble along a wide ridge to a junction with the multi-use Old Springs Trail,►**5** left. Now the dirt road ascends steeply across open ground. Nearing the ridgetop, you pass a single-track trail, right, that climbs toward a fenced-in communication facility on the summit, which is used by the Federal Aviation Administration (FAA) to direct commercial aircraft. Just left of this fork are a few large rocks, a convenient place to sit and rest.

After enjoying the scenery—which includes Mt. Tamalpais, San Pablo Bay, Mill Valley, and Richardson Bay—you continue uphill around the north slope of the 1041-foot summit, which divides the Tennessee and Gerbode valleys.

 **Summit**

 **Great Views**

Swinging right, you come to a four-way junction of three dirt roads and a single-track trail, just east of the FAA facility. Here you turn left on the **Bobcat Trail,** passing a closed trail, left. Your dirt road descends through an unattractive area that was graded for a never-completed boulevard and resembles a gravel pit.

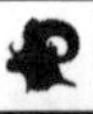

OPTIONS

Hawk Camp

Hawk Camp has three sites that can each hold up to four people. There are picnic tables and a toilet, but no water. No fires are allowed, so if you want to cook, you need a camp stove. For reservations, call (415) 331-1540 between 9:30 A.M. and 4:30 P.M. You must pick up your permit at the visitor center during the above hours. Reservations may be made up to 90 days in advance.

Soon you arrive at a partially-signed junction with the Marincello Trail, left.►6 Continue straight along the Bobcat Trail, a dirt road open to hikers, horses, and bikes, which is now the Bay Area Ridge Trail route. As you descend, you pass a junction with the road to **Hawk Camp,** right, one of three walk-in campgrounds in the headlands.

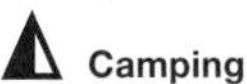

About 0.4 mile past the Hawk Camp turnoff, a trail post with the Bay Area Ridge Trail emblem marks a possibly confusing junction.►7 Here, you stay on the multiuse Bobcat Trail by going straight. (Hikers and equestrians using the Bay Area Ridge Trail turn left then right on the Alta Trail, which is closed to bikes.)

The dirt road begins a long, steady descent to Gerbode Valley. Near the bottom you pass a eucalyptus grove and several plum trees, which mark the site of an old dairy ranch. After a level walk you bear right at a junction with the Rodeo Valley Trail, left, and cross the willow-lined creek draining Gerbode Valley, which passes under the road through a culvert. In about 50 feet, you come to a T-junction with the Miwok Trail you passed at the start of your trip, where you turn left►8 and retrace your route to the parking area.►9

MILESTONES

►1	0.0	Take dirt-and-gravel path north from trailhead
►2	0.1	Right at t-junction on Miwok Trail
►3	0.2	Straight on Miwok Trail as Bobcat Trail branches right
►4	1.2	Right on Miwok Trail at Wolf Ridge Trail junction
►5	1.5	Right on Miwok Trail at Old Springs Trail junction
►6	2.5	Miwok Trail ends at summit; left on Bobcat Trail, then straight as Marincello Trail enters left
►7	3.2	Straight on Bobcat Trail at junction with Alta Trail (Bay Area Ridge Trail hiker/horse route)
►8	5.2	Left on Miwok Trail
►9	5.4	Back at parking area

Muir Woods: Dipsea Trail

TRAIL 2

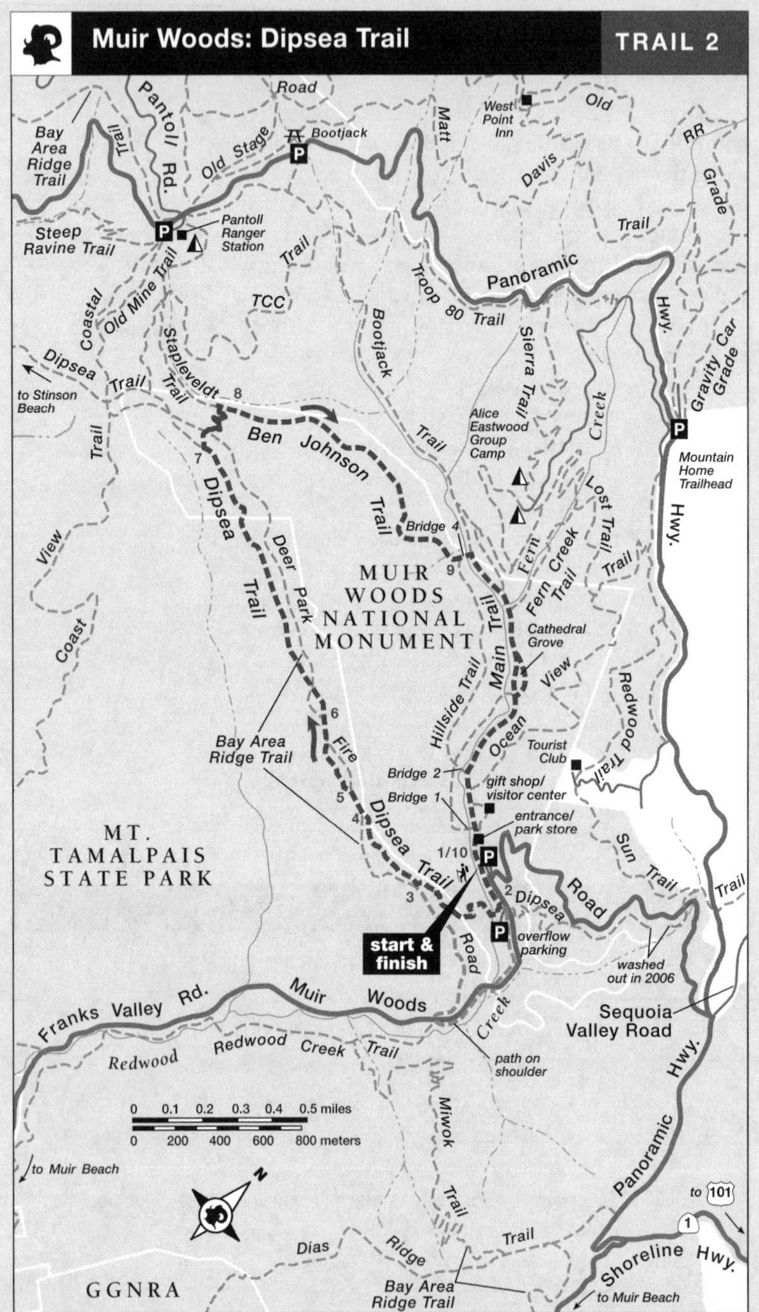

Muir Woods National Monument: Dipsea Trail

This loop climbs across high meadows on a stretch of the famous Dipsea footrace route, then descends through old-growth coast redwoods to the bustle and grandeur of Muir Woods National Monument.

TRAIL USE
Hike
LENGTH
4.0 miles, 3 hours
VERTICAL FEET
±925'
DIFFICULTY
– 1 2 **3** 4 5 +
TRAIL TYPE
Loop
SURFACE TYPE
Dirt, Paved

FEATURES
Stream
Canyon
Birds
Historic
Cool & Shady

FACILITIES
Visitor Center
Park Store
Snack Bar
Restrooms
Water
Phone

Best Time

Spring through fall. In summer expect fog and tourists—parking areas fill by midmorning. In winter, when Redwood Creek may be too deep to cross, use the alternate route described below.

Finding the Trail

From US Hwy. 101 northbound in Mill Valley, take the State Hwy. 1/Mill Valley/Stinson Beach exit (which is also signed for Muir Woods and Mt. Tamalpais). After exiting, stay in the right lane as you go under US 101. At about 1 mile from US 101, get in the left lane, and, at a stoplight, follow Shoreline Hwy. as it turns left.

Continue 2.7 miles to Panoramic Hwy. and turn right. At 0.8 mile on Panoramic Hwy., where the road splits in three directions, turn left down Muir Woods Rd. After 1.6 miles you come to a hairpin turn where Muir Woods Rd. turns left, but you go straight and park in the main parking area for Muir Woods National Monument. If there's a long line of cars, instead turn sharply left on Muir Woods Rd. and go another 100 yards to the overflow parking area, right. If this lot is full, continue south and look for roadside parking (possibly as far south as the Deer Park Fire Rd.). A trail along the west side of Muir Woods Rd. will take you north to the overflow and main parking areas.

From Hwy. 101 southbound in Mill Valley, take the Hwy. 1 North/Stinson Beach exit (which is also signed for Muir Woods and Mt. Tamalpais). After exiting, bear right, go 0.1 mile to a stop sign, and bear left on Hwy. 1. Go 0.5 mile, get in the left lane, and, at a stoplight, follow Shoreline Hwy. as it turns left. Then follow the directions in the second paragraph above.

The trailhead is a paved path on the west side of the main parking area,►1 but if you park at the overflow parking area (or beyond), start from the Dipsea Trail information board at the northwest corner of the overflow parking area.►2 The ranger station at the entrance to Muir Woods National Monument posts current trail conditions; there is a park store with books and maps. Because you will enter Muir Woods National Monument via the "back door," you won't be required to pay admission, but you may leave a suitable donation in the box by the exit path when you reach it.

On weekends and holidays from May through September, consider taking Golden Gate Transit's free Muir Woods shuttle from Marin City to the Muir Woods National Monument entrance. In summer, some Golden Gate Transit shuttles to Muir Woods also depart from the Sausalito ferry terminal.

Trail Description

From the west side of the main parking area,►1 head south on a paved path past restrooms and through a shady grove. In 100 yards you come to the overflow parking area,►2 where the **Dipsea Trail** from Mill Valley enters left. Now on the Dipsea Trail, go straight another 50 feet, then descend right on wooden steps and cross alder-shaded **Redwood Creek** on a low, log footbridge. Although an easy crossing from spring through fall, it is impossible to cross here in winter when the creek flows over the log.

(Check at the ranger station for current conditions and see below for an alternate winter route.)

Safely across the creek, the Dipsea Trail crosses a gravelly flood plain, then ascends on a moderately steep grade toward the ridgeline through a forest of California bay and Douglas-fir. After 0.3 mile, your single-track trail comes alongside the Deer Park Fire Road►**3** but does not join it. Stay right on the Dipsea Trail and climb across open coastal scrub and meadows at the edge of the forest.

Soon this segment of the Dipsea Trail ends at a T-junction.►**4** Turn right and continue west on **Deer Park Fire Road** for 100 yards. As the road bends right, stay straight on another short segment of the Dipsea Trail,►**5** which climbs across a meadow then rejoins the road about 500 feet ahead.

Angle left on the Deer Park Fire Road for about 400 feet, now in forest. As the road bends left, the Dipsea Trail►**6** ascends right at an unsigned junction. Follow this single-track trail through a pine grove and then out into coastal scrub. Just ahead, Deer Park Fire Road crosses your trail, ascending from left to right, but you continue straight. Now the Dipsea Trail begins a long, easy ascent across a wide meadow, edged by Douglas-fir and California bay. After about 0.5 mile you leave the meadow, dip to cross a stream, and then begin a steady climb amid tall conifers. Along the trail, several Douglas-firs have been toppled by winter storms, exposing their roots and opening the shady canopy for sun-loving shrubs such as huckleberry.

On level ground you come to a junction where you turn right on the **Ben Johnson Trail.**►**7** In a few steps you cross Deer Park Fire Road at the upper edge of a magnificent coast redwood forest. Straight ahead, the Ben Johnson Trail plunges steeply via a dozen switchbacks to a sheltered grove and a junction with the Stapleveldt Trail, left.►**8**

Stretching 7.1 miles from Mill Valley to Stinson Beach, the Dipsea Trail is the route of a rugged footrace, held nearly every year since 1905.

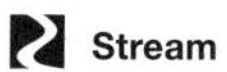
Stream

Turn right and continue down the Ben Johnson Trail, which descends easily across hillsides and gulches as the main canyon of Redwood Creek drops left. After nearly a mile of relative solitude amid the redwoods, you descend past the Hillside Trail, right, and arrive at Bridge 4 across Redwood Creek. A few steps past the bridge is a T-junction with the Bootjack and Main Trails.▶9

Turn right on the **Main Trail**, a paved path that winds between the stately old-growth giants and follows the east bank of Redwood Creek. From here you will share the trail with a steady stream of visitors from all over the world. Split-rail fences line the trail to keep people from trampling the fragile tree roots.

Amid the enormous redwoods, look for shade-loving deciduous trees including California bay, alder, and bigleaf maple. You may notice many dead, mature tanbark oaks, along with young tanbark oak saplings still sprouting.

Along the last mile of this loop, the Camp Eastwood and Fern trails enter left, then Bridges 3

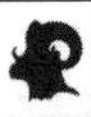

OPTIONS

Winter Detour

When the Dipsea Trail footbridge across Redwood Creek is flooded, one alternative is to hike south to the overflow lot▶2 then detour left and turn right along **Muir Woods Rd.** For the first 0.3 mile, you follow a wide, fenced trail along the east shoulder. Then, after crossing Redwood Creek, you continue south along the left shoulder, facing traffic. Another 0.2 mile ahead you pass a trailhead for Redwood Creek Trail to the left. Here turn right, carefully cross the road, and ascend the **Deer Park Fire Rd.,** a gravel road. About 0.5 mile up the ridge the Dipsea Trail appears on the right; follow either the trail or road 0.3 mile farther to the formal junction▶3 then follow the described route. This variation totals 4.7 miles, with ±965 vertical feet.

A simpler alternative is to hike the last half of this trail in reverse. Enter Muir Woods National Monument and follow the Main Trail 1 mile along Redwood Creek. At Bridge 4, turn left up the Ben Johnson Trail as far as you like, then retrace your route.

and 2 head right to the west side of the creek. In winter these bridges are good places to look for migratory steelhead and salmon.

Just after the Ocean View Trail enters left, the Main Trail joins a wooden boardwalk. Spurs branch left to the gift shop, snack bar, and restrooms, and right to Bridge 1. Continue straight on the Main Trail to the main entrance, park store, and main parking area.►**10**

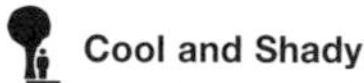

Cool and Shady

To return to the overflow lot, follow the paved path on the west edge of the main parking area past the restrooms, then turn left at the Dipsea Trail junction to the overflow lot. If you parked farther south, walk to the entrance of the overflow lot, then turn right on the gravel path that parallels Muir Woods Road.

MILESTONES

►1	0.0	From west edge of main parking area, take paved path south past restrooms
►2	0.1	Dipsea Trail enters on left; continue straight on Dipsea Trail, which bends right across Redwood Creek
►3	0.4	Deer Park Fire Rd. appears left briefly; stay right on Dipsea Trail
►4	0.6	Dipsea Trail ends at T-junction; turn right on Deer Park Fire Rd.
►5	0.7	Stay left on single-track Dipsea Trail, then angle left on Deer Park Fire Rd.
►6	0.9	Angle right on single-track Dipsea Trail; stay straight 100 yards ahead as you cross Deer Park Fire Rd.
►7	1.7	Right on Ben Johnson Trail; go straight across Deer Park Fire Rd. and descend switchbacks
►8	2.0	Stapleveldt Trail goes left; stay right on Ben Johnson Trail
►9	2.9	Stay straight past Hillside Trail to Bridge 4, then turn right on Main Trail
►10	4.0	Back at ranger station, entrance, and main parking area

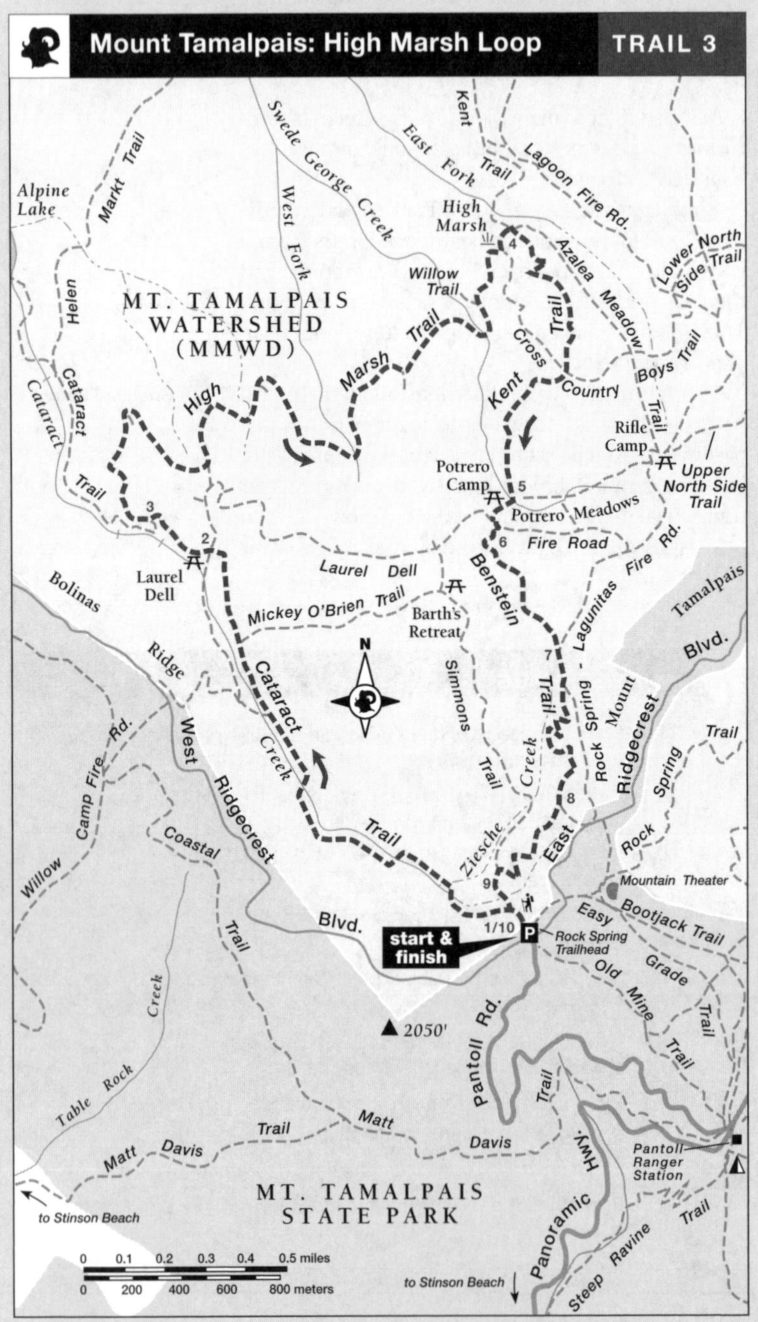
Mount Tamalpais: High Marsh Loop
TRAIL 3
Alpine Lake
Markt Trail
Swede George Creek
West Fork
East Fork
Kent Trail
Lagoon Fire Rd.
High Marsh
Azalea Meadow
Lower North Side Trail
Willow Trail
MT. TAMALPAIS WATERSHED (MMWD)
Helen
High Marsh Trail
Kent Trail
Cross Country Boys Trail
Cataract
Cataract Trail
Rifle Camp
Potrero Camp
Upper North Side Trail
Potrero Meadows Fire Road
Laurel Dell
Bolinas Ridge
Mickey O'Brien Trail
Barth's Retreat
Benstein Trail
Lagunitas - Rock Spring Fire Rd.
Tamalpais Blvd.
Mount Ridgecrest
Rock Spring Trail
Simmons Trail
Cataract Creek
Cataract Trail
Creek
West Ridgecrest Blvd.
Willow Camp Fire Rd.
Coastal Trail
Ziesche Creek
East
Mountain Theater
Easy Grade
Bootjack Trail
start & finish
Rock Spring Trailhead
Old Mine Trail
Trail
Pantoll Rd.
2050'
Creek
Table Rock
Matt Davis Trail
Matt Davis
Hwy.
Trail
Pantoll Ranger Station
MT. TAMALPAIS STATE PARK
to Stinson Beach
Panoramic
Steep Ravine Trail
to Stinson Beach
0 0.1 0.2 0.3 0.4 0.5 miles
0 200 400 600 800 meters
N
1/10 2 3 4 5 6 7 8 9
P

Mount Tamalpais: High Marsh Loop

This beautiful and strenuous loop takes you past a scenic waterfall, beside a freshwater marsh, through areas of chaparral, and into groves of Sargent cypress and forests of Douglas-fir and oak as it explores the rugged canyons and ridges of Marin Municipal Water District (MMWD) lands above Alpine Lake on the north side of Mt. Tamalpais.

TRAIL USE
Hike, Run, Dogs Allowed

LENGTH
5.8 miles, 4–5 hours

VERTICAL FEET
±1400'

DIFFICULTY
– 1 2 3 **4** 5 +

TRAIL TYPE
Loop

SURFACE TYPE
Dirt

FEATURES
Stream
Waterfall
Canyon
Mountain
Birds
Secluded
Cool & Shady

FACILITIES
Restrooms
Picnic Tables

Best Time

All year; Cataract Falls is best in winter and early spring.

Finding the Trail

From US Hwy. 101 northbound in Mill Valley, take the State Hwy. 1/Mill Valley/Stinson Beach exit (which is also signed for Muir Woods and Mt. Tamalpais). After exiting, stay in the right lane as you go under Hwy. 101. At about 1 mile from Hwy. 101, get in the left lane, and, at a stoplight, follow Shoreline Hwy. as it turns left.

Continue 2.7 miles to Panoramic Hwy. and turn right. At 5.4 miles from Hwy. 1, you reach the Pantoll Campground and Ranger Station, left, and Pantoll Rd., right. Turn right, and go 1.4 miles to a T-junction with E. Ridgecrest Blvd. and W. Ridgecrest Blvd. Across the junction is a large paved parking area, shown on the map as the Rock Spring Trailhead. The trailhead is on the north side of the parking area.

From Hwy. 101 southbound in Mill Valley, take the State Hwy. 1 N./Stinson Beach exit (which is also signed for Muir Woods and Mt. Tamalpais). After exiting, bear right, go 0.1 mile to a stop sign, and bear left on Hwy. 1. Go 0.5 mile, get in the left lane, and, at a stoplight, follow Shoreline Hwy. as it turns left. Then follow the directions in the previous paragraph.

Trail Description

From the trailhead,▶1 pass an unsigned spur, right, and descend north on the **Cataract Trail**, a wide dirt-and-gravel path. In about 100 yards you reach a fork, where you veer left to stay on the Cataract Trail. The route takes you gently downhill, through conifers and meadows, and across a wood bridge over **Cataract Creek**, which drains Serpentine Swale and flows into Alpine Lake. Several hundred feet downstream from the bridge, you come to a jumble of big, moss-covered boulders. Although you may see a trail across the creek, left, stay on the creek's right side and follow the Cataract Trail through the boulders. Soon you reach a clearing and another wood bridge, this one over Ziesche Creek.

Stream

Where the route once continued straight, it now turns left, descends a few wooden steps, and then crosses a bridge over Cataract Creek. The trail leads

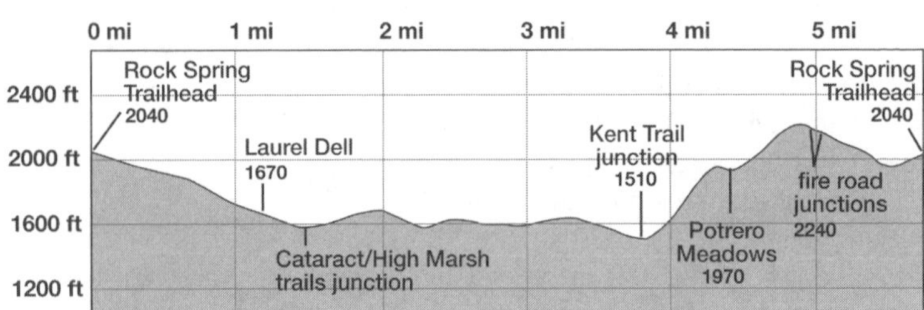

TRAIL 3 Mount Tamalpais: High Marsh Loop Profile

you back into forest. Soon you pass a trail, left, that crosses Cataract Creek via a bridge and heads toward Laurel Dell Road. You continue straight, keeping the creek on your left. Just as you emerge from forest, at the edge of a clearing, you reach a junction with the Mickey O'Brien Trail heading sharply right.

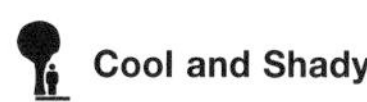

Continue on the Cataract Trail as it branches left and crosses a bridge over a stream. Skirting a large meadow, left, you soon reach restrooms and a junction with Laurel Dell Road. Angle left a few steps to the **Laurel Dell picnic area.▶2**

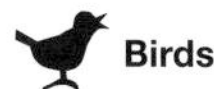

The Cataract Trail leaves the picnic area from its west side, with the creek on your left. During winter and spring, a wonderful waterfall cascades down over the ledge of a rocky cliff, downhill and left. Be patient and cautious: you'll have a great view of the falls soon enough! Soon you come to a junction with the **High Marsh Trail.▶3**

To visit the falls, turn left on the Cataract Trail and walk several hundred feet to a level spot near the base of the falls. Now return to the previous junction▶3 and go straight on the High Marsh Trail, a narrow single track. The trail traverses a grassy hillside with northward views of the Cataract Creek watershed, then wanders amid a shady forest of California bay.

Waterfall

The route now alternates between wooded and open areas. A steep climb brings you to a junction with a short side trail to Laurel Dell Road, uphill and right. Back in forest, the trail pursues a rolling course. Soon you pass a creek bed, which may be dry, and begin a steep climb, passing an unsigned trail heading uphill and right. Descending over rough ground, you drop steeply into a ravine that holds a seasonal creek. The trail soon crosses **Swede George Creek.** If the creek is flowing, look uphill for a series of beautiful miniature waterfalls.

Waterfall

About 140 yards past Swede George Creek, you reach an unsigned fork: stay on the High Marsh

Trail by climbing right on a moderate grade. After topping a ridge, the trail descends and High Marsh comes into view ahead. Your trail curves right, around the edge of the marsh, to a T-junction with the Cross Country Boys Trail. Turn left and skirt High Marsh's southeast edge to a four-way junction▶4 marked by a trail post. Here, the High Marsh Trail ends, the **Kent Trail** runs left-to-right, and the Azalea Meadow Trail continues straight. You turn right onto the Kent Trail.

Secluded

The Kent Trail ascends through forest and chaparral and crosses the Cross Country Boys Trail. Out of the trees, you traverse a manzanita barren, giving you a chance to enjoy a fine view north of Big Rock Ridge, topped by two communication towers, and, beyond it, Burdell Mountain.

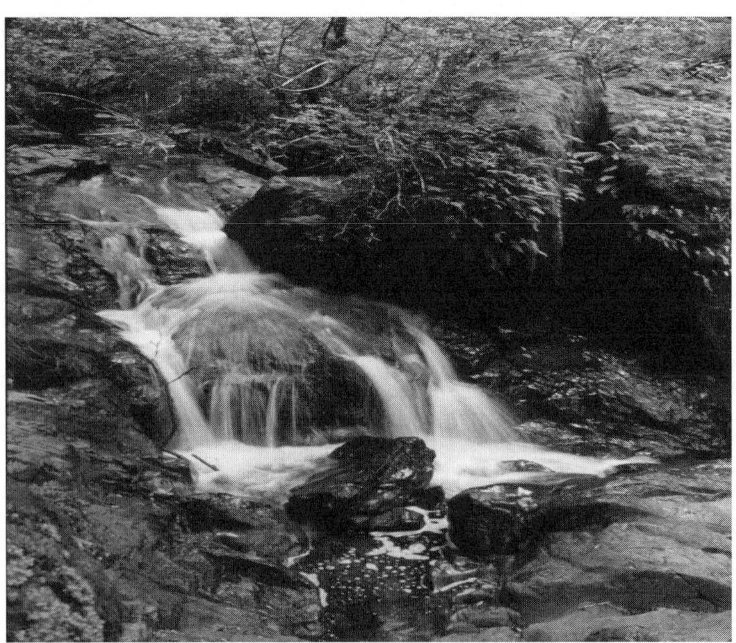

Cataract Creek

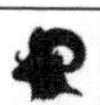

OPTIONS

Kent Trail Scenery

A short (100 yards or so) ramble left on the **Kent Trail** brings you to a scenic bridge over the East Fork of Swede George Creek, where azaleas bloom nearby in midsummer.

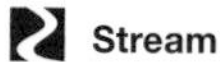

Stream

You now begin a moderate descent, soon finding a lovely stream, the headwaters of Swede George Creek, on your right. Reaching a trail post and a T-junction,▶5 you have **Potrero Meadows** in front of you, toilets to your left, and the **Potrero Camp picnic area,** with tables and fire grates, to your right. Turning right, you follow the trail as it crosses a bridge over the stream and leads, in about 75 feet, to the picnic area. Here you follow a dirt-and-gravel road south and steeply uphill about 100 yards to a T-junction with **Laurel Dell Fire Road.**▶6

Now you turn left onto a dirt road and descend gently for about 150 feet to a junction, right, with the **Benstein Trail.** Turn right and climb moderately on the Benstein Trail, a single track which is closed to bikes and horses. The route climbs over serpentine rock, which may be slippery when wet, through a forest of stunted Sargent cypress, natives of the Coast Ranges of California. Their namesake, Charles Sprague Sargent, founded the Arnold Arboretum at Harvard University and wrote 14 books on North American trees.

Swede George Creek on the north slope of Mt. Tamalpais is named for a mountain man who once had a cabin in the area.

Leaving the cypress behind, you climb amid Douglas-fir and tanbark oak on an ever-steepening grade to reach a ridgetop. Once across the ridge, the Benstein Trail descends gently to a junction with **Rock Spring–Lagunitas Fire Road.**▶7 Bear right and follow the gravel road about 100 yards to a second junction. Bear right on the single-track **Benstein Trail**, which switchbacks down

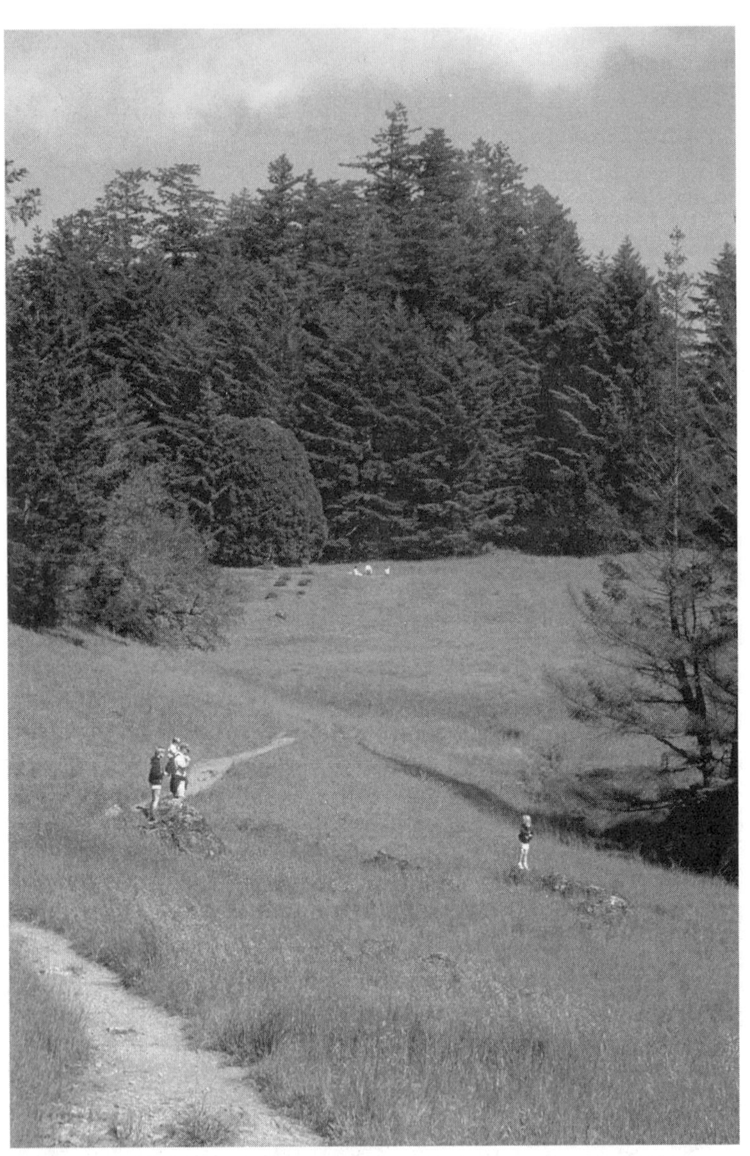

Benstein Trail *crosses Serpentine Swale.*

a wooded slope above **Ziesche Creek.** At a fork with the Benstein Spur Trail,►8 stay right. The Benstein Trail descends via steps and switchbacks to a T-junction with the **Simmons Trail,**►9 where you turn left to return to the **Rock Spring picnic area** and the trailhead.►10

MILESTONES

►1	0.0	Take Cataract Trail north, ignoring spur on right
►2	1.2	Laurel Dell picnic area
►3	1.6	T-junction: Left on Cataract Trail to view falls, then return to junction and go straight on High Marsh Trail
►4	3.8	Right on Kent Trail at four-way junction
►5	4.4	Right at T-junction to Potrero Camp picnic area, then dirt-and-gravel road south to Laurel Dell Rd.
►6	4.5	Left on Laurel Dell Rd., then right on Benstein Trail
►7	5.0	Right on Rock Spring–Lagunitas Rd., then right to stay on Benstein Trail
►8	5.5	Stay right on Benstein Trail at Benstein Spur junction
►9	5.7	Left on Simmons Trail
►10	5.8	Left on Cataract Trail; back at parking area

Mount Tamalpais: Middle Peak

TRAIL 4

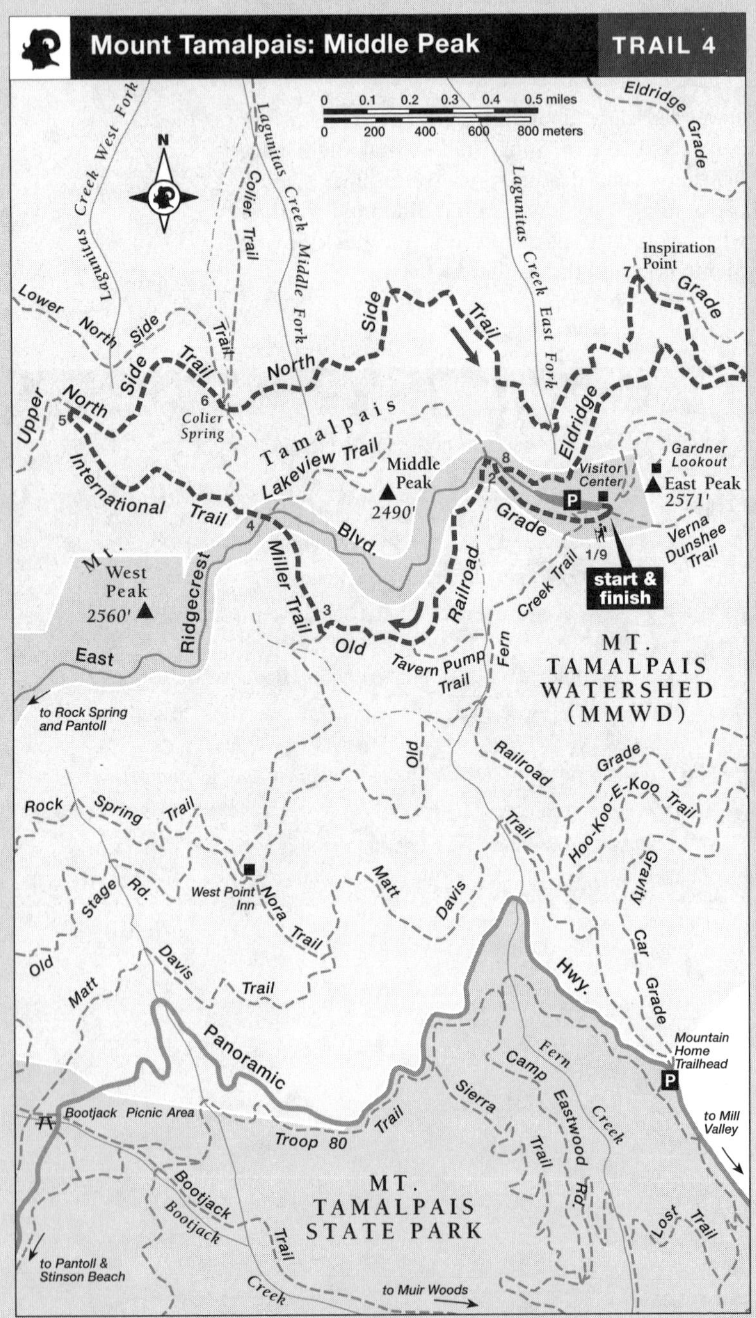

Mount Tamalpais: Middle Peak

This circuit of Middle Peak explores a wonderful variety of terrain, from chaparral cloaking the mountain's upper reaches to redwood groves hidden on its northern side. Along the way, you have fine views of Marin Municipal Water District (MMWD) lands, including Bon Tempe Lake and Lake Lagunitas.

TRAIL USE
Hike, Run, Dogs Allowed

LENGTH
5.1 miles, 3 hours

VERTICAL FEET
±1450'

DIFFICULTY
– 1 2 **3** 4 5 +

TRAIL TYPE
Loop

SURFACE TYPE
Dirt, Paved

FEATURES
Fee
Stream
Canyon
Mountain
Birds
Great Views
Cool & Shady

FACILITIES
Visitor Center
Restrooms
Picnic Tables
Water
Phone

Best Time

All year; expect fog in summer. In winter, if fog blankets the Bay Area, this trail may rise above it.

Finding the Trail

From US Hwy. 101 northbound in Mill Valley, take the State Hwy. 1/Mill Valley/Stinson Beach exit (which is also signed for Muir Woods and Mt. Tamalpais). After exiting, stay in the right lane as you go under Hwy. 101. At about 1 mile from Hwy. 101, get in the left lane, and, at a stoplight, follow Shoreline Hwy. as it turns left.

Continue 2.7 miles to Panoramic Hwy. and turn right. At 5.4 miles from Hwy. 1, you reach the Pantoll Campground and Ranger Station, left, and Pantoll Rd., right. Turn right, and go 1.4 miles to a T-junction with E. Ridgecrest Blvd. and W. Ridgecrest Blvd. Turn right on E. Ridgecrest Blvd. and go 3 miles to the East Peak parking area and a self-registration station, just below East Peak. The trailhead is on the east end of the East Peak parking area, just south of the visitor center and restrooms.

From Hwy. 101 southbound in Mill Valley, take the State Hwy. 1 N./Stinson Beach exit (which is also signed for Muir Woods and Mt. Tamalpais). After exiting, bear right, go 0.1 mile to a stop sign, and bear left on Hwy. 1. Go 0.5 mile, get in the left lane, and, at a stoplight, follow Shoreline Hwy. as it turns left. Then follow the directions in the previous paragraph.

Trail Description

From the trailhead,►1 walk down a narrow paved road, closed to cars, that descends through chaparral below the south edge of the parking area. Several hundred yards from the start, you briefly join East Ridgecrest Boulevard, and pass Eldridge Grade, a dirt road, on your right. About 100 feet farther, you turn left onto **Old Railroad Grade,** a dirt road favored by mountain bikers.►2

A sea of chaparral—manzanita, chamise, buckbrush, and toyon—blankets these upper reaches of the mountain. Soon you pass the Tavern Pump Trail, which heads left and steeply downhill. When you reach the **Miller Trail,**►3 turn right and begin a moderate ascent through manzanita and clumps of native bunchgrass, aided in places by wood and stone steps. After a few steep sections, the Miller

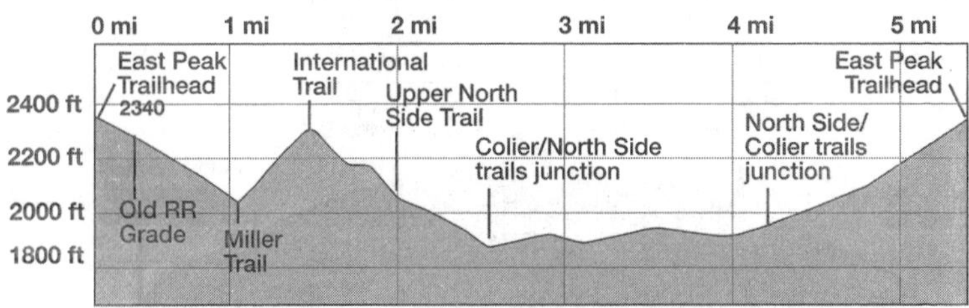

TRAIL 4 Mount Tamalpais: Middle Peak Profile

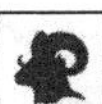

OPTIONS

Mount Tam's East Peak

From the trailhead you can easily climb **East Peak** (2571') via the well-graded **East Peak Trail,** which starts off from the trailhead on a boardwalk just between the restrooms and the snack bar. The rustic fire lookout on the summit is staffed in summer.

Trail arrives at **East Ridgecrest Boulevard,**▶4 which divides the north and south sides of the mountain.

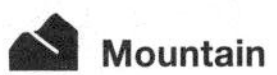

After carefully crossing the paved road, find the **International Trail** heading northwest. Several hundred feet from the road, you reach a junction where the Colier Spring Trail, a shortcut to the North Side Trail, descends right. Your route continues straight through dense forest of Douglas-fir, tanbark oak, California bay, and California nutmeg, dropping in places to lose elevation, leveling in others.

On a rocky, open ridge studded with Sargent cypress, the International Trail ends at a junction with the **Upper North Side Trail**; here you turn right.▶5 The Upper North Side Trail traverses eastward through mixed evergreen forest on an easy grade, soon reaching a junction at **Colier Spring** in a coast redwood grove, where a rest bench awaits.▶6 From here continue straight, now on the gently rolling **North Side Trail.** Once past **Lagunitas Creek Middle Fork,** which flows under the trail through a culvert, you make a gentle climb through open stands of madrone and tanbark oak. At one ridge, your trail makes a sharp right-hand bend and crosses a closed fire trail. Middle Peak, topped by communication towers, is uphill and right.

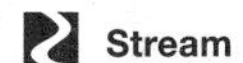

Continuing straight, the route crosses a culvert holding **Lagunitas Creek East Fork,** where waterfalls may tumble over mossy rocks just upstream. After passing a seasonal creek, the trail bends left,

On a clear day you can see San Francisco, Angel Island, the Bay Bridge, the East Bay hills, the Marin Headlands, and the East, Middle, and West summits of Mt. Tamalpais.

affording views of Pilot Knob and Bon Tempe Lake. Soon you reach **Inspiration Point,** a clearing marked by a trail post. Continue straight on the Northside Trail about 100 yards to meet **Eldridge Grade,** a dirt road, where you bear right.►**7**

The road heads eastward, only to reverse field with a sharp right-hand switchback. Now follow the road generally southwest, with the summit of East Peak slightly left and only a few hundred feet above. Eldridge Grade skirts the west side of East Peak, swings right, and soon makes a moderate climb to East Ridgecrest Boulevard. Here you turn left►**8** and retrace your route to the parking area.►**9**

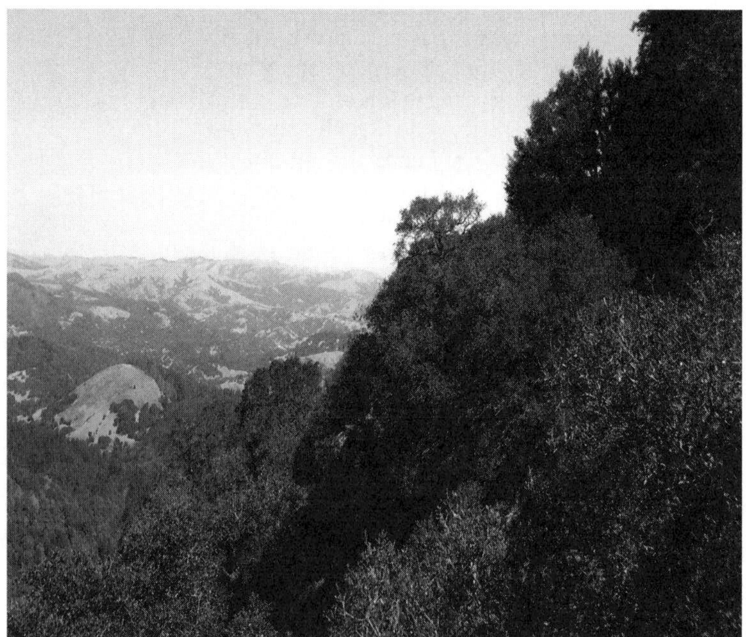

Ben Pease

View north *from Mt. Tam's Middle Peak*

MILESTONES

▶1	0.0	Take closed paved road south and west
▶2	0.2	Merge with E. Ridgecrest Blvd., then left on Old Railroad Grade
▶3	0.8	Right on Miller Trail
▶4	1.1	Cross E. Ridgecrest Blvd., take International Trail
▶5	1.6	Right on Upper North Side Trail
▶6	2.1	Straight on North Side Trail
▶7	3.7	Right on Eldridge Grade
▶8	4.9	Left on E. Ridgecrest Blvd.
▶9	5.1	Back at parking area

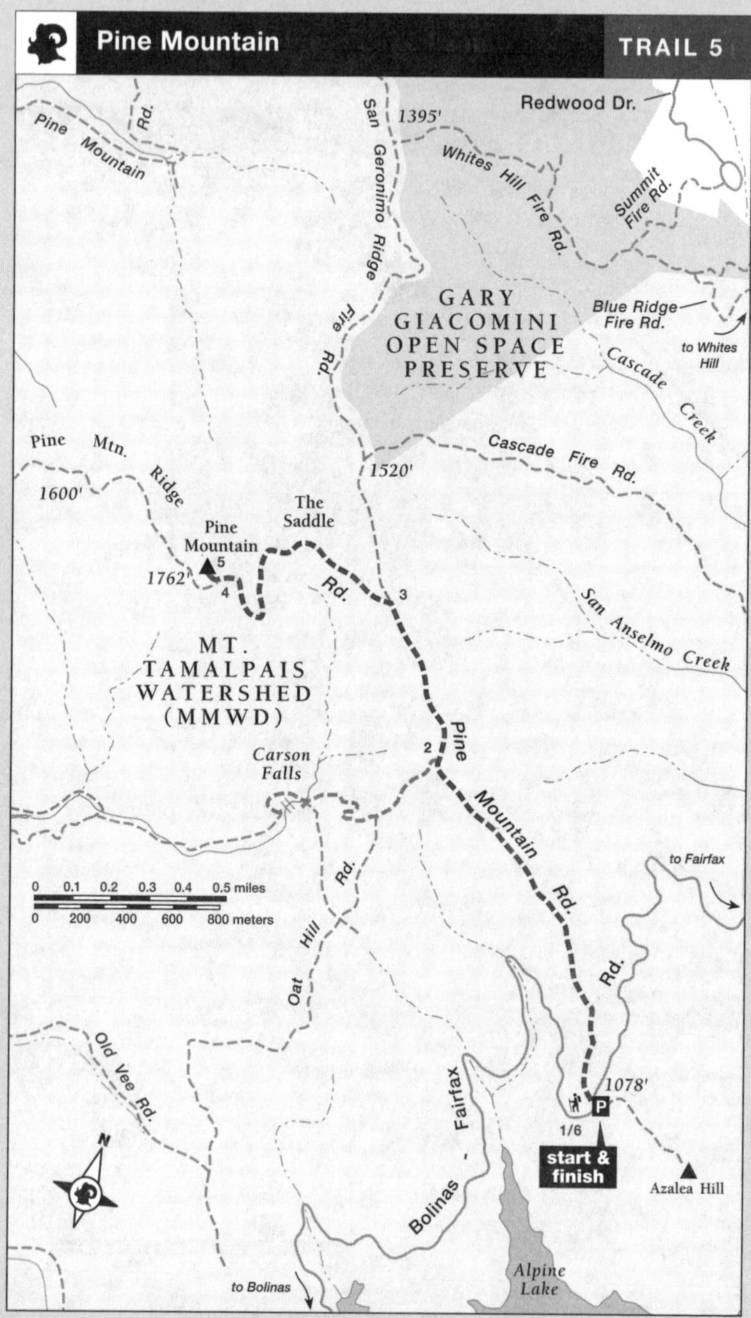
Pine Mountain
TRAIL 5
Redwood Dr.
Pine Mountain
Rd.
San Geronimo Ridge Fire Rd.
1395'
Whites Hill Fire Rd.
Summit Fire Rd.
GARY GIACOMINI OPEN SPACE PRESERVE
Blue Ridge Fire Rd.
to Whites Hill
Cascade Creek
Cascade Fire Rd.
Pine Mtn. Ridge
1600'
1520'
The Saddle
Pine Mountain
1762'
Rd.
San Anselmo Creek
MT. TAMALPAIS WATERSHED (MMWD)
Carson Falls
Pine Mountain Rd.
to Fairfax
0 0.1 0.2 0.3 0.4 0.5 miles
0 200 400 600 800 meters
Oat Hill Rd.
Rd.
Old Vee Rd.
Fairfax - Bolinas
1078'
1/6
start & finish
Azalea Hill
Alpine Lake
to Bolinas

Pine Mountain

This out-and-back route takes you to one of the best vantage points in the Bay Area, where on a clear day your efforts will be rewarded by fantastic views. Along the way, plant lovers can stay busy identifying a variety of trees and shrubs, some found only on the locally prevalent serpentine soil. This area is also a favorite with mountain bikers.

TRAIL USE
Hike, Run, Bike, Dogs Allowed
LENGTH
4.7 miles, 2–3 hours
VERTICAL FEET
±1000'
DIFFICULTY
– 1 2 **3** 4 5 +
TRAIL TYPE
Out & Back
SURFACE TYPE
Dirt

FEATURES
Mountain
Summit
Birds
Great Views
Photo Opportunity
Secluded

FACILITIES
None

Best Time

This route is enjoyable all year.

Finding the Trail

From US Hwy. 101 northbound, take the San Anselmo exit, also signed for San Quentin, Sir Francis Drake Blvd., and the Richmond Bridge. Stay in the left lane as you exit, toward San Anselmo. Follow Sir Francis Drake Blvd. 5.5 miles to a stoplight at Claus Dr. in Fairfax. Jog left onto Broadway and right onto Bolinas Rd., which is heavily used by bicyclists. (Bolinas Rd. soon becomes Fairfax–Bolinas Rd.) Go 3.9 miles to gravel Azalea Hill parking area on the left. The trailhead is on the west side of Fairfax–Bolinas Rd., about 50 feet north of the parking area.

From Hwy. 101 southbound, take the Sir Francis Drake/Kentfield exit and follow the directions above.

Trail Description

After carefully crossing **Fairfax–Bolinas Road,**▶1 you walk north about 50 feet from the parking area to **Pine Mountain Road**, a gated dirt road. A rolling,

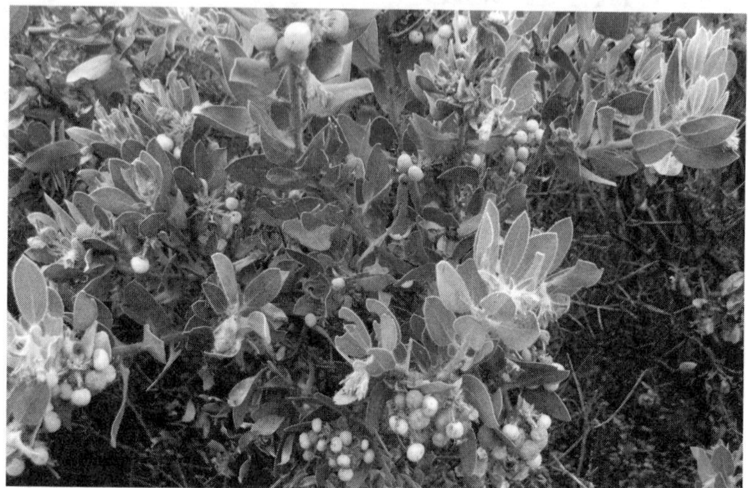

Manzanita, *a hardy, fire-adaptive shrub, is found in dry, rocky areas.*

Look northwest from The Saddle to find Barnabe Mountain, a 1466-foot peak on the edge of Samuel P. Taylor State Park. A route to Barnabe Mountain's summit is described in Trail 6 (page 57).

ridgetop course through scrub affords views of Liberty Gulch, left, and Mt. Tamalpais, behind you to the southeast. The serpentine soil here favors hardy plants such as leather oak and Sargent cypress. You climb on a gentle and then moderate grade to a high point, from where you can see **The Saddle,** a windy gap between Pine Mountain and an unnamed peak to its northeast.

Dropping slightly, you soon pass Oat Hill Road, signed OATHILL RD, on your left.►**2** Gaining elevation over rough but not ankle-twisting ground, you reach a junction with San Geronimo Ridge Fire Road.►**3** You turn left on Pine Mountain Road and begin a moderate ascent, with a deep valley on your left and a grassy hillside rising right. As you near The Saddle, flattened grasses downhill and left attest to the wind's power as it rushes unhindered from the Pacific Ocean through the gap.

From The Saddle, the road swings left and rises on a moderate grade, soon changing to steep. The rough and rocky road eventually levels at a saddle and then climbs to another saddle, where you find

 **Mountain**

 **Great Views**

OPTIONS

Carson Falls

Due south of Pine Mountain lies scenic Carson Falls, a side trip that adds 1.8 miles and ±400 vertical feet to the overall trip. To visit, descend west on **Oat Hill Rd.** 0.3 mile from its junction with Pine Mountain Rd.▶2 Past a grassy saddle, turn right on the Carson Falls Trail, which is hiking-only. A narrow single track descends via switchbacks through a California bay forest to a grassy valley. At a fork, a short trail leads left to an overlook of **Carson Falls,** whereas the main trail crosses **Little Carson Creek** on a log bridge and descends via well-built steps and switchbacks to a second viewpoint below the falls. The pools in the rocky outcrop are home to endangered foothill yellow-legged frog. The new trail provides a safe route for hikers to avoid disturbing the frogs (please stay on trails). After enjoying the falls, retrace your route to Pine Mountain Rd.

an unsigned single-track trail, right.▶4 Turning right, you begin the final push through chaparral to the summit.▶5

Without a doubt, Pine Mountain is one of the best vantage points in the Bay Area. The 360-degree panorama may keep you busy identifying such landmarks as Mt. Tamalpais, Mt. Diablo, the East Bay hills, San Pablo Bay, Big Rock Ridge, Bolinas Ridge, Tomales Bay, and Kent Lake.

After you've had your fill of the scenery, retrace your route to the parking area.▶6

MILESTONES

▶1	0.0	Take Pine Mountain Rd. northwest
▶2	0.9	Oat Hill Rd; straight on Pine Mountain Rd.
▶3	1.4	Left to stay on Pine Mountain Rd.
▶4	2.3	Right on single-track trail
▶5	2.4	Summit of Pine Mountain (1762')
▶6	4.7	Back at parking area

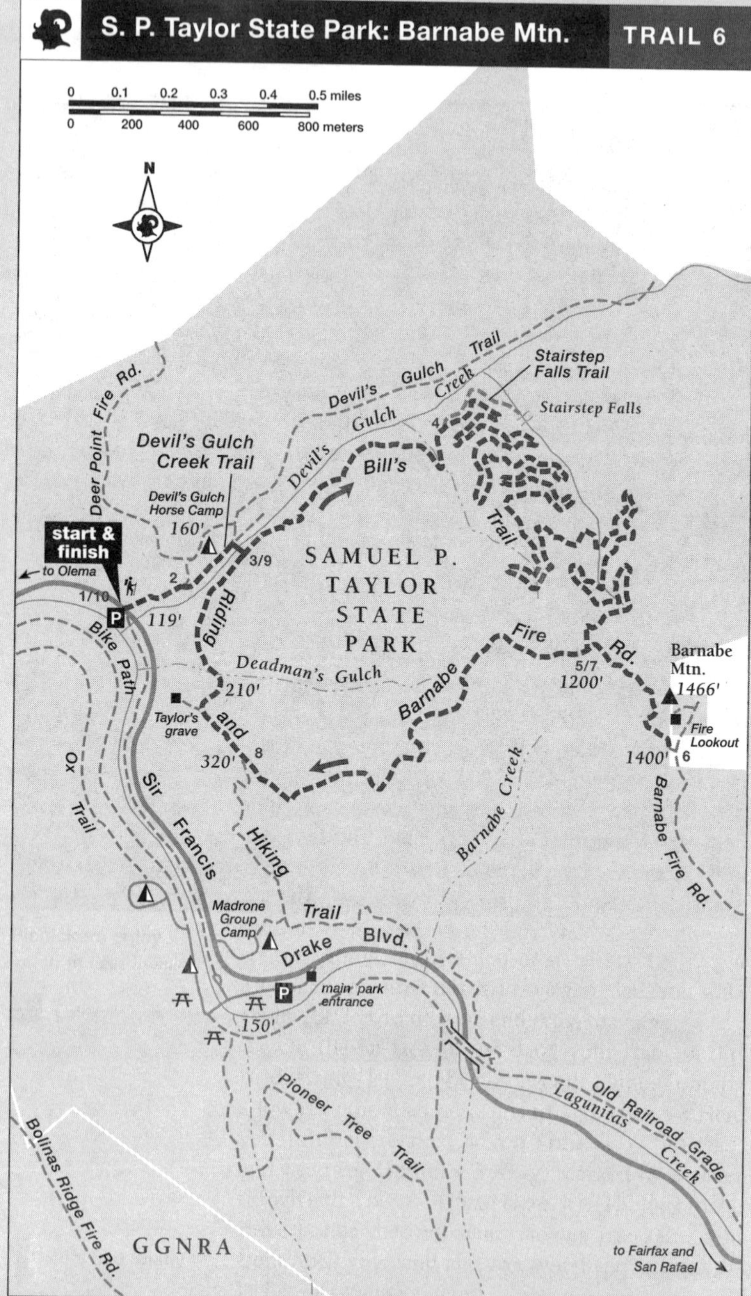
S. P. Taylor State Park: Barnabe Mtn.
TRAIL 6
0 0.1 0.2 0.3 0.4 0.5 miles
0 200 400 600 800 meters
N
Deer Point Fire Rd.
Devil's Gulch Trail
Devil's Gulch Creek
Stairstep Falls Trail
Stairstep Falls
Devil's Gulch Creek Trail
Devil's Gulch Horse Camp
160'
Bill's Trail
start & finish
to Olema
1/10
2
3/9
4
119'
SAMUEL P. TAYLOR STATE PARK
Riding and Hiking Trail
Bike Path
Deadman's Gulch
210'
Taylor's grave
320'
8
Barnabe Fire Rd.
5/7
1200'
Barnabe Mtn.
1466'
Fire Lookout
1400'
6
Barnabe Creek
Barnabe Fire Rd.
Ox Trail
Sir Francis Drake Blvd.
Madrone Group Camp
main park entrance
150'
Pioneer Tree Trail
Old Railroad Grade
Lagunitas Creek
Bolinas Ridge Fire Rd.
GGNRA
to Fairfax and San Rafael

Samuel P. Taylor State Park: Barnabe Mountain

This loop climbs gently through mixed forest, alive with birdsong and brightened by wildflowers, struggles steeply to high ground just below the summit of Barnabe Mountain (1466'), and then descends through open country with wonderful views of west Marin, Point Reyes, and the Tomales Bay area.

TRAIL USE
Hike, Run

LENGTH
6.5 miles, 4 hours

VERTICAL FEET
±1900'

DIFFICULTY
– 1 2 3 **4** 5 +

TRAIL TYPE
Loop

SURFACE TYPE
Dirt, Paved

FEATURES
Stream
Canyon
Mountain
Wildflowers
Birds
Great Views
Secluded

FACILITIES
None

Best Time

All year, but trails may be muddy in wet weather.

Finding the Trail

From US Hwy. 101 northbound, take the San Anselmo exit (also signed for San Quentin, Sir Francis Drake Blvd., and the Richmond Bridge). Stay in the left lane as you exit, toward San Anselmo, crossing over Hwy. 101. After 0.4 mile you join Sir Francis Drake Blvd., with traffic from Hwy. 101 southbound merging on your right. From here, it is 3.6 miles to a stoplight at the intersection with Red Hill Ave. Stay on Sir Francis Drake Blvd. as it first goes straight and then immediately bends left.

At 15.5 miles on Sir Francis Drake Blvd., you pass the main entrance to Samuel P. Taylor State Park. At 16.5 miles you reach a wide turnout, left, opposite a sign reading DEVIL'S GULCH HORSE CAMP. Park here. The Devil's Gulch trailhead is directly across Sir Francis Drake Blvd.▶1

From US Hwy. 101 southbound, take the Sir Francis Drake/Kentfield exit and follow the directions above.

Enjoy the view from the park boundary atop Barnabe Mountain: Mt. Diablo (east), Mt. Tamalpais (southeast), Kent Lake (south), and Big Rock Ridge (northeast).

Trail Description

After carefully crossing Sir Francis Drake Boulevard, you follow a paved one-lane road that heads northeast beside **Devil's Gulch Creek.** Turn right onto **Devil's Gulch Creek Trail,**►2 a single track that descends toward the creek, and follow it to a junction beneath an enormous coast redwood.►3

Turn right and cross a long wooden bridge spanning the creek. Once across, you arrive at a T-junction. Your route, **Bill's Trail,** heads left and begins a long, gentle climb. In 0.7 mile, you reach a junction with the Stairstep Falls Trail,►4 left.

Bearing right from this junction, you climb across a steep hillside that falls away left, and then begin a long series of switchbacks. As you climb, the vegetation changes between shady stands of bigleaf maple, California bay, Douglas-fir, and California nutmeg. Sunlight illuminates weedy patches of poison hemlock, cow parsnip, Italian thistle, and blackberry tangles. Finally leaving the trees behind, you reach a superb vantage point, where the view extends west to the lands of Point Reyes National Seashore and northwest to Tomales Bay. Now you meet the **Barnabe Fire Road.**►5 From here, turn left to continue your ascent of Barnabe Mountain.

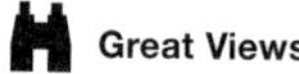

After a leg-stretching climb across a steep, grassy slope dotted with coastal scrub, you reach a T-junction at the state-park boundary.►6 From here, a dirt road goes left and uphill to a fire lookout, and also goes right along the ridge. (Please respect any private property postings.)

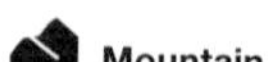

Retrace your route downhill on the Barnabe Fire Road past the junction with Bill's Trail.►7 From here, continue descending on this dirt road, initially steep but then moderate. Far down the mountain, you come to a junction with the **Riding and Hiking Trail,** on which you turn right.►8

Ahead, a short path leads left to **Taylor's grave site,** but your route, the Riding and Hiking

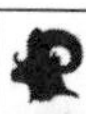

OPTIONS

Stairstep Falls

This slender cascade in a narrow, wooded cleft, is reached by the **Stairstep Falls Trail.** This easy, 0.2-mile spur trail descends across the hillside to a viewing area and rest bench at the foot of the falls. Retrace your steps, and continue up **Bill's Trail,** from which the falls are sometimes audible but never seen.

Trail, bends right. Heading into forest, you follow a rough, eroded road steeply downhill into **Deadman's Gulch.** Your route narrows, veers left, and skirts a grassy hillside. Now with Devil's Gulch Creek downhill and left, you make a steep descent and soon reach the junction with Bill's Trail and the wooden bridge you crossed at the start of this loop.►**9** Here you turn left, cross the bridge, turn left again, and retrace your route to the parking area. Look both ways before crossing the highway!►**10**

Samuel P. Taylor (1827–1896) established the West Coast's first paper mill nearby on the banks of Lagunitas Creek.

MILESTONES

►1	0.0	Take paved road northeast
►2	0.1	Right on Devil's Gulch Creek Trail
►3	0.2	Right across bridge, then left on Bill's Trail
►4	0.9	Trail to Stairstep Falls, left
►5	4.0	Left on Barnabe Fire Rd.
►6	4.3	Park boundary near summit; retrace to previous junction
►7	4.6	Bill's Trail on right; go straight to stay on Barnabe Fire Rd.
►8	5.8	Go right on Riding and Hiking Trail
►9	6.3	Left across bridge, then retrace on Devil's Gulch Trail
►10	6.5	Back at parking area

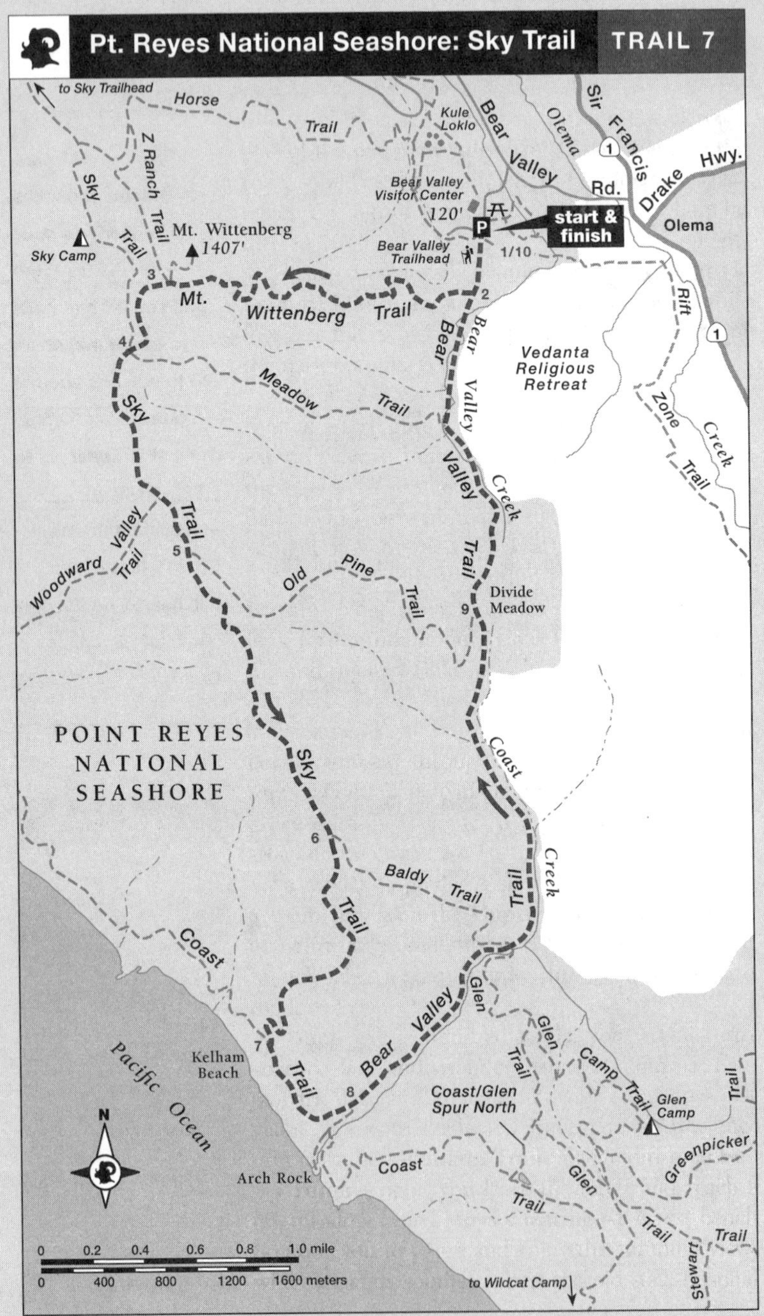
Pt. Reyes National Seashore: Sky Trail
TRAIL 7
to Sky Trailhead
Horse Trail
Z Ranch Trail
Sky Trail
Sky Camp
Mt. Wittenberg 1407'
Kule Loklo
Bear Valley Rd.
Olema
Sir Francis Drake Hwy.
1
Bear Valley Visitor Center 120'
start & finish
Bear Valley Trailhead
Olema
1/10
2
3
4
Mt. Wittenberg Trail
Bear Valley Trail
Bear Valley Creek
Vedanta Religious Retreat
Rift Zone Trail
Creek
Meadow Trail
Sky Trail
Woodward Valley Trail
5
Old Pine Trail
Divide Meadow
9
POINT REYES NATIONAL SEASHORE
Coast Creek
Coast Trail
6
Baldy Trail
Glen Trail
7
Kelham Beach
Pacific Ocean
Glen Camp Trail
Glen Camp
Coast/Glen Spur North
8
Greenpicker Trail
Arch Rock
Stewart Trail
to Wildcat Camp
N
0 0.2 0.4 0.6 0.8 1.0 mile
0 400 800 1200 1600 meters

Point Reyes National Seashore: Sky Trail

This is one of the premier hikes in the Point Reyes area, offering a grand tour of Inverness Ridge and Bear Valley, with the Pacific shoreline thrown in for good measure. The route has something for everyone, including a wonderful array of plant and bird life, and fine views.

TRAIL USE
Hike, Run
LENGTH
10.5 miles, 5–7 hours
VERTICAL FEET
±1650'
DIFFICULTY
– 1 2 3 4 **5** +
TRAIL TYPE
Loop
SURFACE TYPE
Dirt

FEATURES
Stream
Autumn Colors
Wildflowers
Birds
Great Views
Cool & Shady
Camping

FACILITIES
Visitor Center
Restrooms
Picnic Tables
Water
Phone

Best Time

This route is enjoyable all year.

Finding the Trail

From State Hwy. 1 northbound in Olema, just north of the junction with Sir Francis Drake Blvd., turn left on Bear Valley Rd. and go 0.5 mile to the visitor-center entrance road. Turn left and go 0.2 mile to a large paved parking area in front of the visitor center. If this lot is full, there is a dirt parking area ahead and left.

From Hwy. 1 southbound in Point Reyes Station, go 0.2 mile from the end of the town's main street to Sir Francis Drake Blvd. and turn right. Go 0.7 mile and turn left onto Bear Valley Rd. At 1.7 miles you reach the visitor-center entrance road; turn right and follow the directions above.

The Bear Valley trailhead is at the end of the paved visitor-center entrance road, about 150 feet south of the paved parking area.

Trail Description

From the trailhead,▶1 walk south on the **Bear Valley Trail**, a wide dirt road that skirts a broad grassland.

Mt. Wittenberg is named for a rancher who once lived nearby, not for Hamlet's alma mater.

When you reach the **Mt. Wittenberg Trail,▸2** turn right and begin to climb a single track through a dense forest of California bay. Occasional level stretches, some in small meadows, relieve the otherwise constant climbing.

Climbing out of the forest to a grassy saddle,▸3 you pass the Z Ranch Trail and a short trail to Mt. Wittenberg's tree-encircled, viewless summit, both right. As the Mt. Wittenberg Trail rambles down the far side of the saddle, there are fine views north and west across the Point Reyes peninsula. At a junction with the **Sky Trail,▸4** join it by merging left. About 50 feet ahead, you pass the Meadow Trail on your left. Continue on the Sky Trail, enjoy a rolling course through a wonderful Douglas-fir forest.

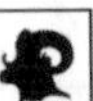

OPTIONS

Sky Camp

Sky Camp, a hike-in campground, is on the Sky Trail, northwest of its junction with the Mt. Wittenberg Trail.▸4 For reservations, call (415) 663-8054 weekdays from 9 A.M. to 2 P.M. Reservations for campsites at Point Reyes can fill up quickly, so you might want to plan ahead.

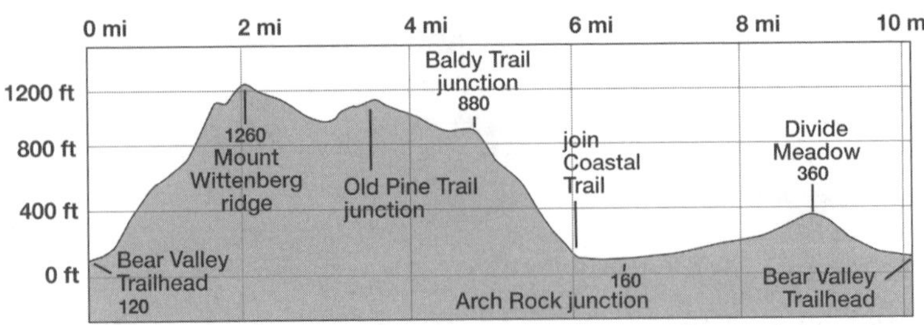

TRAIL 7 Point Reyes National Seashore: Sky Trail Profile

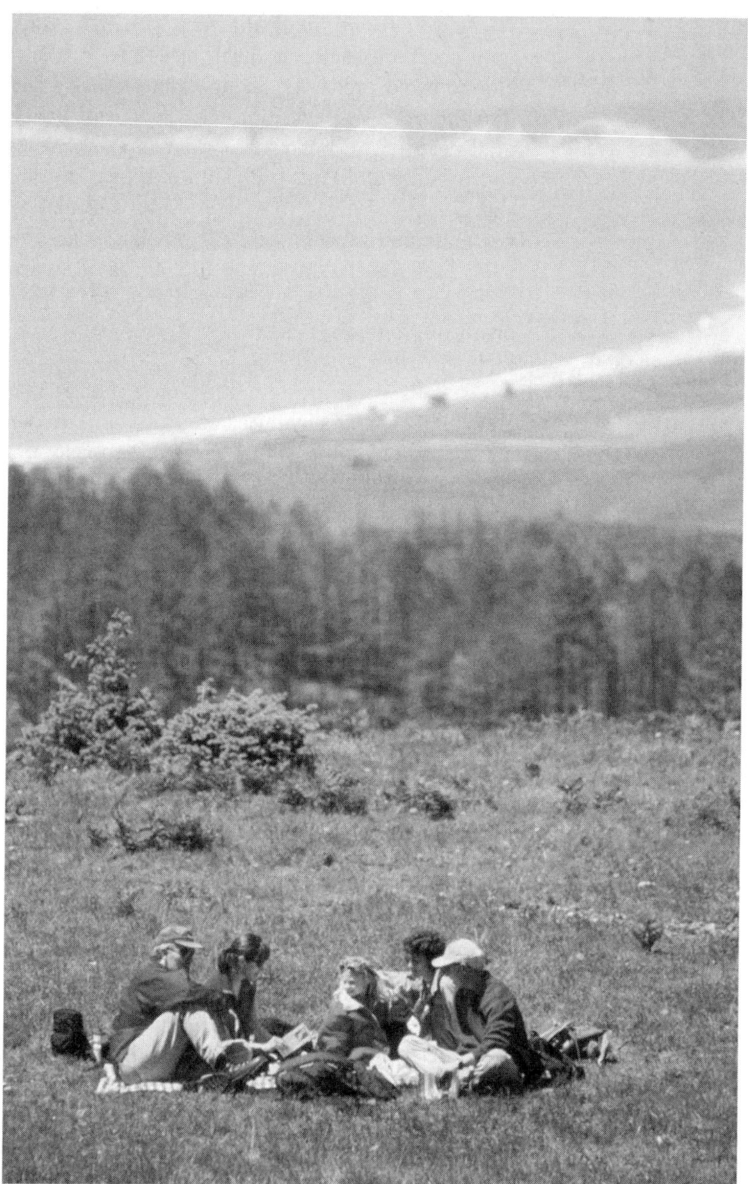

Sky Trail *offers dramatic views of Drakes Bay and Point Reyes.*

As you tromp along the trail, you may scare up a covey of California quail, birds that run and hide to avoid predators, taking flight only as a last resort. From a small clearing, the Woodward Valley Trail heads right, but you continue straight. Next, you pass the Old Pine Trail, left.►5 About 0.8 mile ahead, you emerge from forest and negotiate a moderate descent across a grassy knoll. Passing the Baldy Trail,►6 left, you enter a zone of coastal scrub, where shrubs such as California sagebrush, coyote brush, poison oak, bush monkeyflower, and silver lupine thrive.

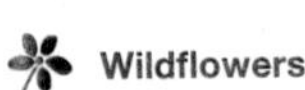

Now the route drops through forest and across a grassy slope. Angle slightly left on the **Coast Trail,**►7 a dirt road along the coastal terrace. Eventually the road swings left into the canyon of **Coast Creek** and you arrive at a junction where the Coast Trail and the spur for **Arch Rock** turn sharply right.►8

From the Arch Rock junction, continue straight on the **Bear Valley Trail**, a dirt road often crowded with hikers. Coast Creek flows vigorously year-round to your right, screened by stands of Douglas-fir, bay, red alder, and California buckeye. About a mile inland, you pass the Baldy Trail on the left and the Glen Trail on the right. From here on, this busy trail is open to bicyclists and (on weekdays) to horses.

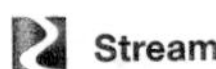

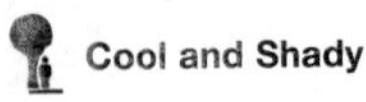

Continuing beside Coast Creek, you ascend gradually to **Divide Meadow,**►9 where there are restrooms and a junction with the Old Pine Trail,

OPTIONS

Shorter Loops and Arch Rock

Along the Sky Trail you can turn left on either the **Meadow, Old Pine,** or **Baldy trails** and then left on the **Bear Valley Trail.** The round-trip distances are then 4.7 miles, 6.9 miles, and 9 miles, respectively.

►8 Visit **Arch Rock** during the spring wildflower bloom for great photos! This side trip adds 0.6 mile to the described route.

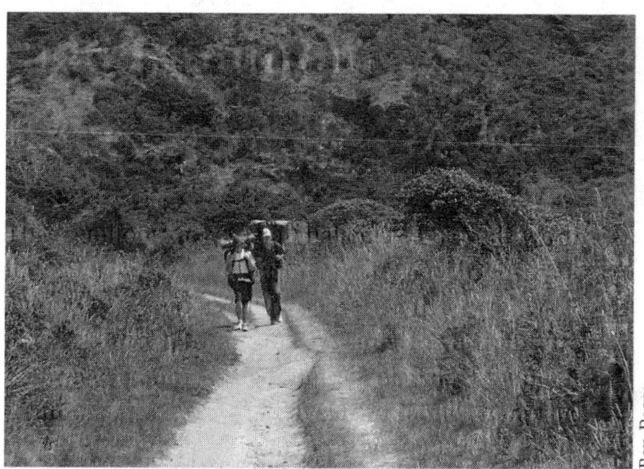

Ben Pease

Backpackers *on the Coast Trail*

both left. The Bear Valley Trail now descends past the headwaters of **Bear Valley Creek.** A rest bench signals a junction with the Meadow Trail. You emerge from the wooded canyon at the junction with the Mt. Wittenberg Trail; continue straight on the Bear Valley Trail and retrace your route to the parking area.►10

MILESTONES

►1	0.0	Take Bear Valley Trail south
►2	0.2	Right on Mt. Wittenberg Trail
►3	2.0	Veer left at junction with trail to Mt. Wittenberg summit
►4	2.4	Merge with Sky Trail; Meadow Trail on left
►5	3.4	Old Pine Trail on left; go straight on Sky Trail
►6	4.8	Baldy Trail on left; go straight on Sky Trail
►7	6.0	Left on Coast Trail
►8	6.5	Coast Trail and side trail to Arch Rock on right; continue straight on Bear Valley Trail
►9	8.9	Ascend Divide Meadow; go straight, and pass Old Pine Trail on left
►10	10.5	Back at parking area

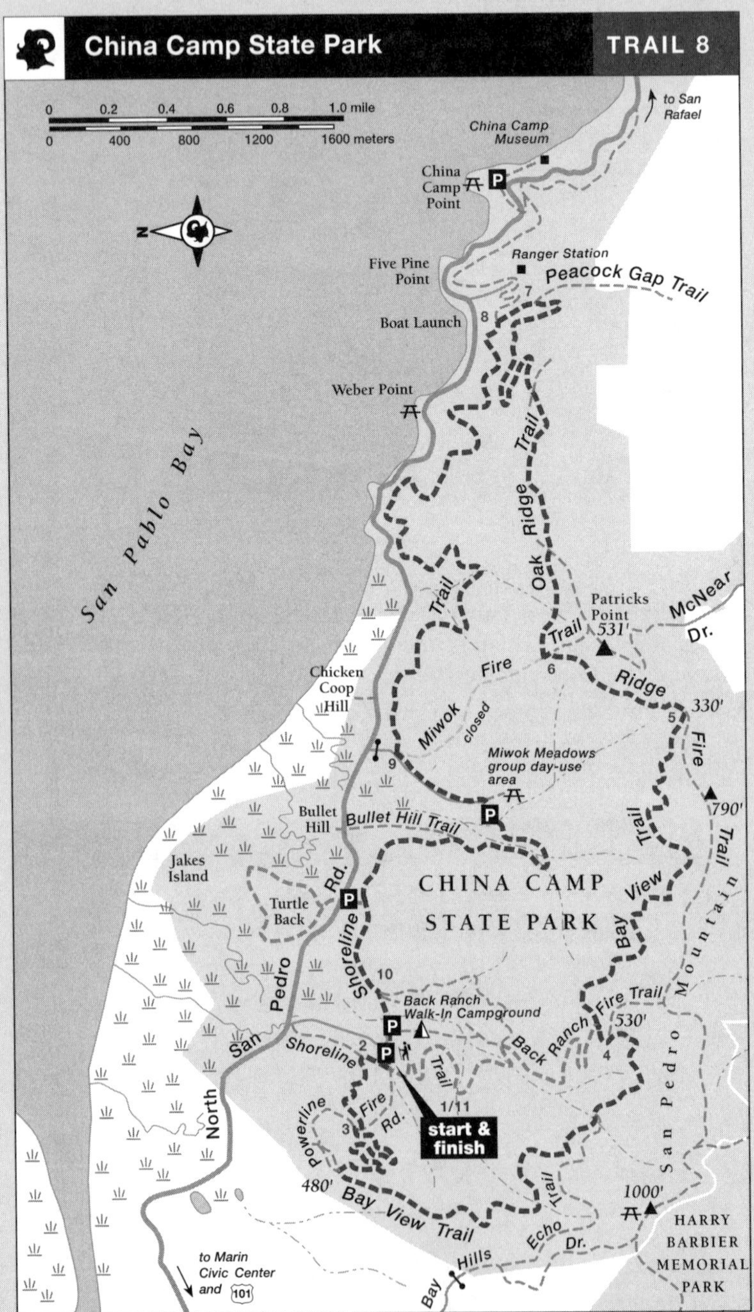
China Camp State Park
TRAIL 8
0 0.2 0.4 0.6 0.8 1.0 mile
0 400 800 1200 1600 meters
to San Rafael
China Camp Museum
China Camp Point
Five Pine Point
Ranger Station
Peacock Gap Trail
Boat Launch
Weber Point
San Pablo Bay
Oak Ridge Trail
Miwok Trail
Miwok Fire Trail
closed
Patricks Point
531'
McNear Dr.
Ridge Fire Trail
330'
790'
Chicken Coop Hill
Miwok Meadows group day-use area
Bullet Hill
Bullet Hill Trail
Jakes Island
Turtle Back
CHINA CAMP STATE PARK
Bay View Trail
Mountain Trail
North San Pedro Rd.
Shoreline Trail
Back Ranch Walk-In Campground
Back Ranch Fire Trail
530'
San Pedro
Powerline Fire Rd.
start & finish
480'
Bay View Trail
Echo Trail
1000'
HARRY BARBIER MEMORIAL PARK
Bay Hills Dr.
to Marin Civic Center and 101

China Camp State Park: Bay View–Shoreline Loop

This loop samples China Camp's wide variety of habitats, from shady groves of coast redwood and California bay to sheltered enclaves where manzanita and madrone hold sway. This route starts and ends barely above sea level but climbs to 600 feet on its course above Miwok Meadows and Back Ranch. The multiuse trails and fire trails of this park are enjoyed by bicyclists and equestrians as well as by hikers and runners. (The closure of the Miwok Trail in 2007, to help prevent the spread of a disease that kills native trees and shrubs, has lengthened the 5.4-mile route described in the first edition of this guide to 8.4 miles; however, there is also an enjoyable 3.1-mile option described on page 69.)

TRAIL USE
Hike, Run, Bike
LENGTH
8.4 miles, 4–5 hours
VERTICAL FEET
±1450'
DIFFICULTY
– 1 2 3 **4** 5 +
TRAIL TYPE
Loop
SURFACE TYPE
Dirt, paved

FEATURES
Fee
Birds
Great Views
Cool & Shady
Camping

FACILITIES
Restrooms
Picnic Tables
Water
Phone

Best Time

All year; in summer this may be one of the few fog-free places close to the Golden Gate.

Finding the Trail

From US Hwy. 101 northbound in San Rafael, take the N. San Pedro Rd. exit, which is also signed for the Marin County Civic Center and China Camp State Park. After exiting, bear right, following the lane marked EAST. After 0.3 mile you join N. San Pedro Rd. Once on it, go 2.9 miles to the Back Ranch Meadows walk-in campground entrance road, right. Go 0.2 mile past the entrance kiosk to the day-use parking area, right. The trailhead is on the west end of the parking area.

From US Hwy. 101 southbound in San Rafael, take the N. San Pedro Rd. exit, which is also signed for the Marin County Civic Center and China Camp

China Camp State Park takes its name from a Chinese fishing village that flourished nearby during the 1880s and 1890s, one of 26 on San Francisco Bay.

State Park. After 0.2 mile, you come to a stop sign. Turn left, go 0.1 mile to a stoplight, and turn left again, onto N. San Pedro Rd. At 0.3 mile, the exit ramp from Hwy. 101 northbound joins on your right. From here, follow the directions above.

Facilities

There are restrooms, water, a phone, and a campground host at the campground parking area, about 0.1 mile ahead on the entrance road. Maps are sold at the ranger station, 1.8 miles ahead on N. San Pedro Rd. opposite the Bullhead Flat picnic area, or at the China Camp museum.

Trail Description

From the west end of the parking area, just past the self-registration station and an information board, you pass through a gap in a split-rail fence and come to a four-way junction.▶1 Here the Powerline Fire Trail goes straight, but you turn right on the multiuse **Shoreline Trail.** After a few hundred yards, you come to a T-junction.▶2 Here the Shoreline Trail goes right, but your route, the multiuse **Bay View Trail,** turns sharply left for a gentle ascent that alternates between open areas and stands of blue oak.

At a T-junction▶3 with the Powerline Fire Trail, a dirt road, you ascend right and in 100 feet turn sharply left on the continuation of the Bay View Trail.

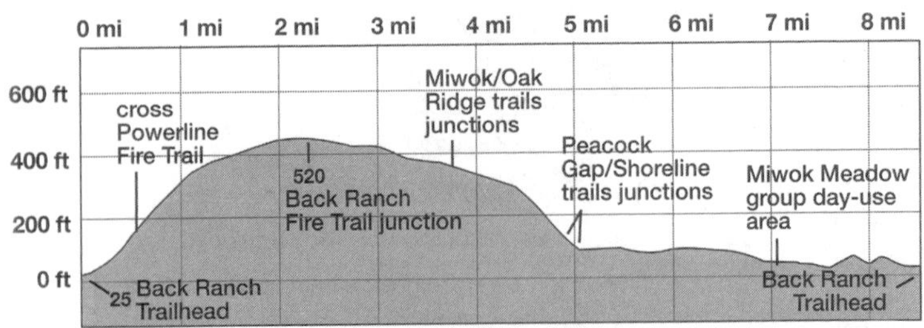

TRAIL 8 China Camp State Park Profile

Several switchbacks bring you to a junction on a wooded ridgetop. Two paths go north along the ridge to the Powerline Fire Trail; ignore these and instead swing sharply left and climb south along the ridge on the Bay View Trail. Just past a picnic table is the first of several vantage points with views east across San Pablo Bay to the East Bay shoreline and Point Pinole.

Using wooden bridges to cross several watercourses, the route wanders in deep shade through a woodland of California bay and occasional stands of coast redwoods. Now on a gentle but rocky uphill grade, you pass a junction with the Echo Trail, right, signed TO BAY HILLS DRIVE. A few feet ahead, you cross another watercourse and enjoy a level walk that follows the folds of a hillside.

 **Great Views**

 **Cool and Shady**

Under a set of power lines is a junction with the Back Ranch Fire Trail,►**4** an eroded dirt road that descends straight (joined for a short distance with the Bay View Trail) and also ascends right. You continue straight, descending past a power-line tower and then bending right into the trees. At an upcoming switchback, you turn right on the continuation of the Bay View Trail.

After slightly more than a mile of mostly level travel, the Bay View Trail ends in a clearing ringed with eucalyptus trees.►**5** There is a confusing welter of trails converging here, some of them unofficial.

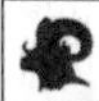

OPTIONS

China Camp Variations

For a 3.1-mile loop, descend the **Back Ranch Fire Trail**►**4** from its junction with the **Bay View Trail.** At a four-way junction with the Shoreline Trail, turn left and follow the **Shoreline Trail** back to the day-use parking area.

The short nature trail around **Turtle Back Hill** offers great views of the hills and salt marshes. Find road-shoulder parking along N. San Pedro Rd., 0.1 mile southeast of the campground entrance road, or cross N. San Pedro Rd. from the Shoreline Trail.

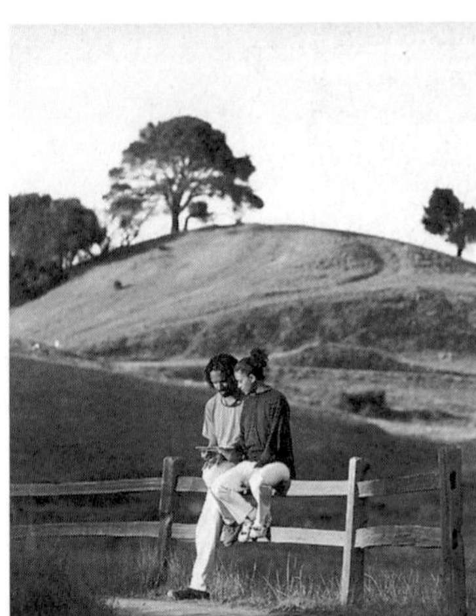

Hikers enjoy a quiet moment *along China Camp State Park's Shoreline Trail.*

You join the **Ridge Fire Trail**, a dirt road, by angling left and climbing.

Once over a little rise, you begin to descend, only to climb again on a moderate grade to a T-junction with the **Miwok Fire Trail.**►**6** Descend left on this dirt road about 100 feet (closed ahead as of this writing), then turn right on the **Oak Ridge Trail**, right. This multiuse single track heads east along a ridgetop, crosses the McNears Fire Trail, and eventually provides terrific views of San Francisco, Angel Island, the Marin Headlands, and perhaps, on a clear day, Mt. Diablo.

Cross the McNears Fire Trail again and stay on the Oak Ridge Trail. Descend via easy switchbacks to a junction with the **Peacock Gap Trail,**►**7** which you join by going straight. At the next junction, turn left on the **Shoreline Trail.**►**8** Follow the trail as it ambles on a mostly level grade through a serene forest, with occasional views of San Pablo Bay. After about 1.5 miles on the Shoreline Trail, you reach a four-way junction with the closed Miwok Fire Trail. Continue straight on the Shoreline Trail, here a dirt road.

Soon the road divides.►**9** One branch goes straight, into the Miwok Meadows group day-use area, which has picnic tables and toilets. The other branch, your

OPTIONS

Back Ranch Meadows Campground

Overnight camping is available in the Back Ranch Meadows Walk-In Campground. There are 30 walk-in family campsites, each with a picnic table, food locker, and fire ring. For camping reservations, call (800) 444-7275. To reserve the Miwok Meadows group day-use picnic area, call Marin District Special Events at (415) 898-4362, extension 23. It has barbeque grills, picnic tables, and chemical toilets (no running water) and can accommodate up to 200 people.

route, marked by a trail post for the Shoreline Trail, angles right into a large dirt parking area.

After about 150 feet, you reach the end of the parking area, where you turn left and find the continuation of the Shoreline Trail, marked by a trail post. Soon level, the route crosses a wood bridge, swings right, and comes into the open. At a junction, right, with the Bullet Hill Trail, you continue straight.

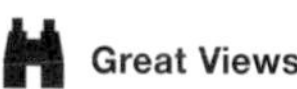

Now the route gains elevation and bends left, running parallel to North San Pedro Road. Just south of Turtle Back Hill, the trail veers away from the road and you continue a level trek over mostly open ground, with woodland left and marshland right. Bear right at an upcoming fork, toward the campground parking area.►**10** Go right across the parking area to the **park entrance road** and follow it 100 yards to the day-use parking area.►**11**

MILESTONES

►1	0.0	West from parking area to four-way junction, then right on Shoreline Trail
►2	0.1	Left on Bay View Trail
►3	0.4	Right on Powerline Fire Trail, then left on Bay View Trail
►4	2.3	Straight on Back Ranch Fire Trail 100 yards, then right on Bay View Trail
►5	3.4	At clearing, angle left on Ridge Fire Trail
►6	3.7	Left on Miwok Fire Trail for 100 feet, then right on Oak Ridge Trail
►7	4.9	Straight on Peacock Gap Trail
►8	5.0	Left on Shoreline Trail
►9	7.1	Miwok Meadows group day-use area; right through dirt parking area to Shoreline Trail
►10	8.4	Right at fork to walk-in campground parking area; right to entrance road
►11	8.4	Back at parking area

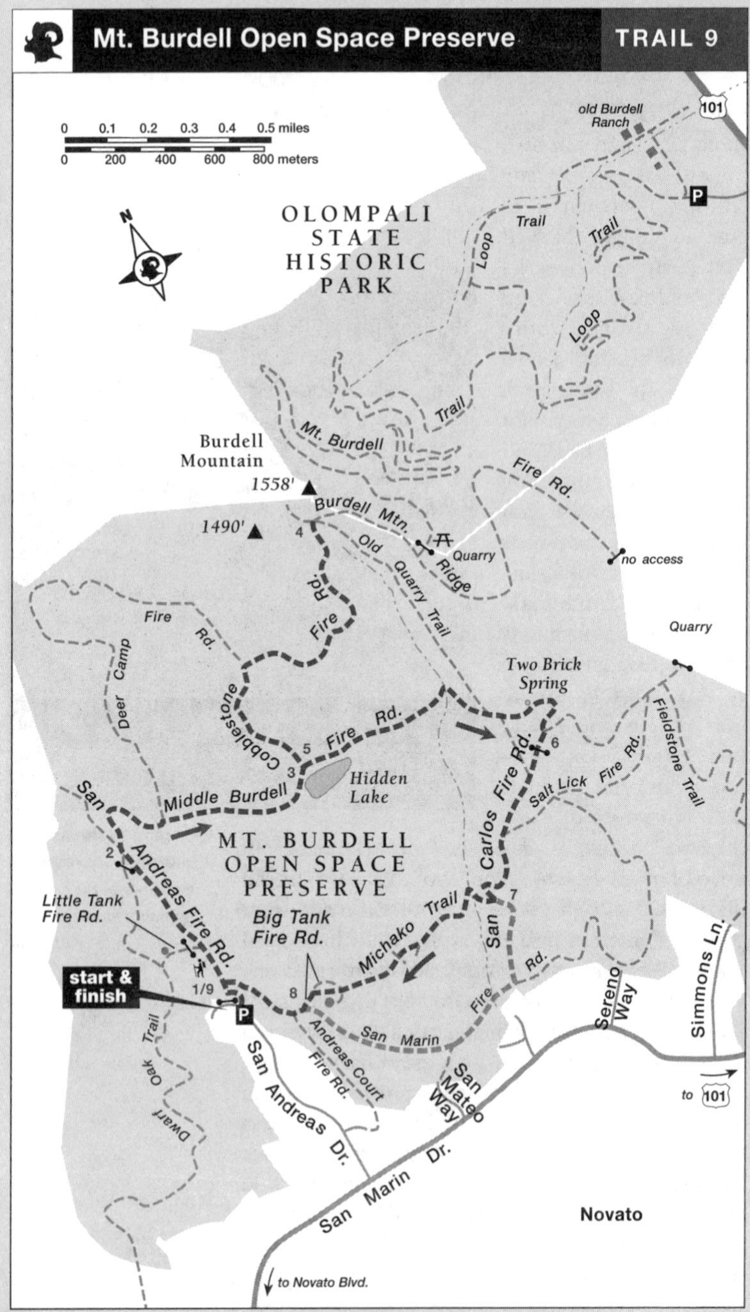

Mt. Burdell Open Space Preserve
TRAIL 9
0 0.1 0.2 0.3 0.4 0.5 miles
0 200 400 600 800 meters
N
OLOMPALI STATE HISTORIC PARK
old Burdell Ranch
101
P
Loop Trail
Loop Trail
Mt. Burdell Trail
Burdell Mountain
1558'
1490'
Burdell Mtn. Ridge Fire Rd.
Old Quarry Trail
Quarry
no access
Quarry
Two Brick Spring
Fire Rd.
Deer Camp Fire Rd.
Cobblestone Fire Rd.
Hidden Lake
Middle Burdell Fire Rd.
San Carlos Fire Rd.
Salt Lick Fire Rd.
Fieldstone Trail
MT. BURDELL OPEN SPACE PRESERVE
San Andreas Fire Rd.
Little Tank Fire Rd.
Big Tank Fire Rd.
Michako Trail
San Marin Fire Rd.
start & finish
1/9
2
3
4
5
6
7
8
P
Dwarf Oak Trail
San Andreas Dr.
San Andreas Court
San Mateo Way
Sereno Way
Simmons Ln.
San Marin Dr.
Novato
to 101
to Novato Blvd.

Mt. Burdell Open Space Preserve

This loop explores the open grasslands, groves, and high ground of Burdell Mountain, a bulky ridge that rises to 1558 feet and dominates the northeast corner of Marin County.

TRAIL USE
Hike, Run, Bike, Child Friendly, Dogs Allowed

LENGTH
5.6 miles, 3–4 hours

VERTICAL FEET
±1200'

DIFFICULTY
– 1 2 3 **4** 5 +

TRAIL TYPE
Loop

SURFACE TYPE
Dirt

FEATURES
Lake
Mountain
Wildflowers
Birds
Great Views
Photo Opportunity

FACILITIES
None

Best Time

Spring wildflowers are a prime attraction; avoid the heat of summer.

Finding the Trail

From US Hwy. 101 in Novato, take the Atherton Ave./San Marin Dr. exit. Go west 2.2 miles on San Marin Dr., turn right onto San Andreas Dr., and go 0.6 mile to where the road makes a sweeping bend to the left. Park on the shoulder and observe the NO PARKING signs.

The trailhead is at the foot of the San Andreas Fire Rd., by the gate just northeast of the parking area. The trailhead stiles are a few steps right of the gate.

Trail Description

From the trailhead,▶1 pass through the stiles and then curve left for about 100 feet to join the **San Andreas Fire Road,** which climbs on a gentle grade. Just beyond an information board, you pass the San Marin Fire Road, right. The San Andreas Fire Road, graded for a development that was never built, ascends to a wide, grassy saddle. Here the single track Dwarf Oak Trail enters on the left, and a faint road continues down the far side of the saddle. You angle right on the **Middle Burdell Fire Road** (part of the Bay Area Ridge Trail).►2 The road wanders through an oak-dotted grassland as it gains elevation. Signs ask visitors to stay on the official trail to avoid habitat damage and aid its restoration.

Where the Deer Camp Fire Road (part of the Bay Area Ridge Trail) goes left, you continue straight on the Middle Burdell Fire Road, climbing moderately over rocky ground. Turning a corner, the road levels and follows the edge of **Hidden Lake,** a large vernal pool. Several stiles allow access through a fence to the water's edge. At a junction,►3 the Middle Burdell Fire Road turns right, and the **Cobblestone Fire Road,** your route to the top of Burdell Mountain, heads left.

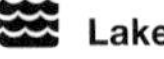

Turning left, you begin climbing on a moderate grade. The route gets steeper and rockier, but you are rewarded by terrific views west toward Big Rock Ridge and Bolinas Ridge, and southeast to San Pablo Bay and the peninsula that holds China Camp State Park. At a fork, the Deer Camp Fire Road comes in on the left, and your route, the Cobblestone Fire Road, veers right.

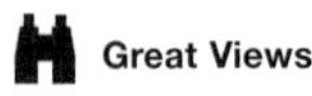

Now the road turns north, trying to find the easiest way up Burdell Mountain The climbing is moderate, with a few level areas to ease your efforts and some groves of bay and coast live oak for shade. Nearing the end of the climb, you come to junctions with the Old Quarry Trail, right, and the paved Burdell Mountain Ridge Fire Road.►4 The preserve's high point lies just ahead, across the road and at the end of a faint single-track trail that climbs north. The true summit of Burdell Mountain (1558') is just beyond the preserve boundary, unreachable on private land.

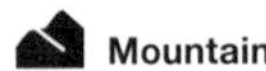

After exploring Burdell Mountain's high ground, retrace your route down the Cobblestone Trail to Hidden Lake and the Middle Burdell Fire Road.►5 Bear left, now on the Middle Burdell Fire Road, and head east over level ground. Dipping into and then out of a small wooded ravine, you soon pass junctions with the Old Quarry Trail, which climbs steeply to the Burdell Mountain Ridge Fire Road, and an unofficial trail heading up the grassy slope, both left. Several hundred feet ahead, the lower part of the Old Quarry Trail descends right.

Continuing straight on the Middle Burdell Fire Road, you pass Two Brick Spring, left, and then amble through a bay grove to a T-junction.▶6 Here the Middle Burdell Fire Road angles left, but your route, the **San Carlos Fire Road,** turns right. After passing through a cattle gate, you enjoy a level, shady walk but soon resume a gentle descent in the open. You pass the Old Quarry Trail, right, and, about 350 feet ahead, the Salt Lick Fire Road, left. Continuing straight and downhill, the San Carlos Fire Road soon veers right, and then makes a sharp left-hand bend, putting you on a southeast course.

Rock walls atop Burdell Mountain mark the preserve boundary. Although reminiscent of New England rock walls, these were built in the 19th century by Chinese laborers who worked in nearby quarries.

At a three-way junction,▶7 where the San Carlos Fire Road continues straight, you turn right onto the **Michako Trail,** a single track that is closed to bikes. Still descending, you pass through an opening in a fence, cross a seasonal creek on rocks, and then find level ground. Just past the creek, a faint trail heads left. Angle right to stay on the Michako Trail. After crossing a swale and a side trail, you meet the faint trail, which rejoins on the left.

The Michako Trail continues across open grassland, soon crossing—and then joining—the **Big Tank Fire Road.**▶8 About 150 feet ahead, you reach a four-way junction with the San Marin and Andreas Court fire roads, both left. Bear right on the **San Marin Fire Road,** which makes an easy descent to close the loop at the San Andreas Fire Road.▶9 Turn left here and retrace your route to the parking area.

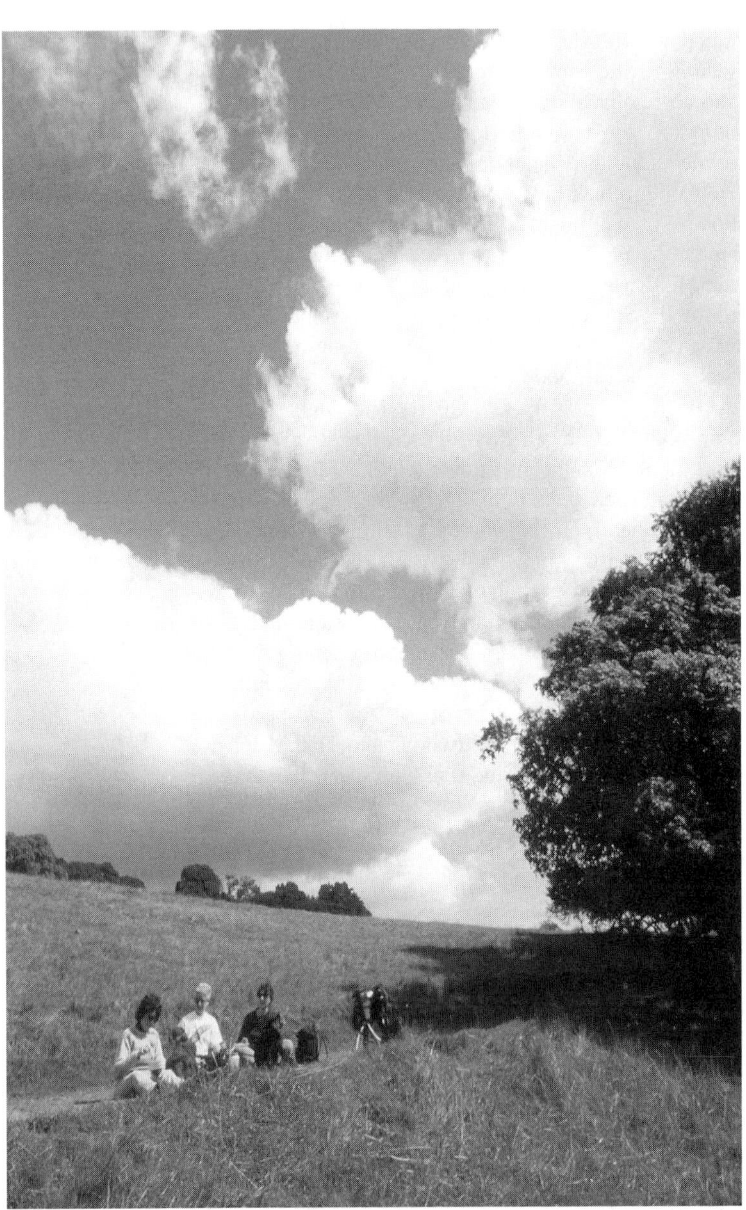

Lunch stop *along the trail in Mt. Burdell Open Space Preserve.*

OPTIONS

Car-Shuttle Hike to Olompali State Historic Park

If you'd like to try a shuttle hike in the area, here's a route that's 7.8 miles one-way. From the junction of the Cobblestone and the Burdell Mountain Ridge fire roads, ►4 turn right and go 0.3 mile on the paved road, then climb left on a dirt road to a gate. Beyond the gate are two picnic tables with views of the Petaluma River and San Pablo Bay. At the picnic tables, turn left on the Mt. Burdell Trail, signed TO PARK ENTRANCE. This single track descends for about 5 miles to the old Burdell Ranch. Auto access to the state park is from southbound Hwy. 101, 2.4 miles south of San Antonio Rd.

MILESTONES

►1	0.0	Take San Andreas Fire Rd. north
►2	0.8	Right on Middle Burdell Fire Rd.
►3	1.5	Left on Cobblestone Fire Rd.
►4	2.5	Burdell Mountain Ridge Fire Rd. and top of mountain, return to junction with Middle Burdell Fire Rd.
►5	3.5	Left on Middle Burdell Fire Rd.
►6	4.3	Right on San Carlos Fire Rd.
►7	4.8	Right on Michako Trail
►8	5.4	Straight on Big Tank Fire Rd.
►9	5.6	Left on San Andreas Fire Rd., back at parking area

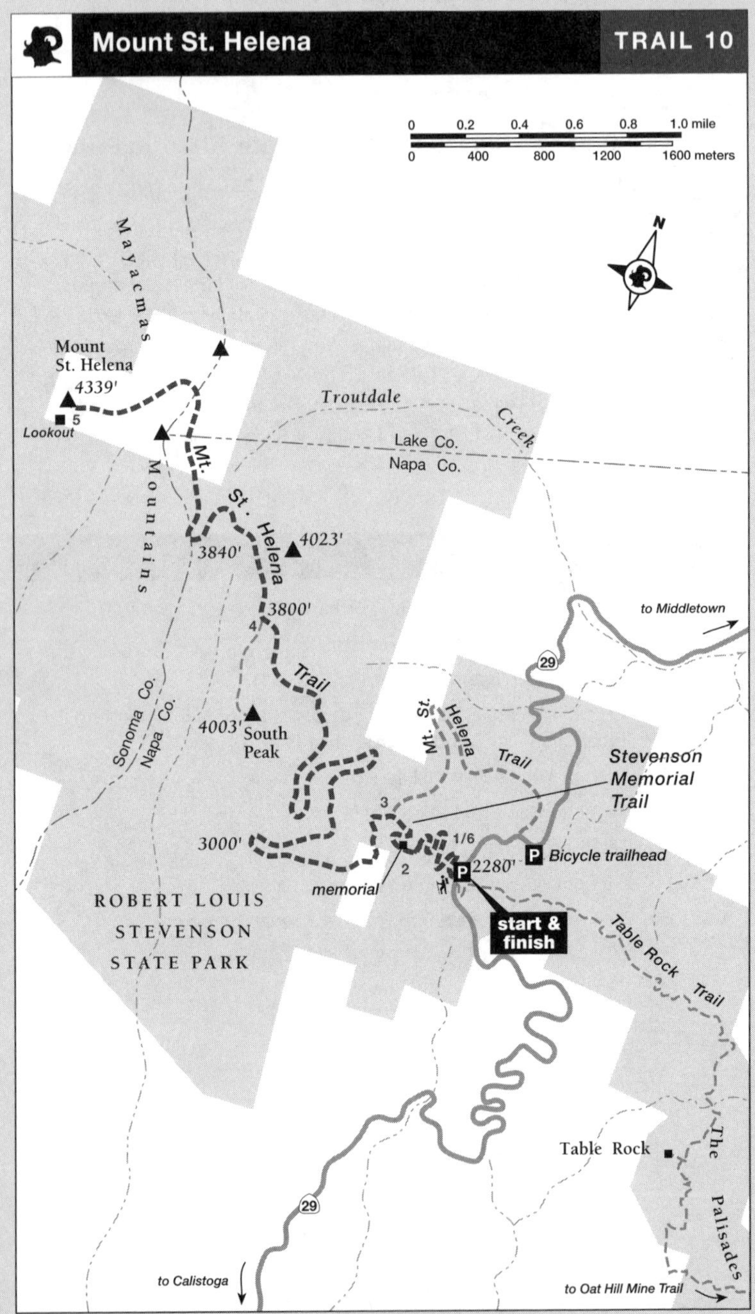
Mount St. Helena
TRAIL 10
0 0.2 0.4 0.6 0.8 1.0 mile
0 400 800 1200 1600 meters
N
Mayacmas
Mountains
Mount
St. Helena
4339'
5
Lookout
Troutdale
Creek
Lake Co.
Napa Co.
Mt. St. Helena Trail
4023'
3840'
3800'
4
4003'
South
Peak
Sonoma Co.
Napa Co.
Mt. St. Helena Trail
to Middletown
29
Stevenson
Memorial
Trail
3
3000'
1/6
2
2280'
P
Bicycle trailhead
memorial
start &
finish
Table Rock Trail
ROBERT LOUIS
STEVENSON
STATE PARK
Table Rock
The Palisades
29
to Calistoga
to Oat Hill Mine Trail

Mount St. Helena

A "must-do" for lovers of high places, this route takes you to the 4339-foot North Peak of Mt. St. Helena, the tallest summit in the North Bay. The route is exposed for much of its length to sun, wind, and weather. Mt. St. Helena is in Robert Louis Stevenson State Park, which is named for the author of *The Silverado Squatters, Treasure Island,* and other books. In 1880 Stevenson, who was recuperating from tuberculosis, lived in a cabin here with his new bride.

TRAIL USE
Hike, Run, Bike
LENGTH
10.6 miles, 4–6 hours
VERTICAL FEET
±2100'
DIFFICULTY
– 1 2 3 4 **5** +
TRAIL TYPE
Out & Back
SURFACE TYPE
Dirt

FEATURES
Mountain
Summit
Birds
Historic
Geologic Interest
Great Views
Steep
Secluded

FACILITIES
Picnic Tables

Best Time

Spring and fall; winter may provide best visibility, but also very cold conditions and even snow; in summer, make sure to get an early start to beat the heat.

Finding the Trail

From the junction of State Hwys. 128 and 29 in Calistoga (at Lincoln Ave.), go northwest 8.7 miles on State Hwy. 29 to a small parking area on the left side of the road at the highway's summit. If this area is full, park in the large area just across the highway, right. The trailhead is on the west side of State Hwy. 29, adjacent to the small parking area. If you need to cross State Hwy. 29, do so carefully!

The trailhead for **bicyclists** is about 0.2 mile northeast of the hiking trailhead, on the north side of State Hwy. 29, at the foot of Mt. St. Helena Trail. Parking is on the south side of the highway, just past this gated fire road.

Trail Description

From the trailhead,►1 hikers ascend a set of wooden steps to the **Stevenson Memorial Trail,** here a wide dirt track, and pass a board with information about the park's namesake. (Bicyclists pedal up the Mt. St. Helena Trail, a well-graded road, for 1.2 miles to join the described route.►3) The trail rises via gentle switchbacks through a shady forest of tanbark oak, madrone, and Douglas-fir. At 0.6 mile, hikers pass a stone marker indicating the site of the **Stevensons' honeymoon cabin,** nothing of which remains.►2 Just past the marker, the route makes a sharp right-hand switchback, and you climb a gently angled slab of loose, volcanic rock via a rough, eroded tread.

Historic Interest

At a junction, hikers turn left on the **Mt. St. Helena Trail.**►3 (Bicyclists join the route here.) The well-built dirt road climbs on a grade that alternates between gentle and moderate, in places affording views of the Napa Valley and the rocky ramparts on Mt. St. Helena's southeast flank.

In a clearing beneath a dramatic, eroded cliff, the road swings sharply right. Here, about 3000 feet above sea level, the route takes on a more isolated, rugged feeling. Stands of manzanita and a few stunted pines cling to the rocky, parched soil. At a wide clearing crossed by power lines, you make a 180-degree turn to the left. Another sharp turn, this one right, aims you almost due north and

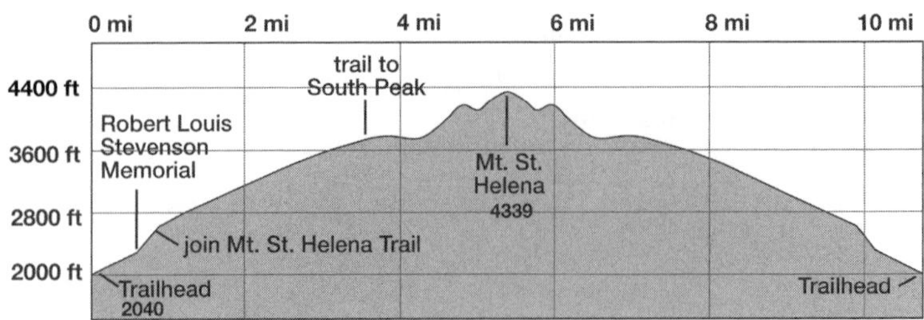

TRAIL 10 Mount St. Helena Profile

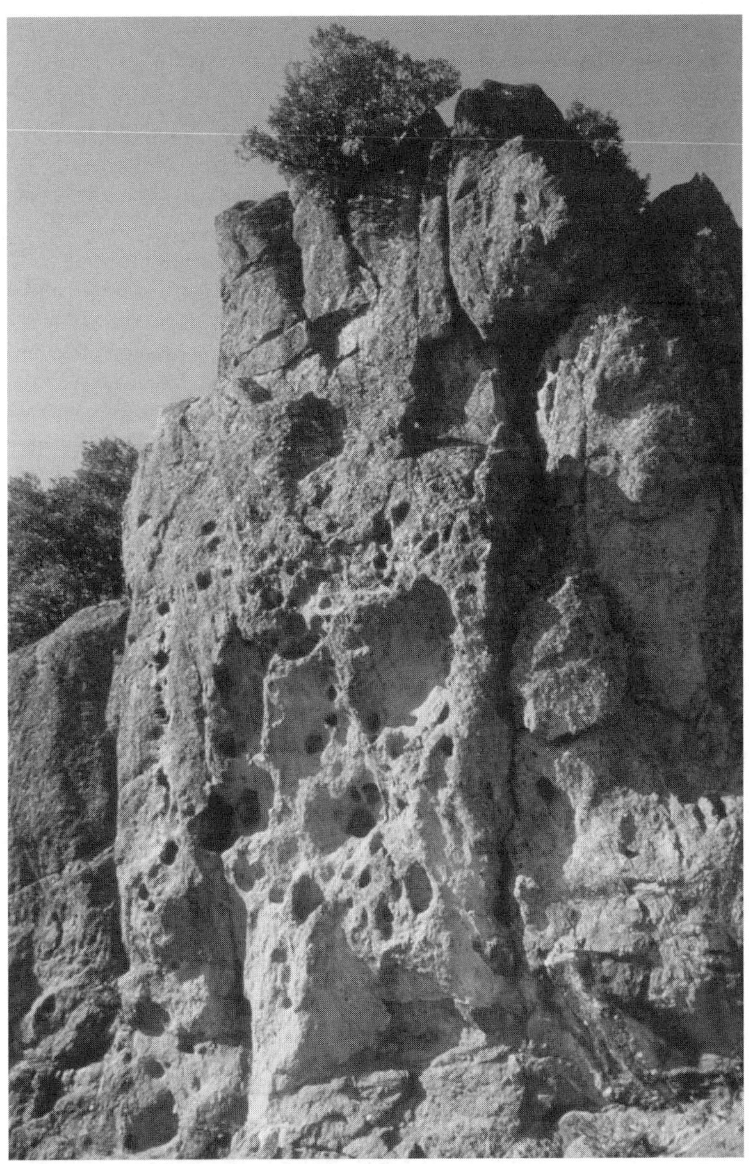

Volcanic rock outcrops *overlook part of the Mt. St. Helena Trail.*

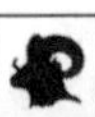

OPTIONS

Nearby Trails

The hiking-only **Table Rock** and **Palisades trails** head southeast from the parking area 2.4 miles to Table Rock, then to the Palisades, and finally, via **Oat Hill Mine Rd.**, to Calistoga.

 Great Views

soon brings you to very eroded ground. Now on a moderate grade, you have sweeping views east and northeast toward the series of ridges and summits that form the border between Napa and Yolo counties; beyond lies the Central Valley.

After a long, steady climb, you pass a junction,▶4 left, with the road to **South Peak** (4003'). Reaching a clearing, you pass another road, left, that heads toward several communication towers. Your route swings left and finds a level course, with **North Peak** in view at last. Soon a turnaround marks the spot where the well-graded road ends and a short, steep, rocky track to North Peak begins.

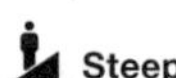

Passing several communication facilities, you arrive at last on the summit of North Peak (4339')▶5—in the Bay Area, only Copernicus Peak on Mt. Hamilton is higher, by a mere 34 feet. On a clear day, the 360-degree views are stunning, taking in all the familiar North Bay summits, plus Mt. Lassen and even Mt. Shasta, 192 miles away.

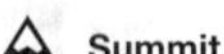

 Great Views

After enjoying the scenery, retrace your route to the parking area.▶6

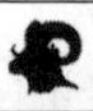

HISTORY

Mount St. Helena

How did **Mt. St. Helena** get its name? *California Place Names* by Erwin Gudde gives no definitive answer but suggests several possibilities. A Russian party climbed the mountain in 1841, and one of its members, Princess Helena de Gagarin, a niece of the Czar, may have bestowed the name in honor of St. Helena, her patron saint.

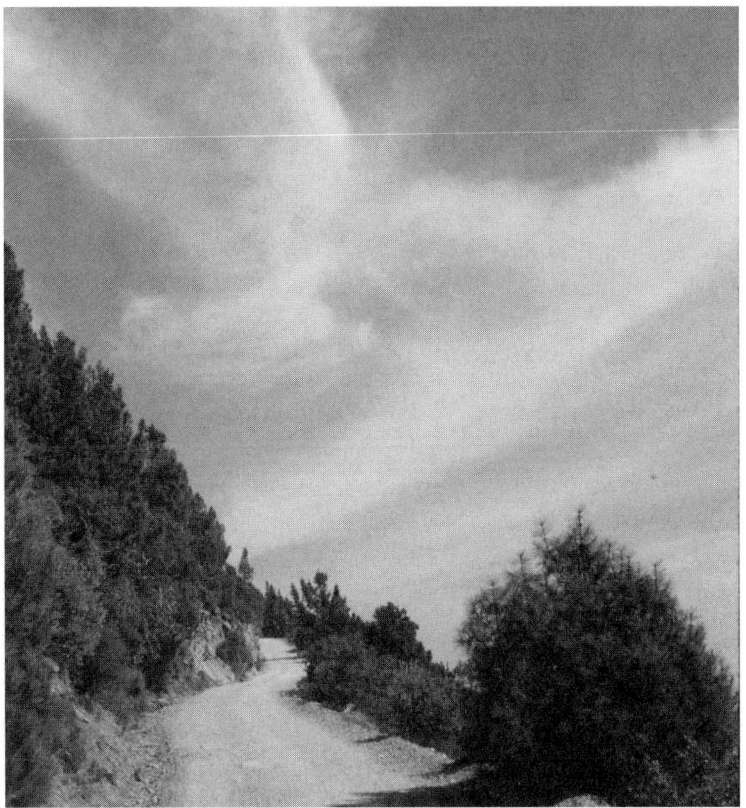

Mt. St. Helena Trail *ascends via long, exposed switchbacks.*

MILESTONES

▶1	0.0	Take steps and then Stevenson Memorial Trail northwest
▶2	0.6	Stevenson memorial
▶3	0.8	Left on Mt. St. Helena Trail
▶4	3.6	Pass junction with road to South Peak on the left
▶5	5.3	Summit of North Peak (4339'), retrace to parking area
▶6	10.6	Back at parking area

Annadel State Park: Lake Ilsanjo

TRAIL 11

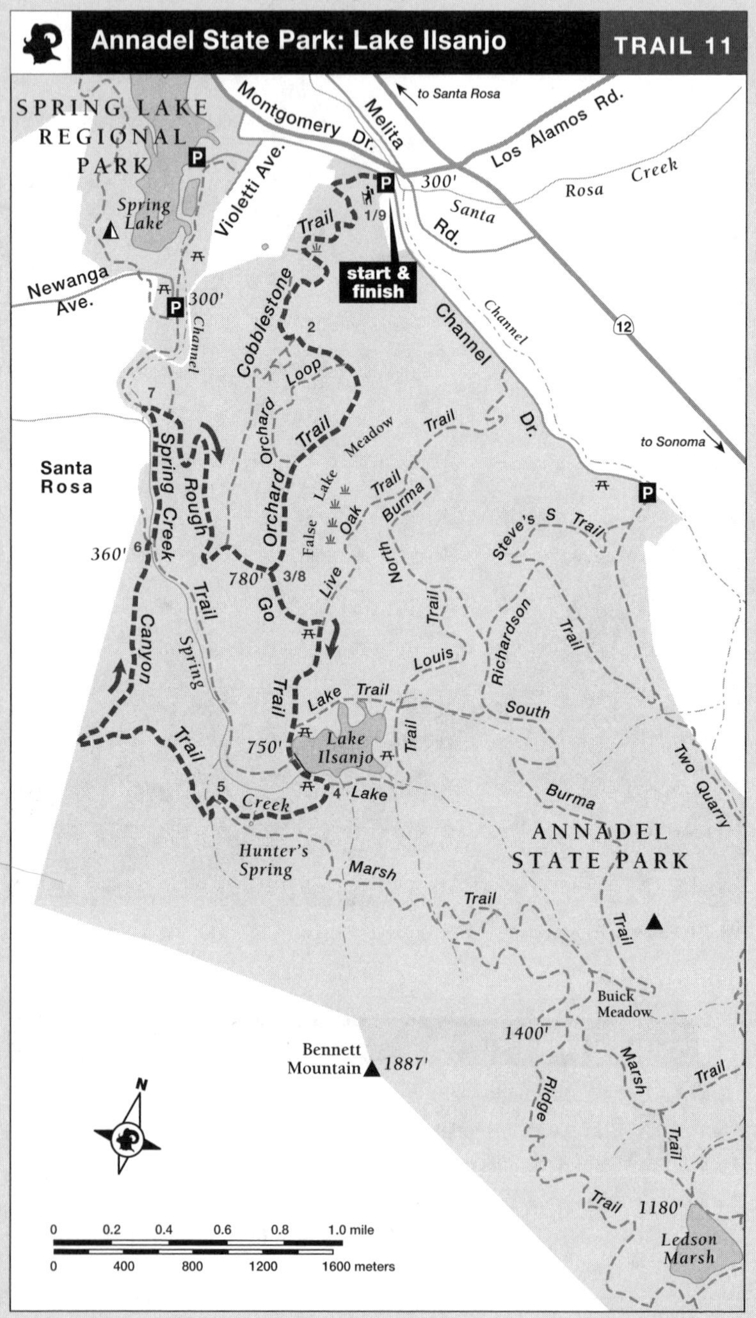

Annadel State Park: Lake Ilsanjo

This semiloop route across the north half of Annadel State Park encounters dense forest, oak savanna, bunch grasses, and a cattail-rimmed lake. Length, not terrain, earns this trip its difficulty rating. Some trails are subject to seasonal closure during wet weather. Please observe all closure signs, and use only named and maintained trails.

TRAIL USE
Hike, Run, Bike

LENGTH
8.8 miles, 5–6 hours

VERTICAL FEET
±1600'

DIFFICULTY
– 1 2 3 **4** 5 +

TRAIL TYPE
Loop

SURFACE TYPE
Dirt

FEATURES
Lake
Autumn Colors
Birds
Wildlife
Secluded
Cool & Shady

FACILITIES
Ranger Station
Restrooms
Picnic Tables
Water

Best Time

Fall through spring, but trails may be muddy during wet weather.

Finding the Trail

From US Hwy. 101 in Santa Rosa, take the exit for Sebastopol/Sonoma/State Hwy. 12 and follow State Hwy. 12 east toward Sonoma. At 1.4 miles, turn left onto Farmers Ln., go 0.8 mile, and turn right onto Montgomery Dr. Go 2.7 miles and turn right onto Channel Dr., signed for Annadel State Park and Spring Lake. Go 0.6 mile to a large dirt-and-gravel parking area, left.

From State Hwy. 12 going northwest from Kenwood to Santa Rosa, turn left on Los Alamos Rd. and go 0.2 mile to Melita Rd. Turn right on Melita Rd. and then immediately left onto Montgomery Dr. Go 0.5 mile to Channel Dr., turn left, and go 0.6 mile to a large, dirt-and-gravel parking area, left.

The trailhead is opposite the east end of the parking area, across Channel Dr. on its south side.

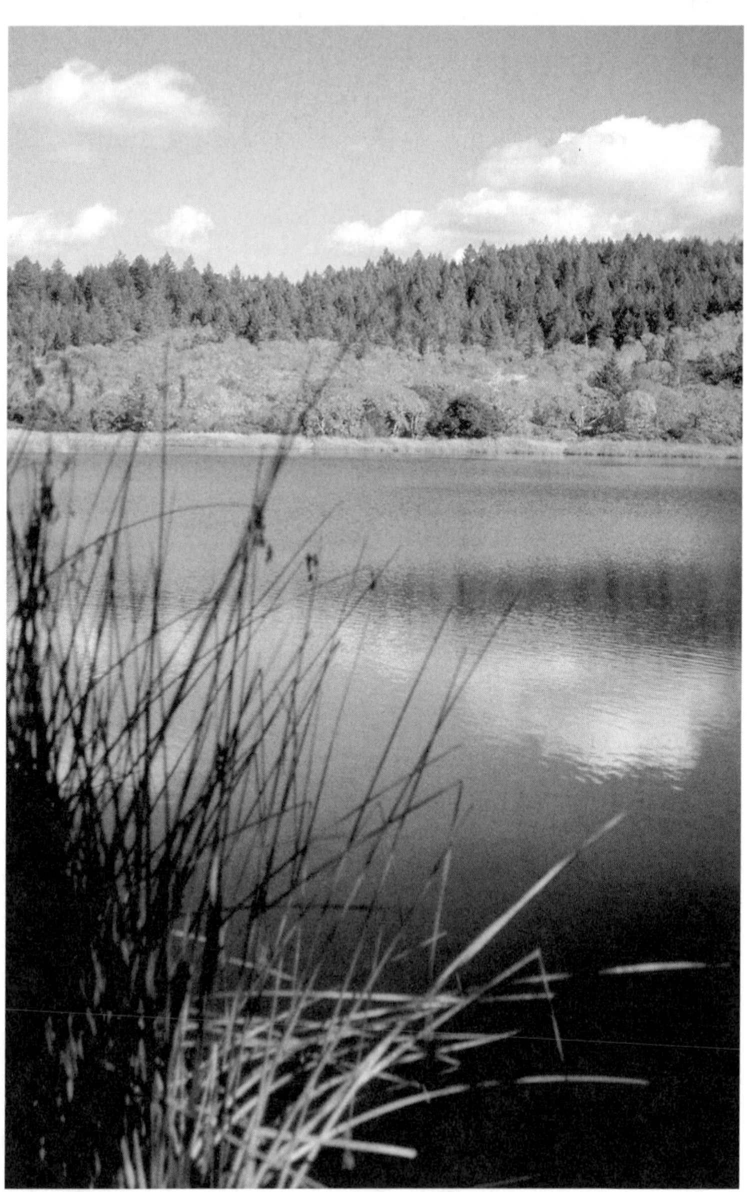

Lake Ilsanjo

Trail Description

From the trailhead, the **Cobblestone Trail**▶1 climbs moderately as it wanders generally south over alternately smooth and rocky terrain, some of which may become muddy during wet weather. Due east, across Highway 12, rises the forested summit of Mt. Hood (2730'), a destination for another day. After traversing an open, grassy field, the route bends sharply left. At a junction where a trail signed TO PARK BOUNDARY branches right, you stay on the Cobblestone Trail as it curves left. Gently gaining elevation and passing a second trail to the park boundary, you enjoy a pleasant stroll through oak groves and across open fields, one holding the few remnants of an old orchard.

Near Hunter's Spring, look for wild turkeys in a dense, fern-floored forest of Douglas-fir, coast live oak, California bay, and bigleaf maple.

Now the Cobblestone Trail▶2 goes right as a dirt road, but you go straight on the **Orchard Trail.** After passing the Loop Trail, right, you make a long traverse, then climb to an open area where manzanita thrives in company with oaks, whose outstretched limbs arch over the trail. Passing the remnants of several cobblestone quarries, you soon reach a fork marked by a trail post, where you stay left, still on the Orchard Trail. Ahead rises Bennett Mountain, at 1887 feet the highest point in Annadel State Park, its slopes dappled in fall with colorful foliage.

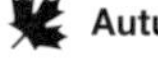

Crossing a beautiful oak savanna, you come to a T-junction with the **Rough Go Trail,**▶3 where you turn left. Climbing on a gentle but rocky grade, the Rough Go Trail soon meets the Live Oak Trail, left, and then bends right. The Rough Go Trail levels, thendescends. Just past a junction with the Lake Trail, left, your route crosses the dam's paved

OPTIONS

More Annadel Trails

Bicyclists and ambitious hikers can explore the shadier east edge of Annadel State Park via the **Marsh** and **Ridge trails** to **Ledson Marsh,** a round-trip that adds about 8 miles to the described route.

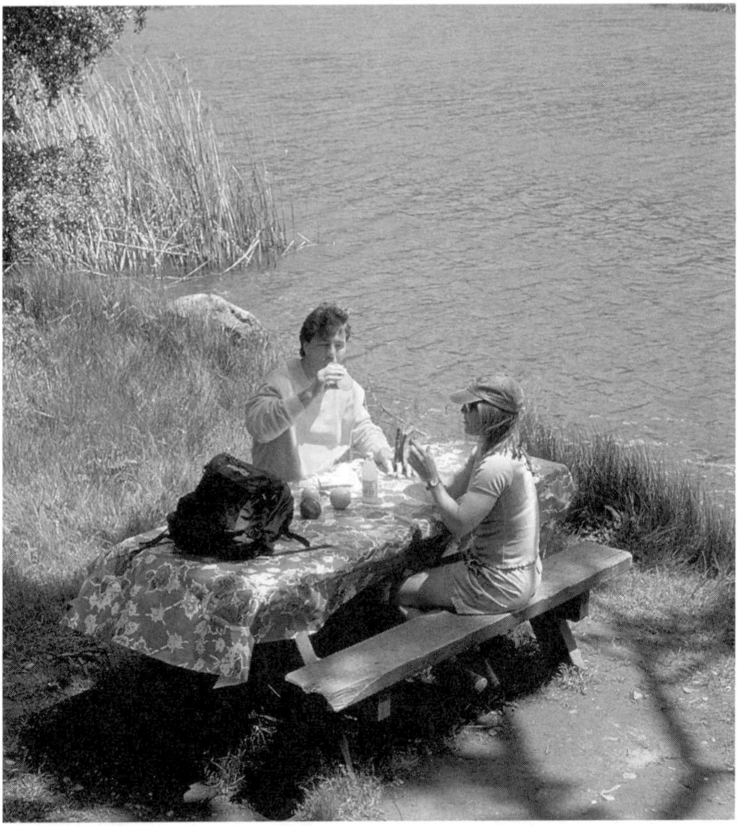

Picnickers enjoy lunch at *Lake Ilsanjo.*

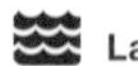 Lake

spillway apron, and 100 feet or so farther it arrives at a T-junction with a dirt road. Turning left, you walk about 200 feet to the lake and cross the dam.

On the far side of the dam, your route, a dirt road, swings left and begins a gentle climb. Topping a low rise, the road descends to a junction.▶4 Here you turn right on the **Canyon Trail,** also a dirt road, and head for **Hunter's Spring,** marked by a water trough and a patch of giant chain fern clinging to the slope beside the trail. The Canyon Trail takes you from open grassland and oak woodland to a north-facing oak-bay woodland.

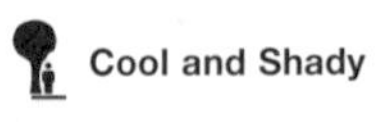 Cool and Shady

Now you reach a junction with a picnic table, left, and a rest bench, right.►5 The dirt road heading left is the Marsh Trail, part of the Bay Area Ridge Trail. You continue straight on the Canyon Trail, now also part of the Bay Area Ridge Trail, in places enjoying a broad view north across Santa Rosa and the Russian River valley. Stay on the trail as it hairpins right, past a gate to private property on the left.

About 1.5 miles from the Marsh Trail, turn sharply right to cross a bridge over **Spring Creek.** Just across the creek, the Canyon Trail ends at a T-junction with the **Spring Creek Trail.**►6 Turning left, you walk along Spring Creek and soon pass a junction where a gravel road heads left to a flood-control dam and levee. Just before the road veers left to cross a wooden bridge, you turn sharply right on the **Rough Go Trail.**►7

An extended climb through rocky grassland brings you to a junction with the **Cobblestone Trail,** left. Continuing straight, you wind uphill past stands of oak and manzanita to the junction with the **Orchard Trail**►8 you arrived at earlier. Now turn left and retrace your route on the Orchard and Cobblestone trails to the parking area.►9

MILESTONES

►1	0.0	From parking area, start up Cobblestone Trail
►2	0.8	Left on Orchard Trail at junction with Cobblestone Trail
►3	2.0	Left on Rough Go Trail
►4	3.0	Right on Canyon Trail
►5	3.6	Straight on Canyon Trail at junction with Marsh Trail
►6	5.2	Left on Spring Creek Trail
►7	5.7	Right on Rough Go Trail
►8	6.9	Left on Orchard Trail
►9	8.8	Back at parking area

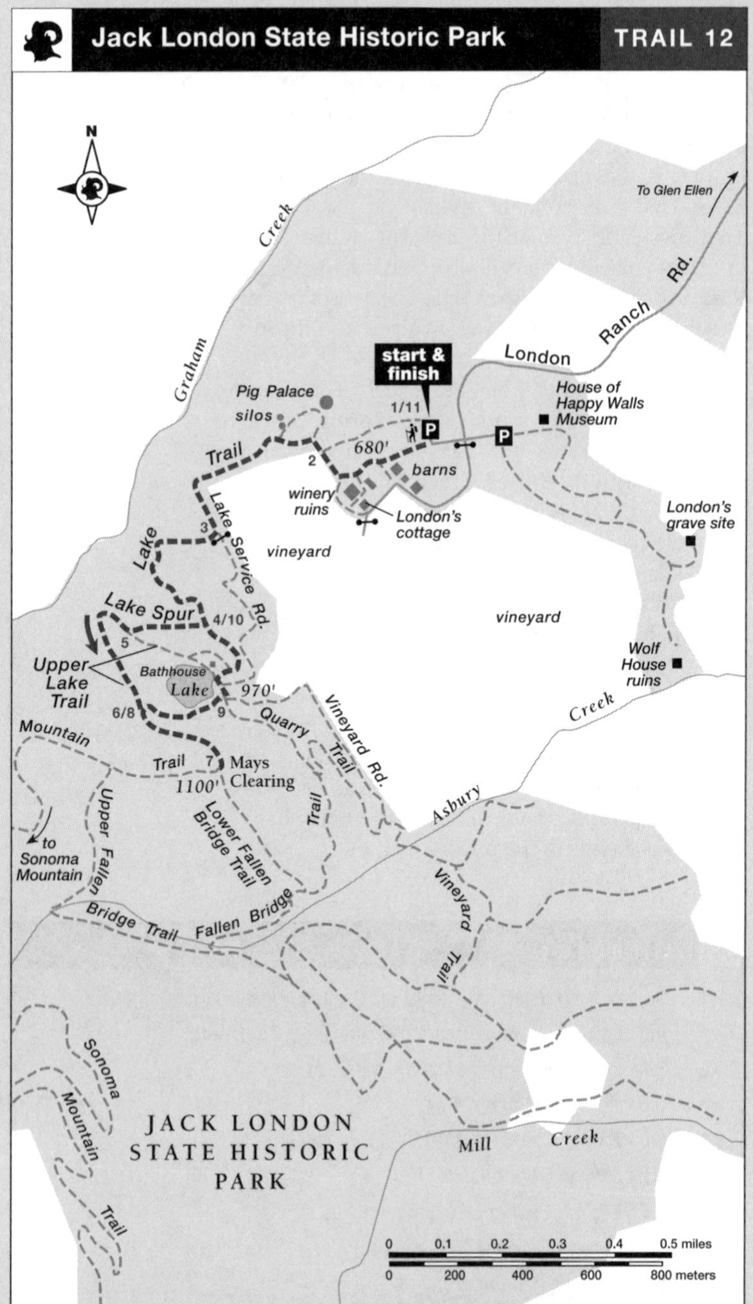
Jack London State Historic Park
TRAIL 12
N
To Glen Ellen
Graham Creek
London Ranch Rd.
start & finish
1/11
Pig Palace
silos
House of Happy Walls Museum
Trail
2
680'
barns
winery ruins
London's cottage
London's grave site
3
Lake
Lake Service Rd.
vineyard
vineyard
Lake Spur
4/10
5
Upper Lake Trail
Bathhouse Lake
970'
Wolf House ruins
Asbury Creek
6/8
9
Quarry Trail
Vineyard Rd.
Vineyard Trail
Mountain Trail
7
Mays Clearing
1100'
Upper Fallen Bridge Trail
Lower Fallen Bridge Trail
to Sonoma Mountain
Bridge Trail
Fallen Bridge
Sonoma Mountain Trail
JACK LONDON STATE HISTORIC PARK
Mill Creek
0 0.1 0.2 0.3 0.4 0.5 miles
0 200 400 600 800 meters

Jack London State Historic Park

Jack London's ranch, a beautiful redwood forest, and a vista point with superb views are the attractions of this semiloop trip that uses the Lake, Upper Lake, and Mountain trails. After your hike, be sure to visit the park's fine visitor center and museum, open daily 10 A.M. to 5 P.M., devoted to the work of its namesake author.

TRAIL USE
Hike, Run, Child Friendly
LENGTH
2.9 miles, 2–3 hours
VERTICAL FEET
±450'
DIFFICULTY
– 1 2 **3** 4 5 +
TRAIL TYPE
Loop
SURFACE TYPE
Dirt, Paved

FEATURES
Fee
Lake
Wildflowers
Birds
Historic
Great Views
Secluded
Cool & Shady

FACILITIES
Visitor Center
Restrooms
Picnic Tables
Water

Best Time

All year, but trails may be muddy in wet weather. In summer, the park closes relatively early, around the same time as the visitor center.

Finding the Trail

From State Hwy. 12 just north of Sonoma Valley Regional Park, take Arnold Dr. southwest to Glen Ellen. At 0.9 mile, Arnold Dr. crosses a bridge over Calabazas Creek and begins to turn left. Here you bear right onto London Ranch Rd., which is heavily used by bicyclists. Go 1.3 miles to the park's entrance kiosk; turn right just past the kiosk into the west parking area.

The trailhead is by an information board on the parking area's southwest side. Equestrians must use a trailhead located a few hundred feet to the right.

Trail Description

Your route begins on a paved path that changes to a dirt-and-gravel road leading through a shady picnic area.▶1 Passing the three stone barns, left, you come

Jack London's adventure books, such as *The Call of the Wild, The Sea Wolf,* and *White Fang,* made him world famous and one of the highest-paid authors of his time.

to a T-junction with another dirt-and-gravel road, part of the Bay Area Ridge Trail. Angle right on the road, soon passing a trail, left, to **London's cottage,** which the author purchased in 1911 and where he died in 1916.

Rising dramatically behind London's vineyard is **Sonoma Mountain,** a long ridge capped by a 2463-foot summit, which is on private land just west of the park boundary.

About 75 feet from the T-junction, you bear right at a fork onto a dirt road, signed LAKE and PIG PALACE. Several hundred feet ahead, the trail from the equestrian trailhead, labeled LAKE TRAIL on the park map, joins from the right.►**2** You continue straight, now on the **Lake Trail.** Follow the road as it curves left, with a beautiful view of the vineyard beyond. When you approach a gate across the road, look for the hiking-only Lake Trail heading downhill and right.►**3** (Bikes and horses must stay on the dirt road to reach the lake and beyond.)

Stream

Veering right onto the Lake Trail, you soon begin climbing through shady forest. Your route turns left at a bench and climbs through a redwood grove. Now you come to a junction signed LAKE SPUR and LAKE TRAIL.►**4** Turn right, gaining elevation on a moderate grade. A short steep pitch leads to a T-junction with the **Upper Lake Trail,**►**5** where you turn right and stay in dense woods. (The left branch takes a shorter route through a meadow to the lake.)

After several hundred yards, your route turns sharply left and wanders amid California bay, tanbark oak, and Douglas-fir, with a meadow just visible below. In a redwood grove, you reach a junction with the **Mountain Trail,** a wide dirt road.►**6**

Cool and Shady

Turning right, you leave the forest and reach a big meadow called **Mays Clearing.**►**7** A rest bench beckons you to pause and enjoy the stunning view, which extends southeast, past the old state-hospital

Great Views

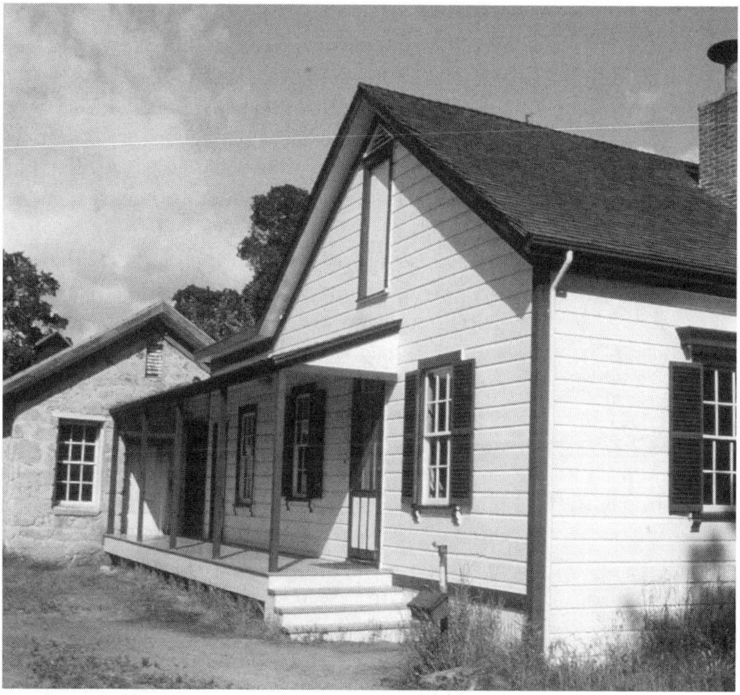

Jack London's cottage *was the author's residence until he died in 1916.*

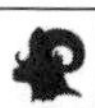

OPTIONS

More Sonoma Mountain Trails

From **Mays Clearing,▸7** ascend the **Mountain Trail** and then the short **Mountain Spur** to just below the 2463-foot summit of **Sonoma Mountain.** This adds 5.1 miles to the described route. Several newly opened trails on former Sonoma State Hospital lands, accessed from the State Park, also warrant exploring.

Wolf House

From the museum, located next to the east parking area, you can walk to London's grave site and the remnants of his elaborate mansion, **Wolf House,** which was destroyed by fire in 1913.

orchards, all the way to Mt. Diablo. In spring, wildflowers abound here, including blue-eyed grass, California buttercup, vetch, and false lupine.

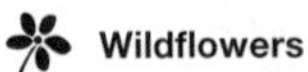
Wildflowers

When you are thoroughly satiated with scenery, retrace your route to the junction of the Upper Lake and Mountain trails.►**8** At this junction, the Mountain Trail makes an almost-180-degree bend to the right, and you follow it downhill on a gentle and then moderate grade. As you approach the **lake,** you pass a path leading left to the stone dam, and then the Quarry Trail, right. Just ahead is a T-junction with a dirt road.►**9** On the park map, the road heading right is labeled VINEYARD ROAD, but here you turn left and walk down the road toward the lake, with the stone dam in front of you.

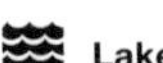
Lake

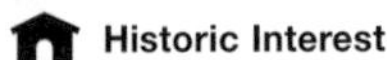
Historic Interest

Once past the dam, you can see **London's bathhouse** and a picnic area with tables, left. Here the dirt road is signed BAY AREA RIDGE TRAIL. A single track to the left of this road is similarly signed. Where the road begins to descend, leave it and bear left on the single track, coming in about 50 feet to a trail post signed with the Bay Area Ridge Trail emblem and the words PARKING LOT, 1 MILE.►**10** This is the **Lake Trail;** follow it downhill to the Lake Spur junction, then retrace your route to the parking area.►**11**

MILESTONES

▶1	0.0	Take paved path to dirt-and-gravel road southwest through picnic area
▶2	0.3	Join Lake Trail from equestrian staging area
▶3	0.6	Right on Lake Trail where dirt road continues straight
▶4	0.9	Right on Upper Lake Trail (Lake Spur on park map)
▶5	1.1	Right on Upper Lake Trail
▶6	1.3	Right on Mountain Trail
▶7	1.5	Mays Clearing
▶8	1.7	Right to stay on Mountain Trail at junction with Upper Lake Trail
▶9	1.9	Left on dirt road (toward lake) at junction with Vineyard Rd., then left on Lake Trail where dirt road begins to descend
▶10	2.0	Straight on Lake Trail
▶11	2.9	Back at parking area

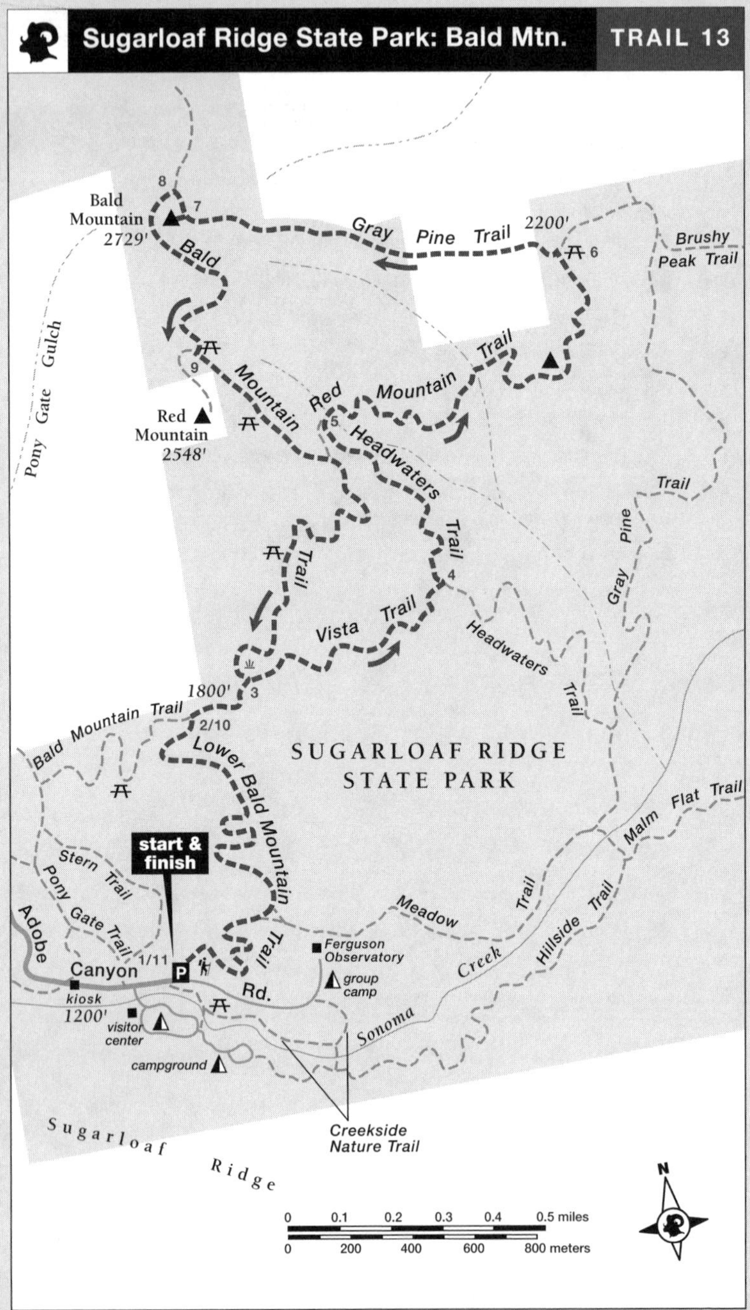
Bald Mountain 2729'
Gray Pine Trail 2200'
Brushy Peak Trail
Bald Mountain Trail
Red Mountain 2548'
Pony Gate Gulch
Red Mountain Trail
Headwaters Trail
Gray Pine Trail
Vista Trail
1800'
Bald Mountain Trail
Lower Bald Mountain Trail
SUGARLOAF RIDGE STATE PARK
Malm Flat Trail
start & finish
Stern Trail
Pony Gate Trail
Meadow Trail
Hillside Trail
Adobe Canyon Rd.
kiosk
1200'
visitor center
Ferguson Observatory
group camp
campground
Sonoma Creek
Creekside Nature Trail
Sugarloaf Ridge
0 0.1 0.2 0.3 0.4 0.5 miles
0 200 400 600 800 meters
N

Sugarloaf Ridge State Park: Bald Mountain

This semiloop route is a challenge, but well worth the effort. A superb array of trees, shrubs, and wildflowers, along with some of the best views in the North Bay, are the rewards for tackling the 1500-foot climb to the summit of Bald Mountain. Camping is available in developed family campsites and a group camp, both near the entrance kiosk. Reservations are required March 15–Oct. 31; first-come, first-served camping is from Nov. 1–March 14. For reservations, call (800) 444-7275.

TRAIL USE
Hike, Run
LENGTH
6.7 miles, 5 hours
VERTICAL FEET
±1900'
DIFFICULTY
- 1 2 3 4 **5** +
TRAIL TYPE
Loop
SURFACE TYPE
Dirt, Paved

FEATURES
Fee
Mountain
Summit
Wildflowers
Birds
Great Views
Camping

FACILITIES
Restrooms
Picnic Tables
Water
Phone

Best Time

This route is best in spring and fall.

Finding the Trail

From State Hwy. 12 just north of Kenwood, take Adobe Canyon Rd. and go northeast 3.4 miles to the Sugarloaf Ridge State Park entrance kiosk. Continue 0.1 mile to a dirt parking area, left. The trailhead is on the northeast corner of the parking area.▶1

Trail Description

The **Lower Bald Mountain Trail,** a single track, heads east from the parking area and wanders gently uphill through a serpentine grassland dotted with native bunchgrass, chaparral, and wildflowers, including blue-eyed grass, yarrow, bluedicks, lupine, vetch, and blow wives. At a junction with the **Meadow Trail,** veer left and soon begin a moderate uphill climb via a series of switchbacks in a densely wooded area. Just short of the 1-mile point, your trail merges with the **Bald Mountain Trail,** part of

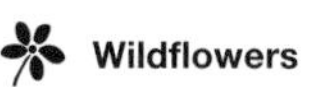

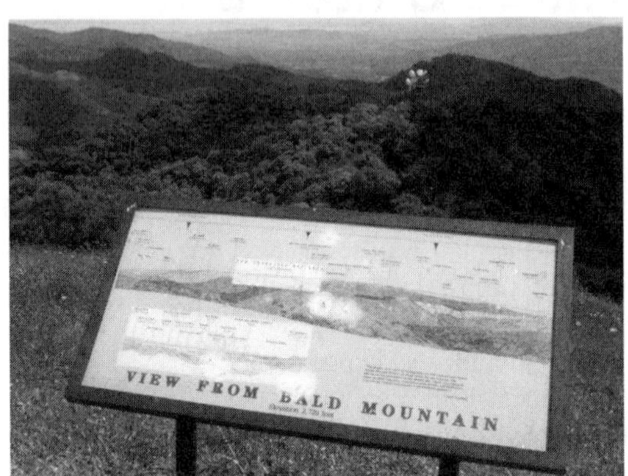

Atop Bald Mountain *two display panels help you identify landmarks to the north and south.*

the Bay Area Ridge Trail.►**2** Bearing right on this paved road, you follow it steadily uphill on a moderate grade. Where the road angles sharply left, you turn right onto the single track **Vista Trail.►3**

The Vista Trail skirts a seasonal wetland, passes a fern-draped spring, and then climbs across a steep, grassy slope that affords views of Sonoma Creek and Sugarloaf Ridge, both right. A short, steep descent brings you to a junction with the **Headwaters Trail.►4** Bearing left, you walk in the shade of Douglas-fir and coast live oak. Reaching **Sonoma Creek** but staying on its west side, the trail bends left and rises on a moderate grade. After struggling uphill over rough ground, the trail at last reaches a T-junction with the **Red Mountain Trail,►5** a single track. Here you turn right and cross a branch of Sonoma Creek.

On a rolling course, the trail heads generally eastward to cross a larger branch of Sonoma Creek via a wooden bridge. Eventually the trail enters a side canyon and switchbacks up to a knoll. Suddenly

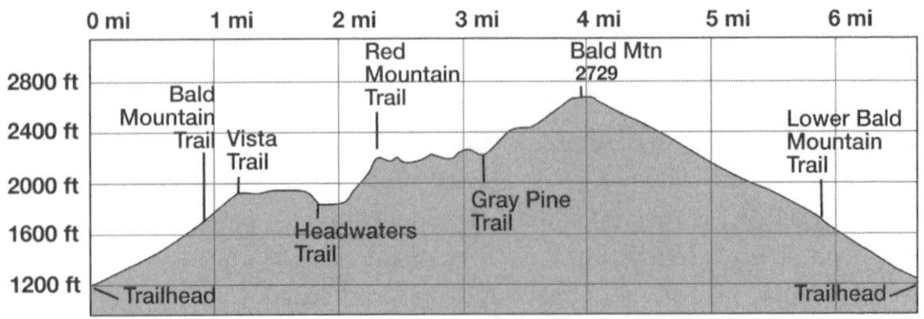

TRAIL 13 Sugarloaf Ridge State Park: Bald Mountain Profile

you are atop a manzanita barren—the sandy, rocky soil is perfect for these hardy, pioneering plants. From here you have a wonderful 360-degree view that, at last, reveals your goal, the summit of Bald Mountain, slightly north of west.

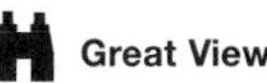
Great Views

Descending north from the knoll, you meet the **Gray Pine Trail,** a dirt road, at a T-junction.►6 Now turning left, you ramble uphill on a moderate grade. After several steep pitches, you leave the Gray Pine Trail where it bends right, and continue west over windswept open ground a few hundred feet to the top of **Bald Mountain** (2729').►7

On a clear day, the views from Bald Mountain are extraordinary, ranging from the Sierra Nevada to Point Reyes, and from Snow Mountain, north of Clear Lake, to San Francisco.

When it is time to head down, retrace your route to the Gray Pine Trail, turn left onto it, and follow it steeply downhill to a T-junction with the **Bald Mountain Trail,** a dirt road.►8 Here you turn left, climb briefly, and then circle the west side of Bald Mountain to a T-junction with a paved road.►9 Turning left, you head downhill on a gentle and then moderate grade into forest. After passing the junction with the Vista Trail, continue downhill on the Bald Mountain and **Lower Bald Mountain** trails,►10 retracing your route to the parking area.►11

MILESTONES

►1	0.0	Take Lower Bald Mountain Trail east, then north
►2	0.9	Right on Bald Mountain Trail (paved)
►3	1.2	Right on Vista Trail
►4	1.8	Left on Headwaters Trail
►5	2.3	Right on Red Mountain Trail
►6	3.2	Left on Gray Pine Trail
►7	3.9	Summit of Bald Mountain (2729')
►8	4.0	Left at T-junction with Bald Mountain Trail (dirt)
►9	4.4	Left at T-junction with Bald Mountain Trail (paved)
►10	5.8	Left at junction with Lower Bald Mountain Trail
►11	6.7	Back at parking area

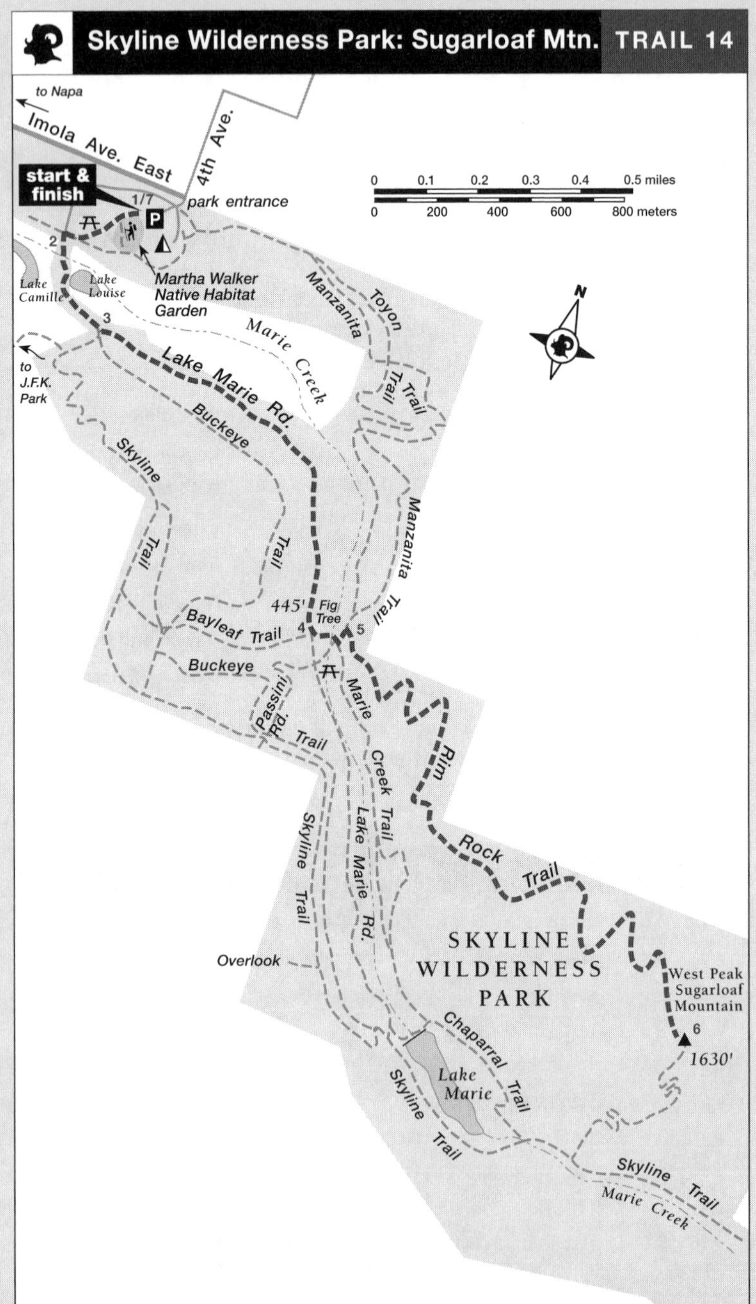

Skyline Wilderness Park: Sugarloaf Mtn.
TRAIL 14
to Napa
Imola Ave. East
4th Ave.
start & finish
1/7
park entrance
0 0.1 0.2 0.3 0.4 0.5 miles
0 200 400 600 800 meters
2
Lake Camille
Lake Louise
Martha Walker Native Habitat Garden
3
Manzanita
Toyon
Marie Creek
N
to J.F.K. Park
Lake Marie Rd.
Trail
Trail
Buckeye
Skyline
Trail
Trail
Manzanita Trail
445'
Fig Tree
Bayleaf Trail
4
5
Buckeye
Passini Rd.
Trail
Marie
Rim
Creek Trail
Skyline Trail
Lake Marie Rd.
Rock
Trail
SKYLINE WILDERNESS PARK
Overlook
West Peak Sugarloaf Mountain
6
1630'
Chaparral Trail
Lake Marie
Skyline Trail
Skyline Trail
Marie Creek

Skyline Wilderness Park: Sugarloaf Mountain

This hike climbs to the highest point in Skyline Wilderness Park, which was created in the late 1970s from surplus Napa State Hospital land. Most trails—but not the Rim Rock Trail—are open to hikers, equestrians, and bicyclists. Maintenance is a volunteer effort by the Skyline Park Citizens Association—some trails may be in better shape than others, and long pants are advised.

TRAIL USE
Hike, Run
LENGTH
6.0 miles, 4 hours
VERTICAL FEET
±1700'
DIFFICULTY
– 1 2 3 **4** 5 +
TRAIL TYPE
Out & Back
SURFACE TYPE
Dirt, Paved

FEATURES
Fee
Mountain
Wildflowers
Birds
Great Views
Secluded

FACILITIES
Restrooms
Picnic Tables
Water

Best Time

Spring and fall, especially when spring wildflowers are at their peak; park is closed on Thanksgiving and Christmas.

Finding the Trail

From State Hwy. 29 in Napa, take the Imola Ave./Lake Berryessa/State Hwy. 121 North exit and go east 2.9 miles on Imola Ave. to the Skyline Wilderness Park entrance, right. Bear right and go about 200 feet to a paved parking area. The trailhead is on the southwest corner of the parking area.

Facilities

A campground adjacent to the parking area hosts RVs year-round. Also in the park are picnic and barbecue areas, an activity center, a cookhouse, a social center for meetings and indoor parties, and an equestrian arena.

Trail Description

Martha Walker Native Habitat Garden is a volunteer effort established in 1986 to honor its namesake, a local botanist, teacher, and journalist.

Walk downhill from the parking area▸1 on a dirt path and then climb generally southwest, keeping the fenced **Martha Walker Native Habitat Garden** on your left. The garden, which was created in 1986 by California Native Plant Society volunteers on the site of the old state-hospital dump, honors a well-loved local botanist, teacher, and journalist.

After cresting a low rise, angle southwest through a picnic area and soon join a paved service road. Turn right and descend gently to a four-way junction.▸2 Turn left on a gravel road signed LAKE MARIE ROAD TRAILS. Your route crosses a bridge over **Marie Creek,** briefly jogs left on a paved driveway for Napa State Hospital's Camp Coombs, and then angles right on a shady gravel road. Passing between two reservoirs—**Lake Louise,** left, and **Lake Camille,** right—the road soon bends left to a reach a junction,▸3 where the Skyline Trail (part of the Bay Area Ridge Trail) turns sharply right.

Wildflowers

You continue straight on **Lake Marie Road,** climbing past an old orchard, left. In the grassy areas beside the trail are spring bloomers such as lupine, yarrow, bluedicks, and Ithuriel's spear. Soon you pass a bench and a watering trough for horses. Nearby is a cave gouged from the hillside, one of several that might have been dug as part of the hospital's water supply or perhaps as the beginnings of mine shafts. Your route ascends moderately across a long meadow dotted with oaks and California buckeyes.

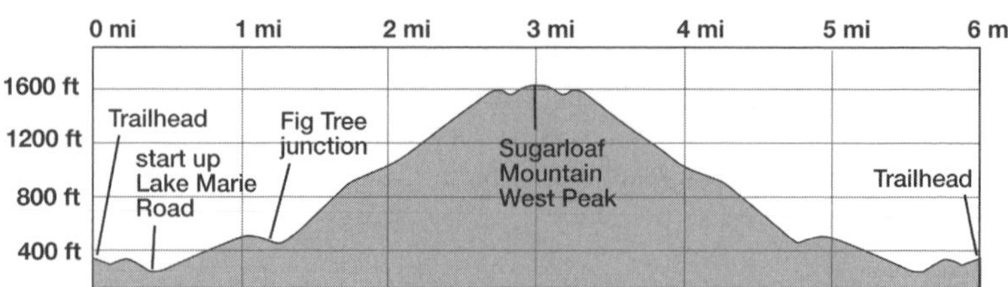

TRAIL 14 Skyline Wilderness Park: Sugarloaf Mountain Profile

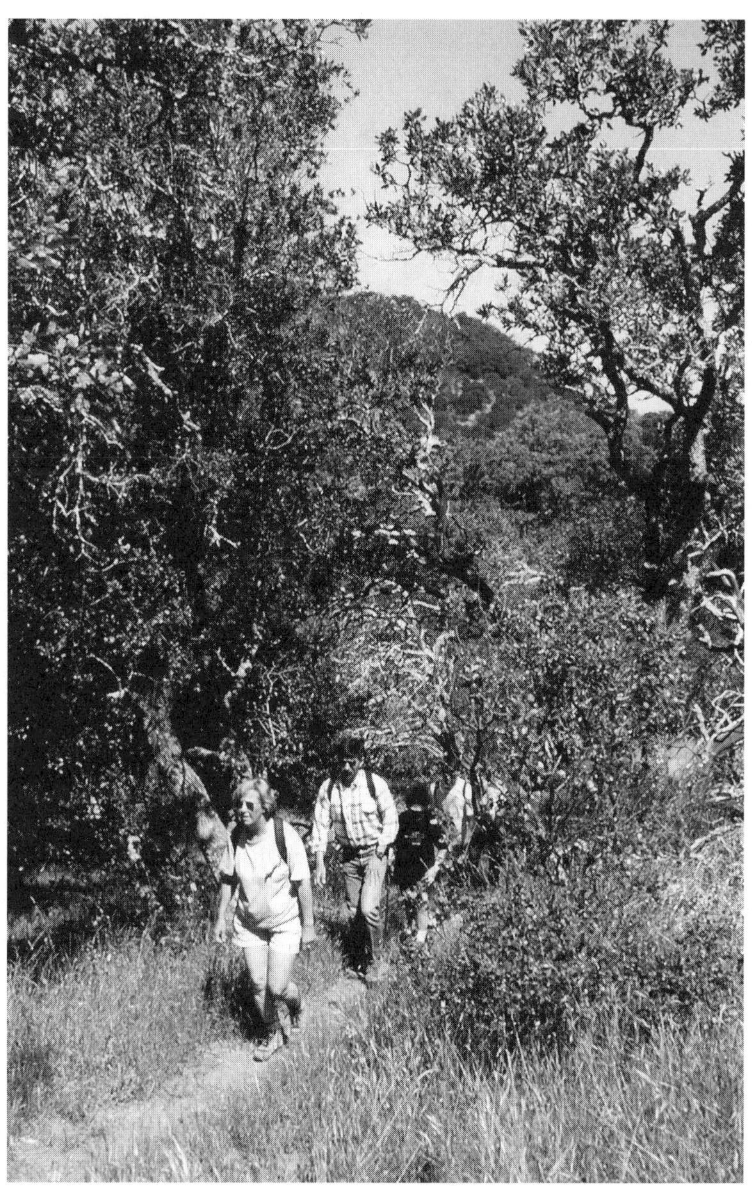

The Rim Rock Trail *ascends through oak woodlands to the top of Sugarloaf Mountain.*

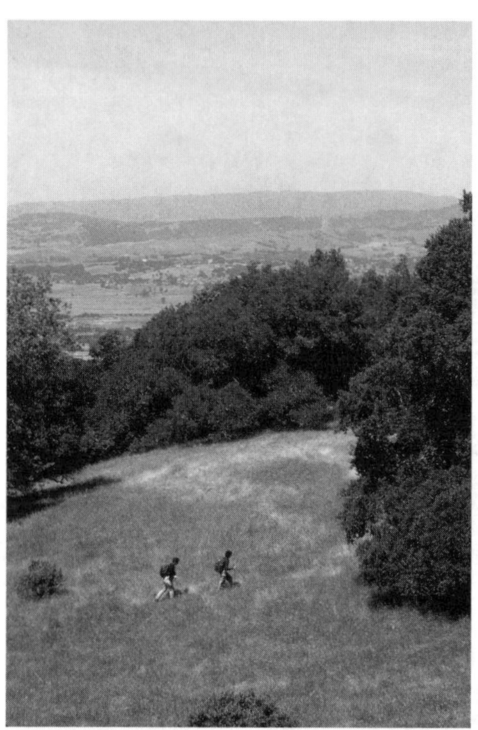

Hikers ascending Sugarloaf Mountain *enjoy views of the Napa Valley and surrounding mountains.*

After leveling, the road descends on a moderate grade and comes to a junction with the Bayleaf, right. On the left is one of the park's most remarkable features, a **giant fig tree** whose branches droop to the ground, enclosing a room-sized area.▶4

Just past the fig tree, you pass an unsigned trail, left. About 150 feet ahead are picnic tables and a toilet. Leave Lake Marie Road at the picnic area and turn left onto a single-track trail, heading toward **Marie Creek.** A bridge provides an easy way across the creek, and about 60 feet farther you come to a junction with the Marie Creek Trail, right. Continue straight, passing two signs, one for the Manzanita and Toyon trails, the other for your route, the Rim Rock Trail. In about 15 feet, where the trail starts to bend left, you come to another junction, this one unsigned.▶5 Here you turn right onto the **Rim Rock Trail,** which passes through a gap in a rock wall. At a HIKING ONLY sign, the trail bears right and begins to switchback up a south-facing slope. The route eventually curves east, following a tributary of Marie Creek, far below and right. The grade eases as you reach the head of a canyon, but then rises steeply via a series of switchbacks. The habitat beside the trail alternates between grassland, chaparral, and oak-bay woodland. In rocky areas you may find a succulent plant called common dudleya, which sports yellow-to-red flowers in late spring and early summer.

The route zigzags up a grassy hillside, then crosses a knoll topped by a grove of bay and coast live oak. A meadow provides a view east to the East Peak of Sugarloaf Mountain (1686'), which is topped with communication towers. You climb the next knoll to a clearing centered around a low boulder. This undistinguished spot, ringed by oaks, is the 1630-foot summit of **Sugarloaf Mountain's West Peak,** the highest point in the park.►6 (From here, the Rim Rock Trail continues to the Skyline Trail, but the descent is too steep and eroded to recommend.)

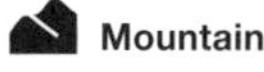

After you have enjoyed relaxing on the summit, retrace your route to the parking area.►7

OPTIONS

Loop Return

If you'd like a different return route, from the fig tree junction,►4 ascend the **Bayleaf Trail** to the **Skyline Trail** (part of the Bay Area Ridge Trail), then turn right on the Skyline Trail to return to Lake Marie Rd.►3

MILESTONES

►1	0.0	Take dirt path south to T-junction, right on paved road
►2	0.2	Left onto dirt road, across bridge, then left on paved road
►3	0.4	Straight on Lake Marie Rd. at junction with Skyline Trail
►4	1.2	Left past fig tree, across bridge, straight at junction with Marie Creek Trail
►5	1.3	Right on Rim Rock Trail, right again at fork
►6	3.0	Sugarloaf Mountain's West Peak; retrace to parking area
►7	6.0	Back at parking area

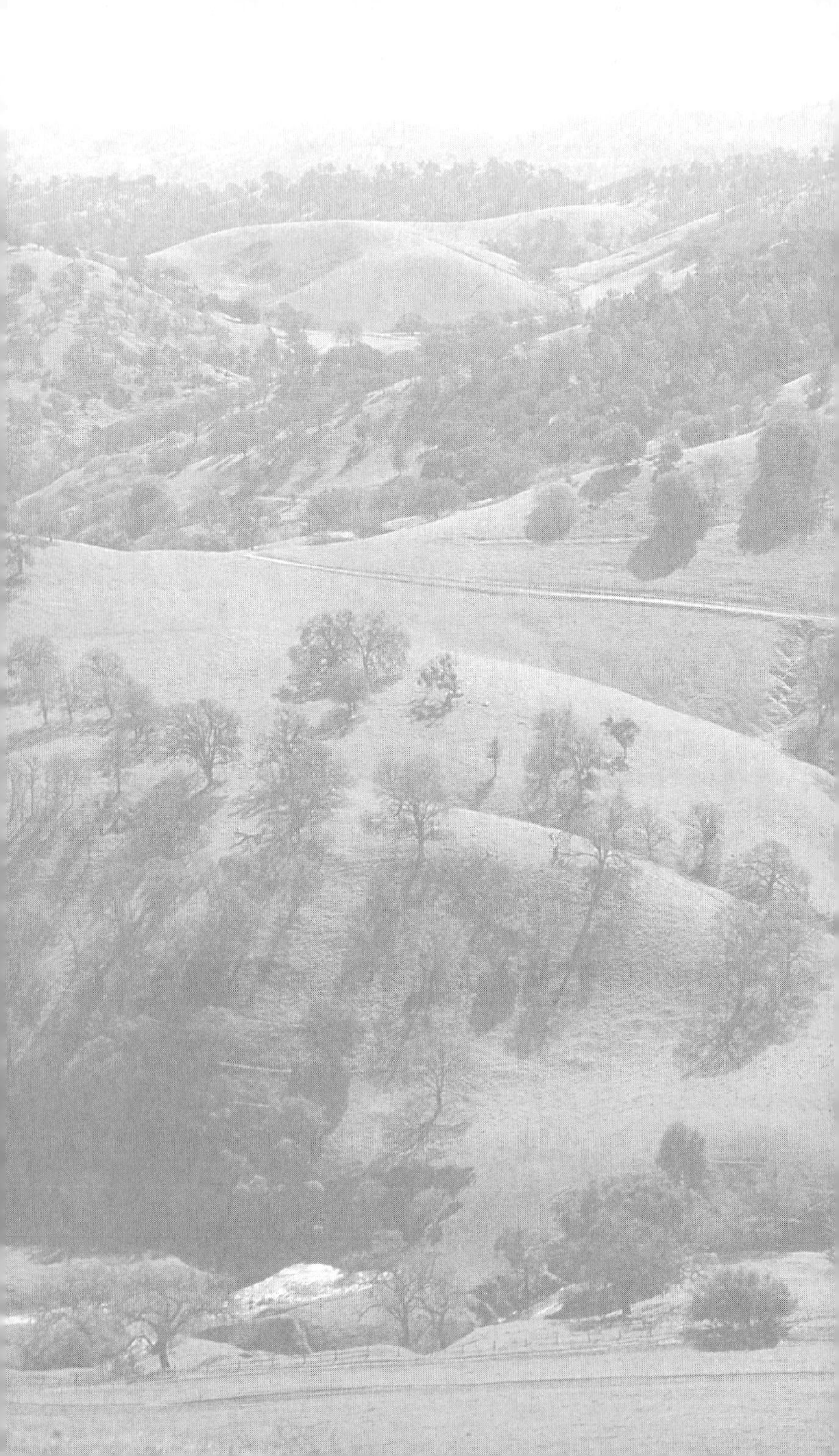

CHAPTER 2

East Bay

15. Wildcat Canyon Regional Park: San Pablo Ridge
16. Tilden Regional Park: Wildcat Peak
17. Sibley Volcanic Regional Preserve: Round Top Loop
18. Redwood Regional Park: East Ridge
19. Briones Regional Park: Briones Crest
20. Black Diamond Mines Regional Preserve: Stewartville Loop
21. Mount Diablo State Park: Grand Loop
22. Morgan Territory Regional Preserve: Bob Walker Ridge
23. Coyote Hills Regional Park: Red Hill
24. Dry Creek Pioneer Regional Park: High Ridge Loop
25. Pleasanton Ridge Regional Park
26. Sunol Regional Wilderness: Maguire Peaks
27. Mission Peak Regional Preserve: Mission Peak

East Bay

The East Bay extends eastward from San Francisco Bay to the edge of the Central Valley, and southeast from the Carquinez Strait and Suisun Bay to the foothills of Mt. Hamilton. Its two counties, **Alameda** and **Contra Costa**, are home to some 2.5 million people.

In 1934, during the Great Depression, Alameda County residents interested in preserving open space voted to create California's first regional park district, and to tax themselves five cents per $100—not an inconsiderable sum at the time—to pay for it. The resounding success of the East Bay Regional Park District led to its expansion, some 30 years later, into Contra Costa County, and to the creation of similar open space districts all over the Bay Area.

Among the East Bay Regional Park District's earliest parks were Tilden and Redwood regional parks, in the Oakland and Berkeley hills. Built as part of the federal public works programs, they included numerous trails and developed recreation areas such as lawns and picnic grounds, a model that continues today. EBRPD leases many of its pastoral parks to nearby cattle ranches, so you may encounter (usually sweet-tempered) cows along the trail.

East of the Caldecott Tunnel, the skyline of Walnut Creek and Concord is dominated by the lofty summit of Mt. Diablo. Although surrounded by sprawling suburbs, Mt. Diablo State Park and adjacent EBRPD parks have preserved a significant area of open space between San Francisco Bay and the Central Valley. Similar large areas of public lands provide respite from the industrial parks of Hayward and the suburbs of Fremont, ranging from the modest but scenic Coyote Hills to lofty Mission Peak and Pleasanton Ridge. Threaded through the East Bay parklands are more than 1,000 miles of trails for hiking, bicycling, walking, jogging, and horseback riding.

See Appendix 2 for agency contact information (page 314) and Appendix 6 for maps (page 321).

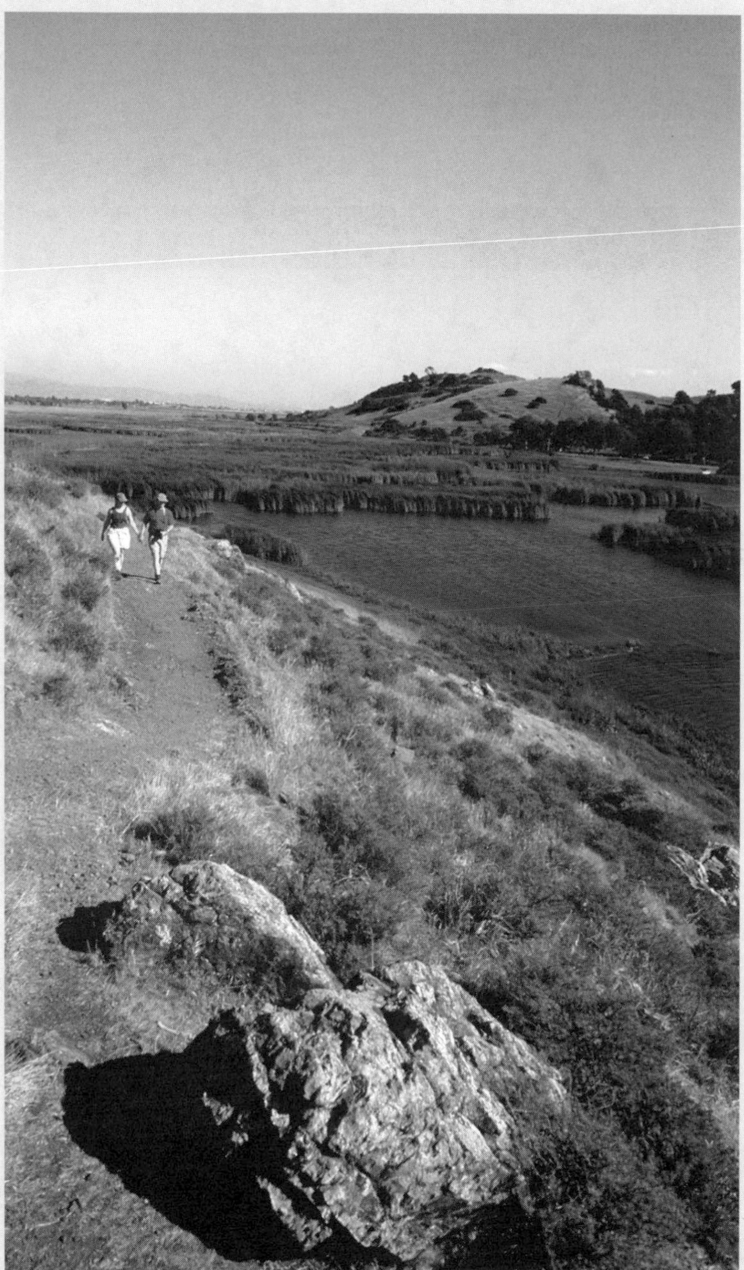

Coyote Hills Regional Park *(Trail 23)*

OVERVIEW MAP

East Bay

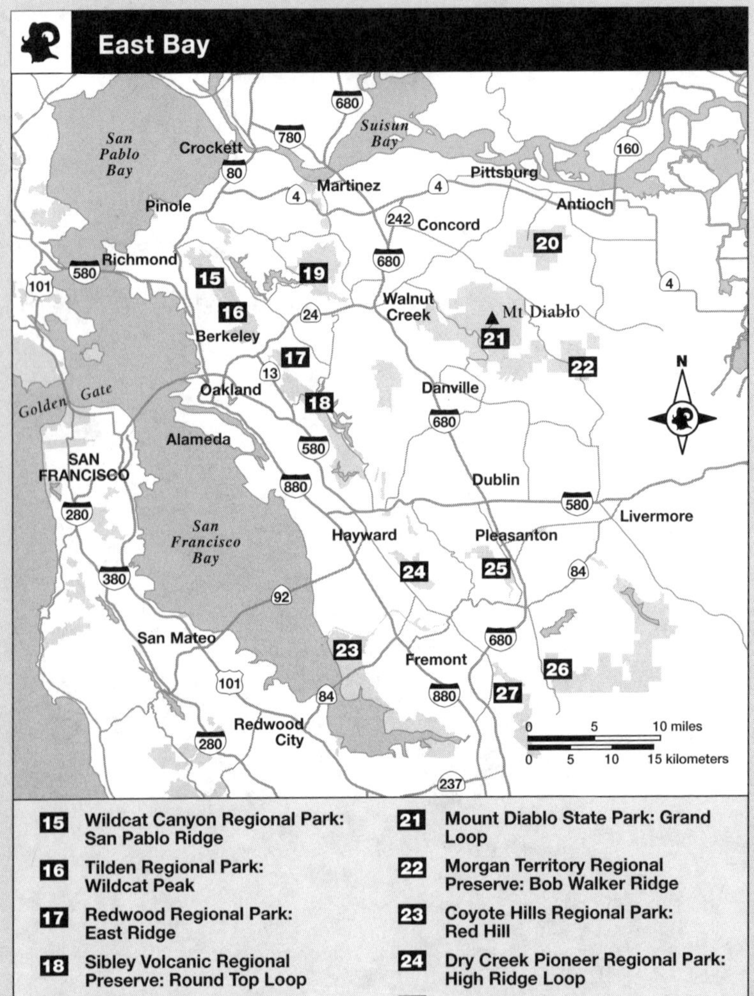

15 Wildcat Canyon Regional Park: San Pablo Ridge

16 Tilden Regional Park: Wildcat Peak

17 Redwood Regional Park: East Ridge

18 Sibley Volcanic Regional Preserve: Round Top Loop

19 Briones Regional Park: Briones Crest

20 Black Diamond Mines Regional Preserve: Stewartville Loop

21 Mount Diablo State Park: Grand Loop

22 Morgan Territory Regional Preserve: Bob Walker Ridge

23 Coyote Hills Regional Park: Red Hill

24 Dry Creek Pioneer Regional Park: High Ridge Loop

25 Pleasanton Ridge Regional Park

26 Sunol Regional Wilderness: Maguire Peaks

27 Mission Peak Regional Preserve: Mission Peak

East Bay

TRAIL	Difficulty	Length	Type	USES & ACCESS	TERRAIN	FLORA & FAUNA	OTHER
15	4	7.0	Loop	Hiking, Running, Biking, Dogs Allowed	River or Stream, Canyon, Summit	Wildflowers, Birds, Wildlife	Great Views, Photo Opportunity
16	3	3.3	Loop	Hiking, Running, Child Friendly	River or Stream, Canyon, Mountain, Summit	Birds	Great Views
17	2	1.8	Loop	Hiking, Running, Child Friendly, Dogs Allowed	—	Birds	Geologic Interest, Great Views
18	3	6.0	Loop	Hiking, Running, Dogs Allowed, Fee	River or Stream	Birds	Great Views
19	4	6.8	Loop	Hiking, Running, Biking, Dogs Allowed, Fee	Lake or Shore, Summit	Wildflowers, Birds	Great Views, Photo Opportunity
20	4	7.6	Loop	Hiking, Running, Biking[1], Dogs Allowed, Fee	Mountain	Wildflowers, Birds	Historic, Geologic Interest, Secluded, Camping
21	5	6.5	Loop	Hiking, Running, Biking[1], Fee	Mountain, Summit	Wildflowers, Birds	Historic, Great Views, Photo Opportunity, Steep, Camping
22	4	5.9	Loop	Hiking, Running, Biking[1], Dogs Allowed	Canyon	Autumn Colors, Birds	Great Views, Secluded
23	2	1.0	Loop	Hiking, Running, Biking[1], Child Friendly, Dogs Allowed, Fee	Lake or Shore, Summit	Wildflowers, Birds	Great Views, Photo Opportunity
24	4	5.7	Loop	Hiking, Running, Biking[1], Dogs Allowed, Fee	Lake or Shore, Summit	Birds, Wildlife	Great Views, Secluded
25	5	12.3	Loop	Hiking, Running, Biking, Dogs Allowed	River or Stream, Canyon, Summit	Wildflowers, Birds	Great Views, Photo Opportunity, Secluded
26	4	5.9	Loop	Hiking, Running, Biking[1], Dogs Allowed, Permit Required	Canyon, Summit	Wildflowers, Birds	Great Views, Secluded
27	5	6.3	Out & Back	Hiking, Running, Biking, Dogs Allowed	Mountain	Birds	Great Views, Steep

USES & ACCESS
- Hiking
- Running
- Biking
- Child Friendly
- Dogs Allowed
- Fee
- Permit Required

TYPE
- Loop
- Out & Back
- Point to Point

DIFFICULTY
- 1 2 3 4 5 +
less more

TERRAIN
- River or Stream
- Waterfall
- Lake or Shore
- Canyon
- Mountain
- Summit

FLORA & FAUNA
- Autumn Colors
- Wildflowers
- Birds
- Wildlife

OTHER
- Historic
- Geologic Interest
- Great Views
- Photo Opportunity
- Secluded
- Cool & Shady
- Camping
- Steep

[1] *Bicyclists use described alternate trails or trailheads*

East Bay

TRAIL 15

Hike, Run, Bike, Dogs Allowed
7.0 miles, Loop
Difficulty: 1 2 3 **4** 5

This loop takes you from the lowlands of Wildcat Creek to the high, open slopes of San Pablo Ridge, rewarding you with some of the best views in the Bay Area, including a 360-degree panorama from an old Nike missile site.

TRAIL 16

Hike, Run, Child Friendly
3.3 miles, Loop
Difficulty: 1 2 **3** 4 5

This scenic loop takes you from the Tilden Park Environmental Education Center to the summit of Wildcat Peak, with terrific views of the Bay Area and a variety of plants and birds to keep things interesting throughout.

TRAIL 17

Hike, Run, Child Friendly, Dogs Allowed
1.8 miles, Loop
Difficulty: 1 **2** 3 4 5

This delightful loop circles Round Top, one of the highest peaks in the Oakland and Berkeley hills and a volcanic area that will be of interest to geology buffs.

TRAIL 18

Hike, Run, Dogs Allowed
6.0 miles, Loop
Difficulty: 1 2 **3** 4 5

This loop pairs a vigorous hike along an exposed ridge with a secluded downhill ramble in the shade of tall redwoods, ending at well-loved picnic areas. The redwood forest along Redwood Creek, though merely a shadow of its former old-growth self, is nevertheless majestic.

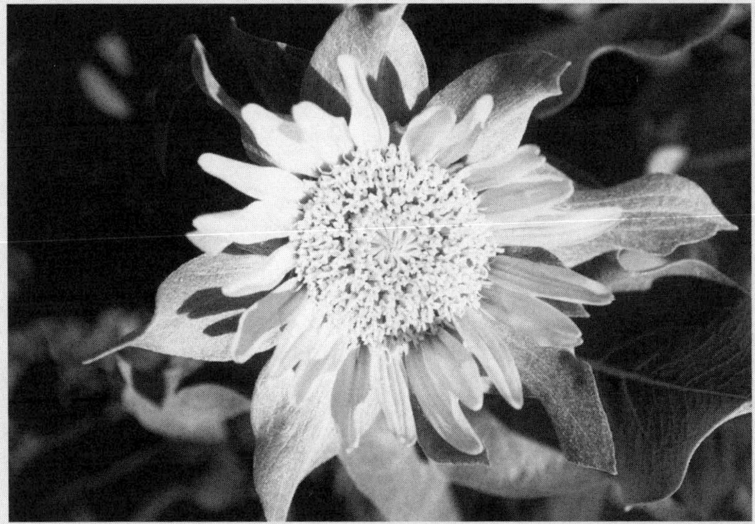

Mules ear *is a large, showy yellow flower found in East and South Bay grasslands.*

Briones Regional Park: Briones Crest 141

This rambling loop offers a great introduction to the south half of this expansive park, an area of rolling hills, high ridges, and forested canyons. The rewards for climbing along the Briones Crest include spring wildflowers and 360-degree views.

TRAIL 19

Hike, Run, Bike, Dogs Allowed

6.8 miles, Loop

Difficulty: 1 2 3 **4** 5

Black Diamond Mines Regional Preserve: Stewartville Loop.......... 147

The Star Mine and the Stewartville town site are reminders of the late 19th century, when these hills bustled with miners prying coal from deep underground. Grassy valleys dotted with grazing cows and sweeping vistas from high ridgetops are other echoes of the Old West.

TRAIL 20

Hike, Run, Bike, Dogs Allowed

7.6 miles, Loop

Difficulty: 1 2 3 **4** 5

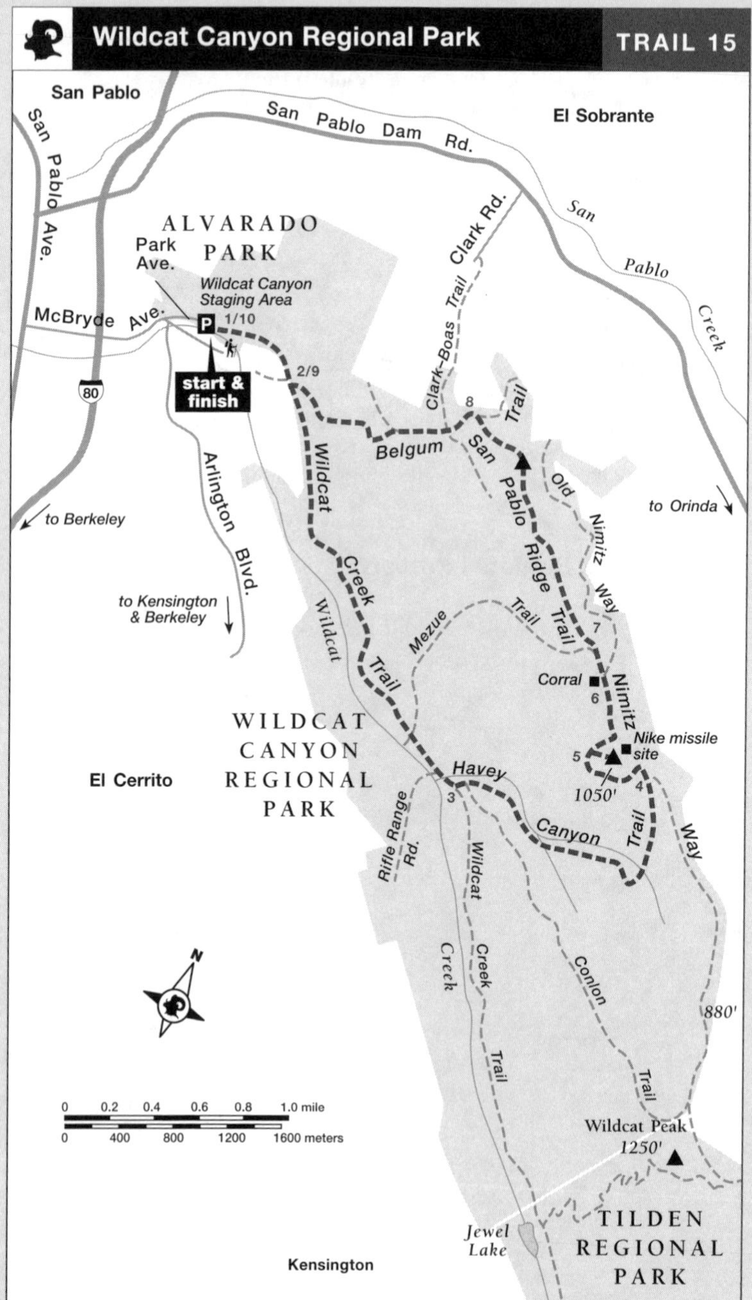

Wildcat Canyon Regional Park
TRAIL 15
San Pablo
El Sobrante
San Pablo Dam Rd.
San Pablo Ave.
San Pablo Creek
ALVARADO PARK
Park Ave.
Wildcat Canyon Staging Area
McBryde Ave.
1/10
2/9
start & finish
80
Clark Rd.
Clark-Boas Trail
8
Trail
Belgum
San Pablo Ridge Trail
Old Nimitz Way
Wildcat Creek Trail
to Berkeley
to Orinda
Arlington Blvd.
to Kensington & Berkeley
Wildcat
Mezue Trail
7
Corral
6
Nimitz
Nike missile site
5
4
1050'
WILDCAT CANYON REGIONAL PARK
El Cerrito
Havey Canyon Trail
3
Rifle Range Rd.
Wildcat Creek Trail
Way
Wildcat Creek
Conlon Trail
880'
0 0.2 0.4 0.6 0.8 1.0 mile
0 400 800 1200 1600 meters
Wildcat Peak
1250'
Jewel Lake
TILDEN REGIONAL PARK
Kensington

Wildcat Canyon Regional Park: San Pablo Ridge

This loop takes you from the lowlands of Wildcat Creek to the high, open slopes of San Pablo Ridge. You are rewarded for your efforts by some of the best views in the East Bay, including a 360-degree panorama from an old Nike missile site. Exposed to sun and wind for much of the way, this hike is best done when spring wildflowers bloom or after summer's heat has abated, when the hills are golden brown.

TRAIL USE
Hike, Run, Bike, Dogs Allowed

LENGTH
7.0 miles, 3–4 hours

VERTICAL FEET
±1700'

DIFFICULTY
– 1 2 3 **4** 5 +

TRAIL TYPE
Loop

SURFACE TYPE
Dirt, paved

FEATURES
Stream
Canyon
Summit
Wildflowers
Birds
Wildlife
Great Views
Photo Opportunity

FACILITIES
Restrooms
Picnic Tables
Water

Best Time

Spring and fall; Havey Canyon Trail is closed to bikes and horses in wet weather.

Finding the Trail

From Interstate 80 eastbound in Richmond, take the Solano Ave. exit, which puts you on Amador St. Go 0.4 mile north to McBryde Ave. Turn right and follow McBryde Ave. 0.2 mile, staying in the left lane as you approach a stop sign. (Use caution at this intersection; traffic from the right does not stop.) Continue straight, now on Park Ave., for 0.1 mile to the Alvarado Staging Area, left. The trailhead is at the far east end of the parking area.

From I-80 westbound in San Pablo, take the McBryde Ave. exit, turn left onto McBryde, go over the freeway, and follow the directions above from the intersection of McBryde and Amador.

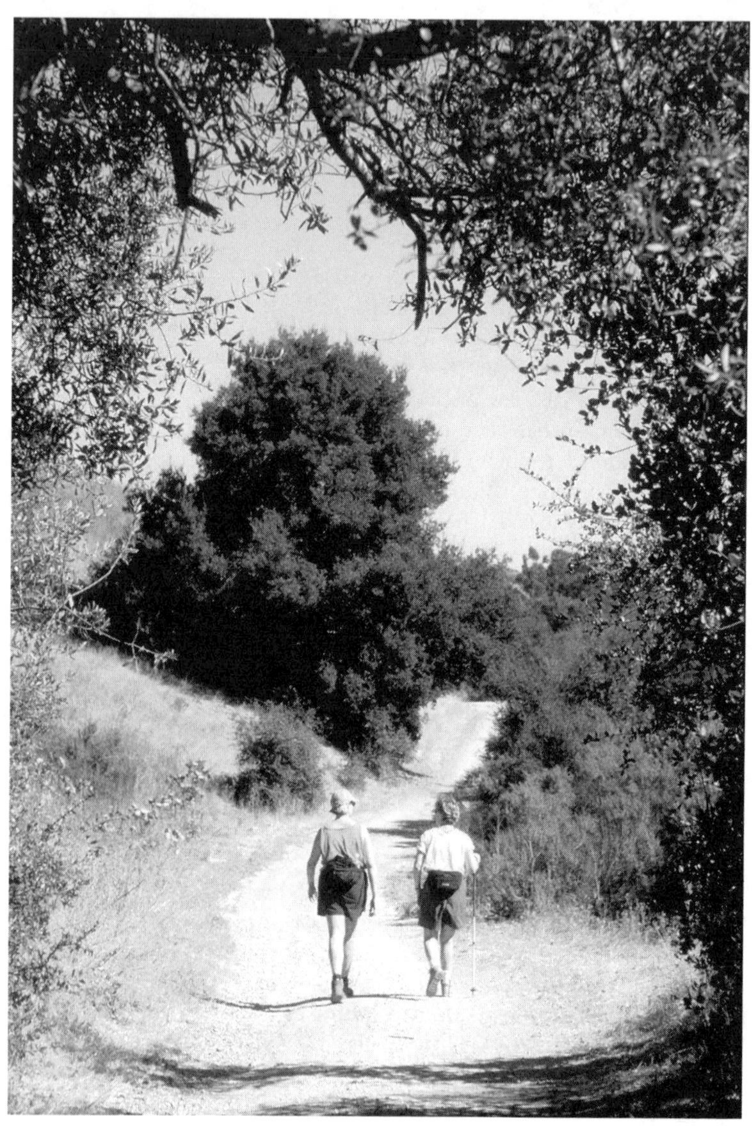

Wildcat Canyon Trail *ascends along Wildcat Creek to Tilden Regional Park.*

Trail Description

The remnant of Wildcat Canyon Road, closed in the early 1980s by landslides, leads you east from the parking area.►1 Renamed the **Wildcat Creek Trail,** the road, paved here but later dirt, runs southeast up the canyon all the way to the Environmental Education Center in Tilden Regional Park.

Visit Wildcat Creek by turning right at the first Mezue Trail junction and walking downhill about 100 yards on a dirt path.

As you climb gently, you pass the Belgum Trail, left,►2 on which you will return. Continue straight, alternating on dirt and pavement, parallel to **Wildcat Creek,** right. The route jogs right, across an old parking area, and then traverses a hillside overlooking a wooded valley, right. At a junction with the Mezue Trail, left, are a drinking fountain and a watering trough for animals.

Continuing straight, the Wildcat Canyon Trail soon descends to tree-shaded Wildcat Creek and a junction with Rifle Range Road, then climbs to a junction with the **Havey Canyon** and **Conlon trails.**►3 Here you turn left up wooded **Havey Canyon Trail,** following a tributary of Wildcat Creek. (This trail is sometimes closed to equestrians during wet weather; if so, return to the Mezue Trail and use it to climb to the San Pablo Ridge Trail.) After most of your climbing is done, the route

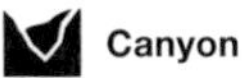

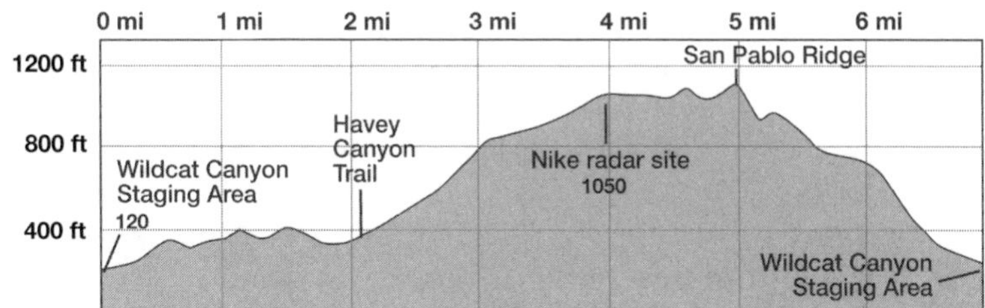

TRAIL 15 Wildcat Canyon Regional Park: San Pablo Ridge Profile

abruptly breaks into the open and turns northward across the grassy flank of San Pablo Ridge.

 **Great Views**

Nimitz Way is named for Chester W. Nimitz, the admiral who commanded the Pacific Fleet during World War II.

At a saddle, you reach a T-junction with **Nimitz Way,▸4** a popular route shared by hikers, horseback riders, bicyclists, in-line skaters, and joggers. Turn left on this old paved road. You wind uphill on a gentle grade across hillsides decorated in spring by colorful wildflowers. Where the road crests, turn right on a spur road to **an abandoned Nike missile site,▸5** a relic of the Cold War, that is perched on the ridgetop. You will be rewarded with a rest bench, 360-degree views, and a chance to reflect on the fact that, for most people, Nike is a name no longer associated with the fear of nuclear war.

Soon the pavement ends, and Nimitz Way continues northwest as a dirt road, with San Pablo Reservoir to the right and far below. You come to a cattle pen and a fork.▸6 Old Nimitz Way descends right, but you bear left on the Mezue Trail. In about 100 yards or so, stay right on the **San Pablo Ridge Trail** as the Mezue Trail drops left.▸7

Heading northwest, the route climbs up and over several steep crests of San Pablo Ridge, then plunges steeply northwest to a junction with the **Belgum Trail.▸8** Turning left on this dirt road, you climb to a low saddle and pass a dirt road, left, and the Clark-Boas Trail, right. Ahead, another road ascends right, toward Monte Cresta gate. Here stay on the Belgum Trail by bearing left. The route now makes a well-graded descent via S-bends to a forest of coast live oak, California bay, and eucalyptus, with a few palm trees thrown in for good measure.

OPTIONS

Trails from San Pablo Ridge

Nimitz Way leads southeast to Tilden Regional Park, and from there you can use the **East Bay Skyline/Bay Area Ridge Trail** to connect to other regional parks along Skyline Blvd.

These trees are all that remain of the **Grande Vista Sanitarium**, which was here from 1914 to the 1940s. A short paved road descends to the Wildcat Creek Trail.►**9** Turn right and retrace your route to the parking area.►**10**

MILESTONES

►1	0.0	Take Wildcat Creek Trail (paved) east
►2	0.4	Belgum Trail on left; go straight
►3	2.1	Left on Havey Canyon Trail
►4	3.6	Left on Nimitz Way
►5	4.0	Road to Nike missile site on right
►6	4.4	Left on Mezue Way
►7	4.5	Right on San Pablo Ridge Trail
►8	5.7	Left on Belgum Trail
►9	6.6	Right on Wildcat Creek Trail
►10	7.0	Back at parking area

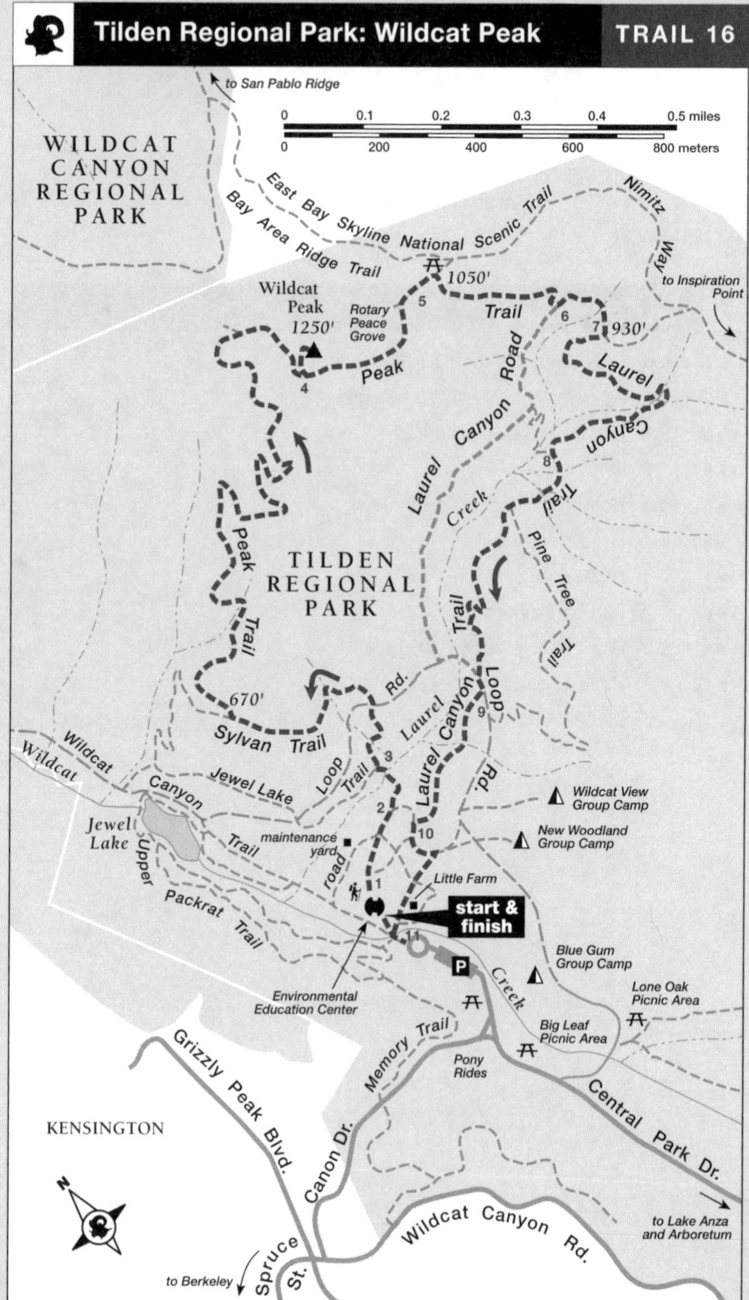
Tilden Regional Park: Wildcat Peak
TRAIL 16
to San Pablo Ridge
0.5 miles
800 meters
WILDCAT CANYON REGIONAL PARK
East Bay Skyline National Scenic Trail
Bay Area Ridge Trail
Nimitz Way
to Inspiration Point
Wildcat Peak 1250'
Rotary Peace Grove
1050'
930'
Peak Trail
Laurel Canyon Road
Laurel Canyon Trail
Laurel Creek
Pine Tree Trail
TILDEN REGIONAL PARK
Peak Trail
670'
Sylvan Trail
Laurel Canyon Rd.
Loop Trail
Laurel Canyon Loop Rd.
Wildcat Canyon Trail
Jewel Lake Trail
Jewel Lake
Upper Packrat Trail
maintenance yard
road
Wildcat View Group Camp
New Woodland Group Camp
Little Farm
start & finish
Environmental Education Center
Blue Gum Group Camp
Creek
Lone Oak Picnic Area
Big Leaf Picnic Area
Memory Trail
Pony Rides
Grizzly Peak Blvd.
Canon Dr.
Central Park Dr.
KENSINGTON
Wildcat Canyon Rd.
to Lake Anza and Arboretum
to Berkeley
Spruce St.

Tilden Regional Park: Wildcat Peak

This scenic loop hike takes you from the Tilden Park Environmental Education Center to the summit of Wildcat Peak via the Jewel Lake, Sylvan, Peak, and Laurel Canyon trails. Terrific views of the Bay Area and a variety of plants and birds keep this route interesting throughout.

TRAIL USE
Hike, Run, Child Friendly
LENGTH
3.3 miles, 1–2 hours
VERTICAL FEET
±900'
DIFFICULTY
– 1 2 **3** 4 5 +
TRAIL TYPE
Loop
SURFACE TYPE
Dirt

FEATURES
Stream
Canyon
Mountain
Summit
Birds
Great Views

FACILITIES
Visitor Center
Restrooms
Picnic Tables
Water
Phone

Best Time

This route is accessible all year, but trails may be very muddy in wet weather.

Finding the Trail

From Interstate 80 in Berkeley, take the University Ave. exit and go east 2.1 miles to Oxford St. Turn left and go 0.7 mile to Rose St. Turn right and go one block to Spruce St. Turn left and follow Spruce St. 1.8 miles to an intersection with Grizzly Peak Blvd. and Wildcat Canyon Rd. Cross the intersection and immediately turn left from Wildcat Canyon Dr. onto Canon Dr. There is a sign here for NATURE TRAIL, PONY RIDE, WILDCAT CANYON. Go downhill 0.3 mile to a junction with Central Park Dr. Turn left and go 0.1 mile to a large parking area.

The trailhead is behind the Environmental Education Center, which is a short walk north from the parking area on a paved path.

Trail Description

From the back deck of the **Environmental Education Center▸1** walk north across the lawn and get on the

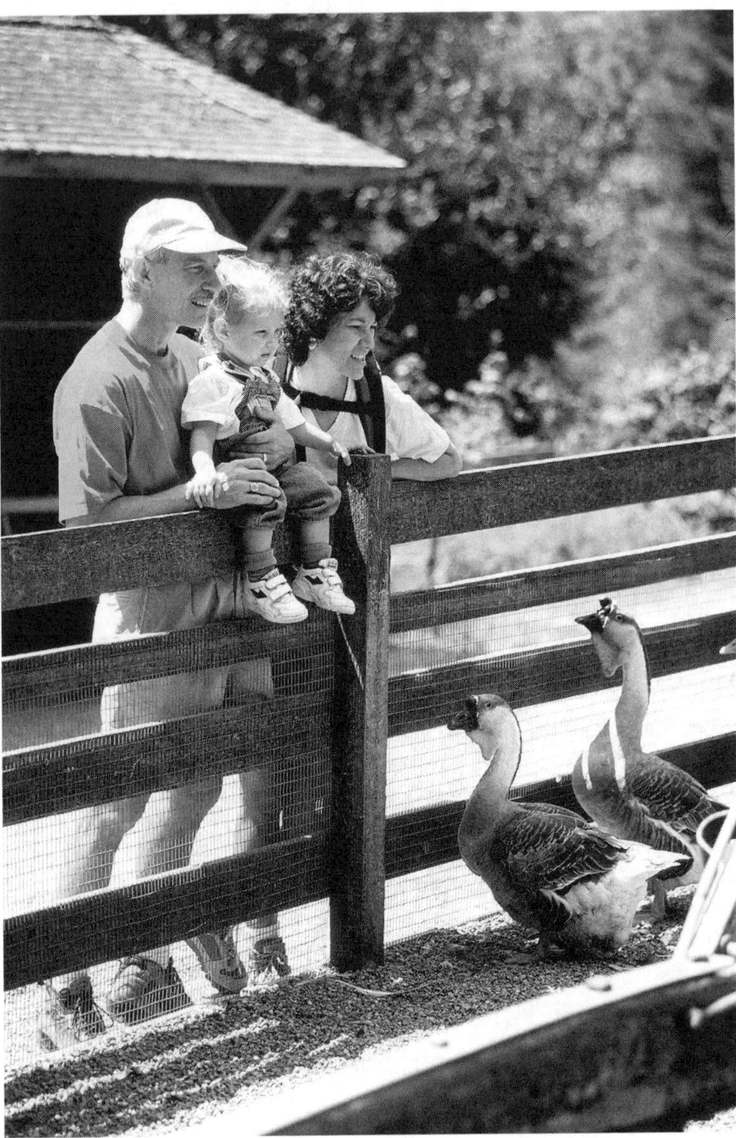

Kids and geese *meet at the Environmental Education Center in Tilden Regional Park, the starting point for the hike up Wildcat Peak.*

OPTIONS

Wet-Weather Descent

The Laurel Canyon Trail may be difficult in wet weather. A more-sure-footed alternative from the intersection of the Peak Trail and Laurel Canyon Rd.▶6 is to turn right and descend **Laurel Canyon Rd.** to Loop Rd. Turn left on **Loop Rd.**, go about 100 yards, and then follow the described route from where the Laurel Canyon Trail joins on the right.

Jewel Lake Trail, which you follow for about 100 yards to a dirt road. Cross it and walk about 50 yards on a wide dirt path to a trail post and a junction. Both the Jewel Lake and Sylvan trails are left; the Laurel Canyon and Pine Tree trails are right.

Turn left and follow the Jewel Lake Trail as it crosses two small streambeds on wooden planks, and then a larger streambed on a wooden bridge. Just after the bridge, you walk up a few wooden steps and reach a junction.▶2 Turn right on the **Sylvan Trail** and climb gently through forest. Reaching Loop Road, a multiuse trail, you cross it and find the continuation of the Sylvan Trail heading northwest through a dense eucalyptus forest. After about 0.5 mile you veer right on the **Peak Trail.**▶3

Landmarks visible from Wildcat Peak include Mt. Tamalpais, Mt. Diablo, the Golden Gate Bridge, Alcatraz and Angel islands, and San Pablo and Briones reservoirs.

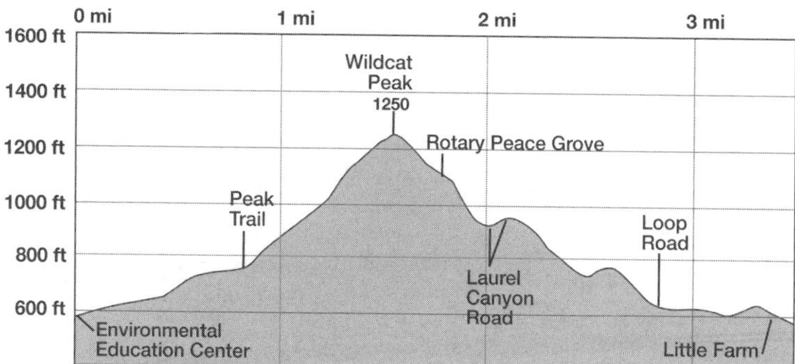

TRAIL 16 Tilden Regional Park: Wildcat Peak Profile

The Peak Trail climbs moderately along the edge of a steep canyon, rising from the eucalyptus forest into native oak–bay woodland and chaparral. Several long switchbacks rise almost to the ridgetop. At a T-junction,▶**4** turn left and climb about 100 yards to the summit of **Wildcat Peak** (1250'), where there are stone benches and a fine view of the Golden Gate, San Francisco Bay, and the neighboring cities.

Great Views

After spending time on the summit, retrace your route to the previous junction, then angle left on the Peak Trail, now a dirt road. East and below the summit of Wildcat Peak is the **Rotary Peace Grove,** a planting of giant sequoias honoring people who have made "outstanding contributions to world peace."▶**5** Because these trees are out of their habitat, they will never attain giant status like their cousins in Yosemite and Sequoia national parks.

Tilden's child-friendly trails are labeled with whimsical pictures—a duck for the Jewel Lake Trail, a tree for the Sylvan Trail, a summit for the Peak Trail, and a bay leaf for the Laurel Canyon Trail.

About 70 yards past the Rotary Peace Grove, near a stand of eucalyptus, veer right on the **single-track Peak Trail,** leaving the dirt road (which joins Nimitz Way in about 30 yards or so). After a steep, brushy section the trail levels, crosses an open hillside, and then drops to **Laurel Canyon Road.**▶**6** Turn left, go about 300 yards, and reach the start of the **Laurel Canyon Trail,** on which you turn right.▶**7**

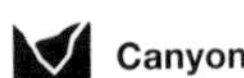
Canyon

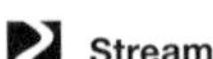
Stream

The narrow, single track descends along the steep edge of **Laurel Canyon** to where a bridge takes you to the south side of **Laurel Creek,** where you may find thimbleberries and blackberries in summer. Descending into a shady forest, you angle left at a junction with a trail to Laurel Canyon Road, right.▶**8** Past a marshy meadow, the Pine Tree Trail heads left, but you descend straight on the Laurel Canyon Trail, on a rolling course to **Loop Road.**▶**9** Here you turn left and walk about 100 feet to the continuation of the Laurel Canyon Trail, right and marked by a trail post. This single track makes an easy descent through eucalyptus and coast live oak to a dirt road.►10 Turn left and follow this road past an unsigned dirt road heading right. Just ahead is the fence at the corner of **Little Farm,** which is an animal-petting area that delights kids and adults alike. Here turn right and go about 0.2 mile downhill through the Little Farm to the Environmental Education Center, right.►11

MILESTONES

►1	0.0	Start up Jewel Lake Trail, then stay left on this trail as Laurel Canyon and Pine Tree trails go right
►2	0.1	Right on Sylvan Trail
►3	0.5	Right on Peak Trail
►4	1.4	Left at T-junction to summit of Wildcat Peak (1250'), then retrace to previous junction and go straight on Peak Trail
►5	1.6	Pass Rotary Peace Grove on left, then right on single-track Peak Trail
►6	1.9	Left on Laurel Canyon Rd.
►7	2.0	Right on Laurel Canyon Trail
►8	2.4	Left to stay on Laurel Canyon Trail
►9	2.8	Left on Loop Rd., then right on Laurel Canyon Trail
►10	3.1	Left on dirt road to Little Farm fence, then right
►11	3.3	Back to visitor center

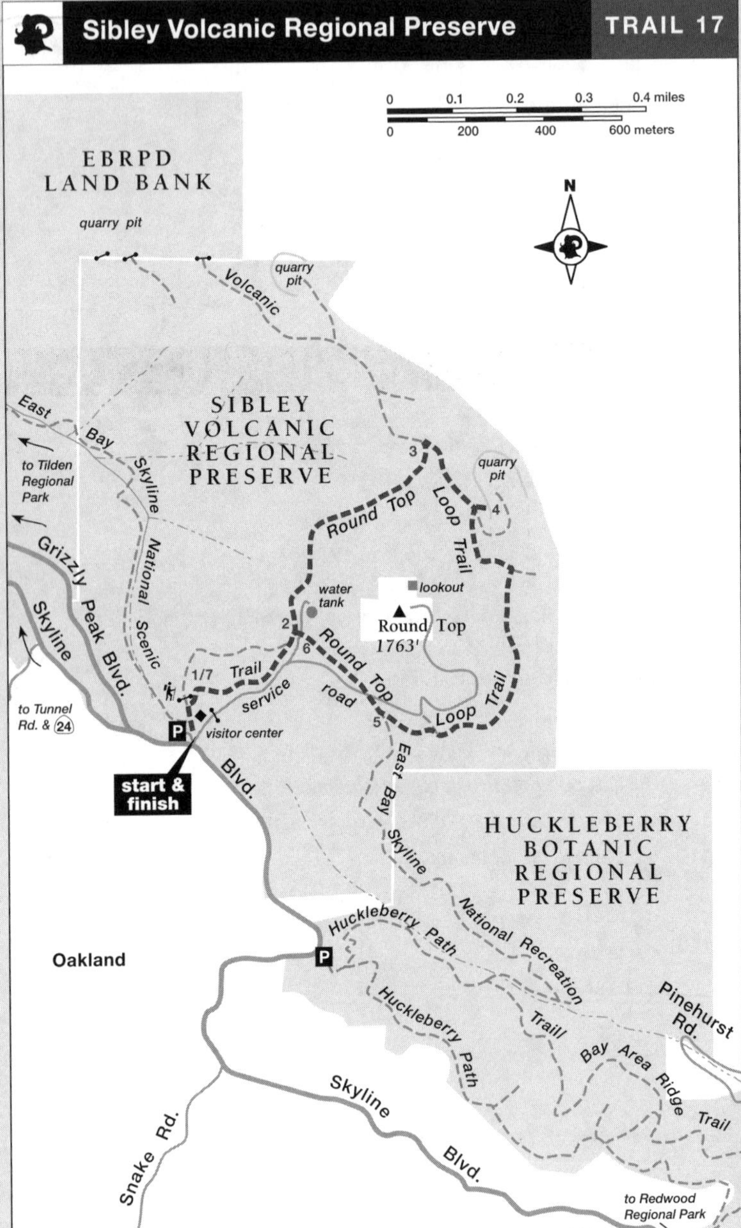
Sibley Volcanic Regional Preserve
TRAIL 17
0
0.1
0.2
0.3
0.4 miles
0
200
400
600 meters
N
EBRPD LAND BANK
quarry pit
quarry pit
Volcanic
SIBLEY VOLCANIC REGIONAL PRESERVE
East Bay Skyline National Scenic Trail
to Tilden Regional Park
Grizzly Peak Blvd.
Skyline Blvd.
3
quarry pit
4
Round Top Loop Trail
water tank
lookout
Round Top 1763'
2
6
1/7
service road
5
visitor center
P
start & finish
to Tunnel Rd. & 24
East Bay Skyline National Recreation Traill
HUCKLEBERRY BOTANIC REGIONAL PRESERVE
Huckleberry Path
P
Oakland
Huckleberry Path
Pinehurst Rd.
Bay Area Ridge Trail
Skyline Blvd.
Snake Rd.
to Redwood Regional Park
Shepherd Canyon Rd.

Sibley Volcanic Regional Preserve: Round Top Loop

This delightful loop circles Round Top, an extinct volcano and one of the highest peaks in the Oakland and Berkeley hills. Old quarries expose volcanic soils that will be of interest to geology buffs. The EBRPD brochure and map, available free at the visitor center, describes points of interest along the self-guiding Volcanic Trail, which is marked by numbered posts along the trail.

One of the oldest East Bay regional parks, the preserve was dedicated in 1936, just two years after the district was formed. Originally called Roundtop, it is named for Robert Sibley, director and president of EBRPD from 1948 to 1958. The preserve was enlarged to its present size by additions of old Kaiser Sand and Gravel quarry sites.

TRAIL USE
Hike, Run, Child Friendly, Dogs Allowed
LENGTH
1.8 miles, 1–2 hours
VERTICAL FEET
±400'
DIFFICULTY
– 1 **2** 3 4 5 +
TRAIL TYPE
Loop
SURFACE TYPE
Dirt

FEATURES
Birds
Geologic Interest
Great Views

FACILITIES
Visitor Center
Restrooms
Water

Best Time

This route is enjoyable all year.

Finding the Trail

From State Hwy. 24 just east of the Caldecott Tunnel, take the Fish Ranch Rd. exit and go uphill one mile to Grizzly Peak Blvd. Turn left and go 2.5 miles to Skyline Blvd. Turn left and go 0.1 mile to the preserve entrance on the left. The trailhead is just west of the visitor center.

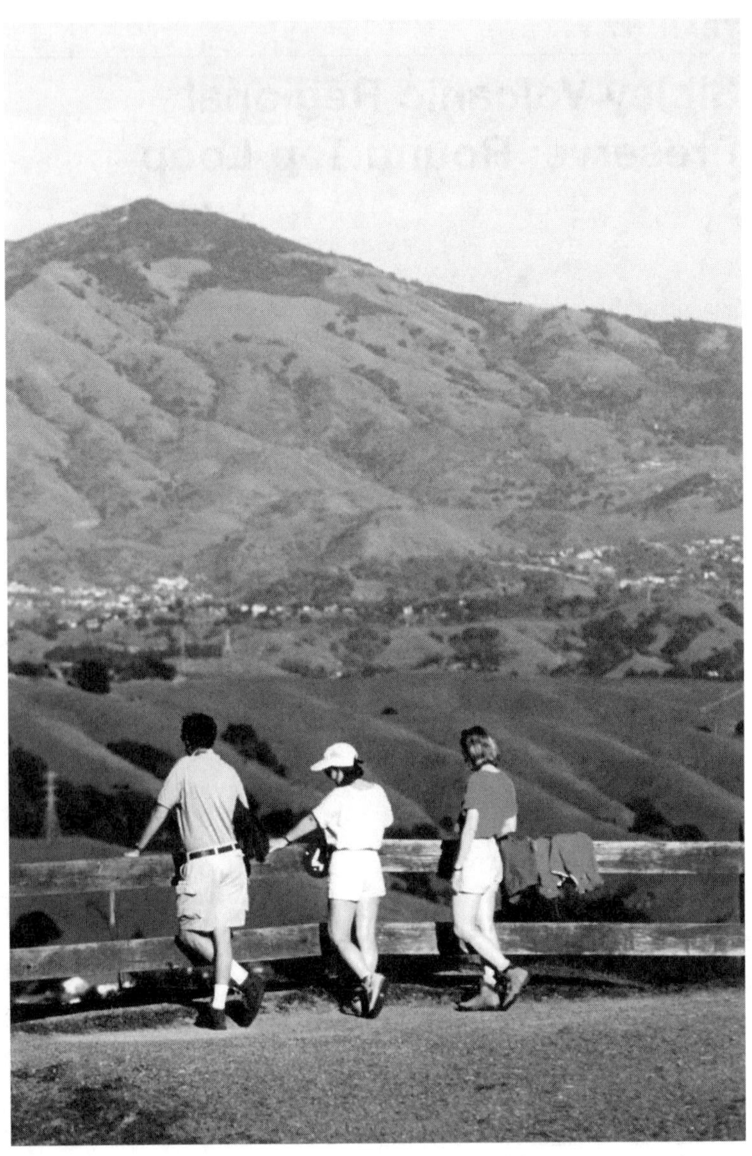

At the quarry overlook *in Sibley Volcanic Regional Preserve hikers gaze east toward Mt. Diablo.*

Trail Description

Before starting on the trail, be sure to visit the preserve's open-air **visitor center**, which has exhibits explaining the area's volcanic past, as well as its plant and wildlife communities. After you have earned your geological credentials, head north from the west side of the visitor center on a paved road.▶1 Just before a gate, turn right on the **East Bay Skyline National Scenic Trail**, which is also part of the Bay Area Ridge Trail. This single track climbs through a wooded area above a steep embankment. Soon, another trail from the visitor center joins on the left, and then you descend to a four-way junction.▶2 Turn left on the wide gravel road, the **Round Top Loop Trail**, which heads north through a cattle gate and then northeast into the volcanic area.

As you hike around Round Top (1763'), remember that it once was an active volcano and that the surrounding hills were created by unimaginable forces acting along nearby fault lines.

A mostly level walk over rocky ground takes you around the west and north sides of Round Top to a T-junction.▶3 Here, the Volcanic Trail heads left down an open, quarried ridge, but your route, the Round Top Loop Trail, bends sharply right and climbs. Soon you come to a wonderful viewpoint, just off the trail and above a **quarry pit**,▶4 with Mt. Diablo looming on the eastern skyline. Quarry operations here from the 1930s to the 1960s dug into the side of Round Top, exposing the basalt lava interior of the volcano, to the delight of geologists.

 Great Views

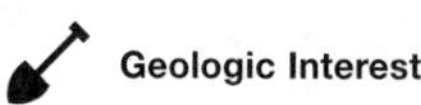

Continue following the Round Top Loop Trail as it makes a rising traverse across the grassy east side of Round Top. A side trail, left, offers access to another east-facing viewpoint. The Round Top Loop Trail, now a single track, passes through a cattle gate, then descends steeply through an area of young pines into a more mature, stately forest.

On the peak's south side, stay on the Round Top Loop Trail by angling left at an unsigned fork. Soon you reach a junction,▶5 where the East Bay Skyline/Bay Area Ridge Trail, a route to Huckleberry Regional Preserve and Redwood Regional Park,

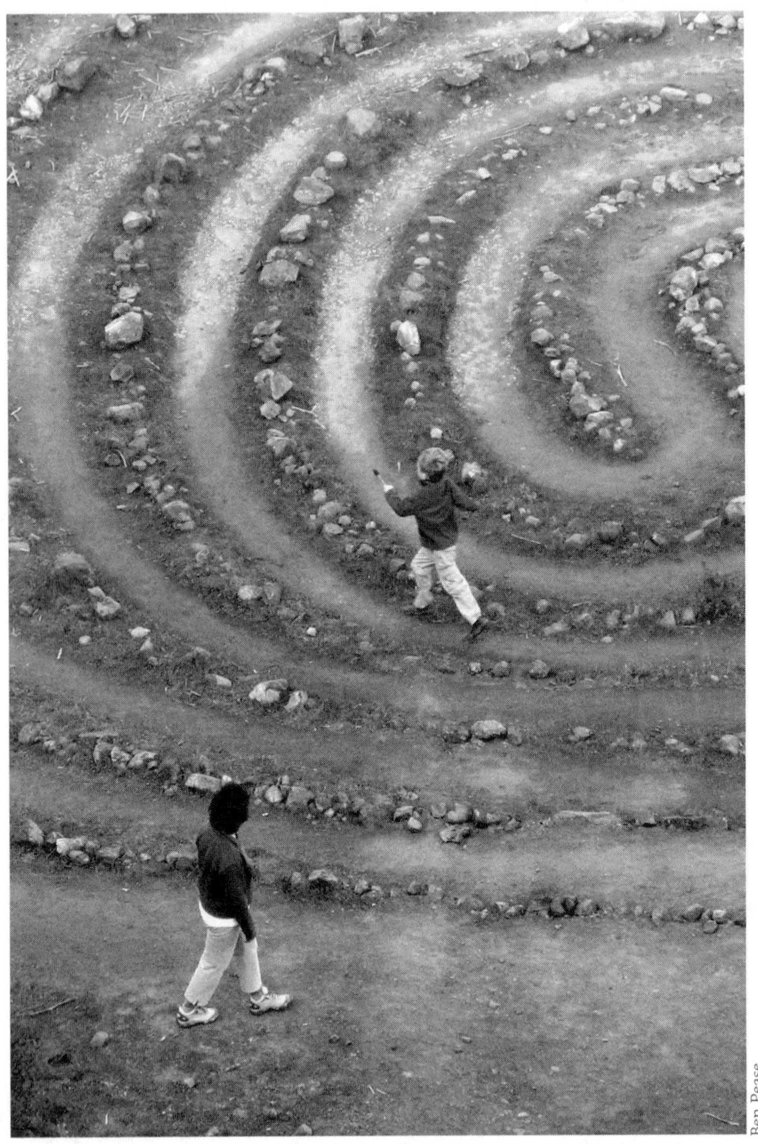

Ben Pease

A labyrinth *in the quarry pit is a magnet for visitors.*

merges from the left. Continue straight and in about 125 feet arrive at Round Top Road. Cross the road and follow the Round Top Loop Trail, soon crossing a paved road leading steeply uphill to an EBMUD water tank▶6. Just ahead is the four-way junction with the gravel road to the volcanic area. Here continue straight—staying left at an upcoming fork—and retrace your route to the parking area.▶7

Because of its bulk and shape, Mt. Diablo could be mistaken for a volcano, but it was formed instead by a mass of rock pushing upward through sedimentary layers.

MILESTONES

▶1	0.0	Start north on paved trail; right on East Bay Skyline Trail
▶2	0.2	Left on Round Top Loop Trail, a gravel road
▶3	0.6	Right at T-junction to stay on Round Top Loop Trail
▶4	0.7	Quarry overlook; then resume Round Top Loop Trail
▶5	1.4	Straight on East Bay Skyline Trail; cross paved Round Top Rd.
▶6	1.6	Cross paved road to EBMUD water tank; cross Round Top Loop Trail; left at next fork
▶7	1.8	Back at parking area

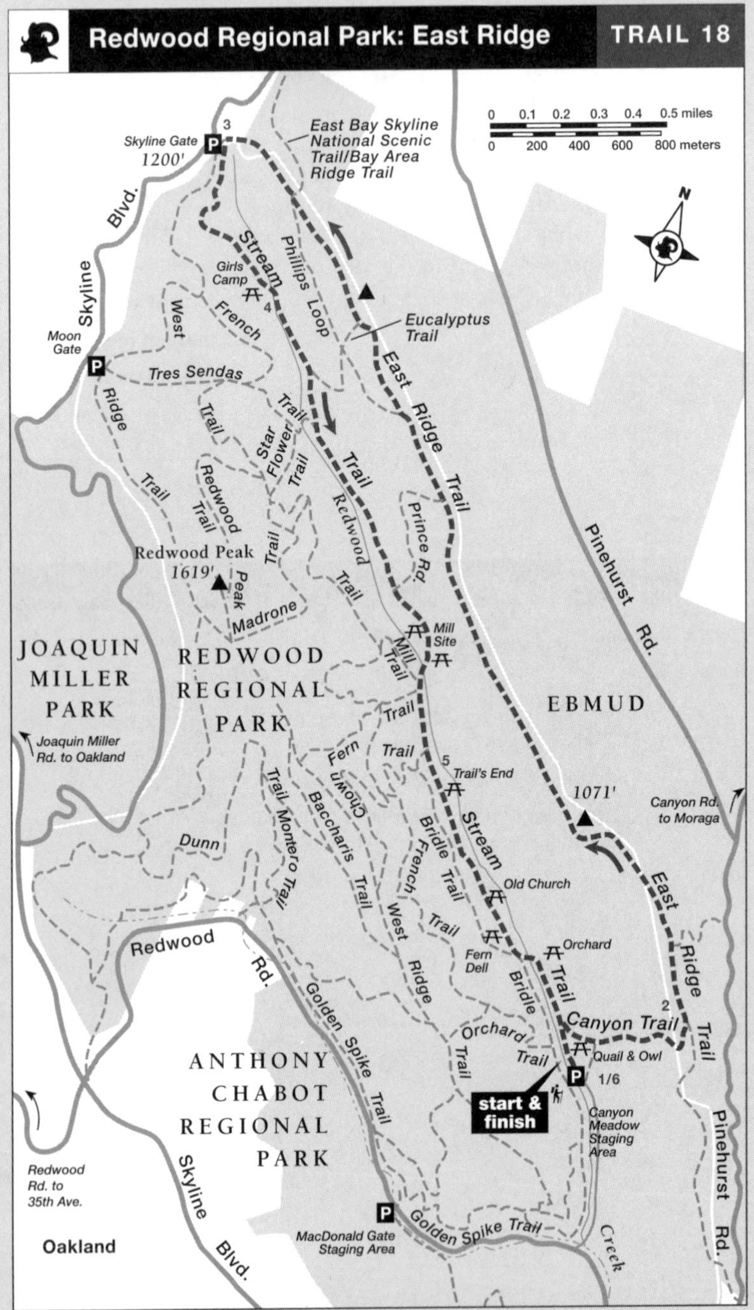
Redwood Regional Park: East Ridge
TRAIL 18
East Bay Skyline National Scenic Trail/Bay Area Ridge Trail
Skyline Gate 1200'
Skyline Blvd.
Moon Gate
Girls Camp
Stream
Phillips Loop
French
West
Tres Sendas
Eucalyptus Trail
East Ridge Trail
Ridge Trail
Trail
Star Flower Trail
Redwood Trail
Trail
Prince Rd.
Redwood Peak 1619'
Peak
Madrone
Mill Site
Mill Trail
Pinehurst Rd.
JOAQUIN MILLER PARK
REDWOOD REGIONAL PARK
EBMUD
Joaquin Miller Rd. to Oakland
Fern Trail
Trail
Trail's End
1071'
Canyon Rd. to Moraga
Chown
Baccharis Trail
Montero Trail
Dunn
Bridle Trail
French Trail
West Ridge
Stream
Old Church
Orchard
Fern Dell
Bridle Trail
Redwood Rd.
Golden Spike Trail
Orchard Trail
Canyon Trail
Quail & Owl
start & finish
1/6
Canyon Meadow Staging Area
ANTHONY CHABOT REGIONAL PARK
Redwood Rd. to 35th Ave.
Skyline Blvd.
Oakland
MacDonald Gate Staging Area
Golden Spike Trail
Creek
0 0.1 0.2 0.3 0.4 0.5 miles
0 200 400 600 800 meters
N

Redwood Regional Park: East Ridge

This loop, using the East Ridge and Stream trails, pairs a vigorous hike along an exposed ridge with a secluded downhill ramble in the shade of tall redwoods, an unbeatable combination. Views from the East Ridge Trail of the surrounding East Bay parklands are superb, and the redwood forest along Redwood Creek, though merely a shadow of its former old-growth self, is nevertheless majestic. As a bonus, water is available not only at the trailhead but also at Skyline Gate and at picnic areas along the Stream Trail.

TRAIL USE
Hike, Run, Dogs Allowed

LENGTH
6.0 miles, 3–4 hours

VERTICAL FEET
±950'

DIFFICULTY
– 1 2 **3** 4 5 +

TRAIL TYPE
Loop

SURFACE TYPE
Dirt, Paved

FEATURES
Fee
Stream
Birds
Great Views

FACILITIES
Restrooms
Picnic Tables
Water
Phone

Best Time

This route is enjoyable all year.

Finding the Trail

From Interstate 580 southbound in Oakland, take the 35th Ave. exit, turn left and follow 35th Ave. east into the hills. After 0.8 mile 35th Ave. becomes Redwood Rd., and at 2.4 miles it crosses Skyline Blvd., where you stay in the left lane and go straight. At 4.6 miles from Interstate 580 you reach the park entrance; turn left and go 0.5 mile to the Canyon Meadow Staging Area.

From I-580 northbound in Oakland, take the Warren Freeway/Berkeley/State Hwy. 13 exit and go 0.9 mile to the Carson St./Redwood Rd. exit. From the stop sign at the end of the exit ramp, continue straight, now on Mountain Blvd., 0.2 mile, and bear right onto Redwood Rd. Go 3.2 miles to the park

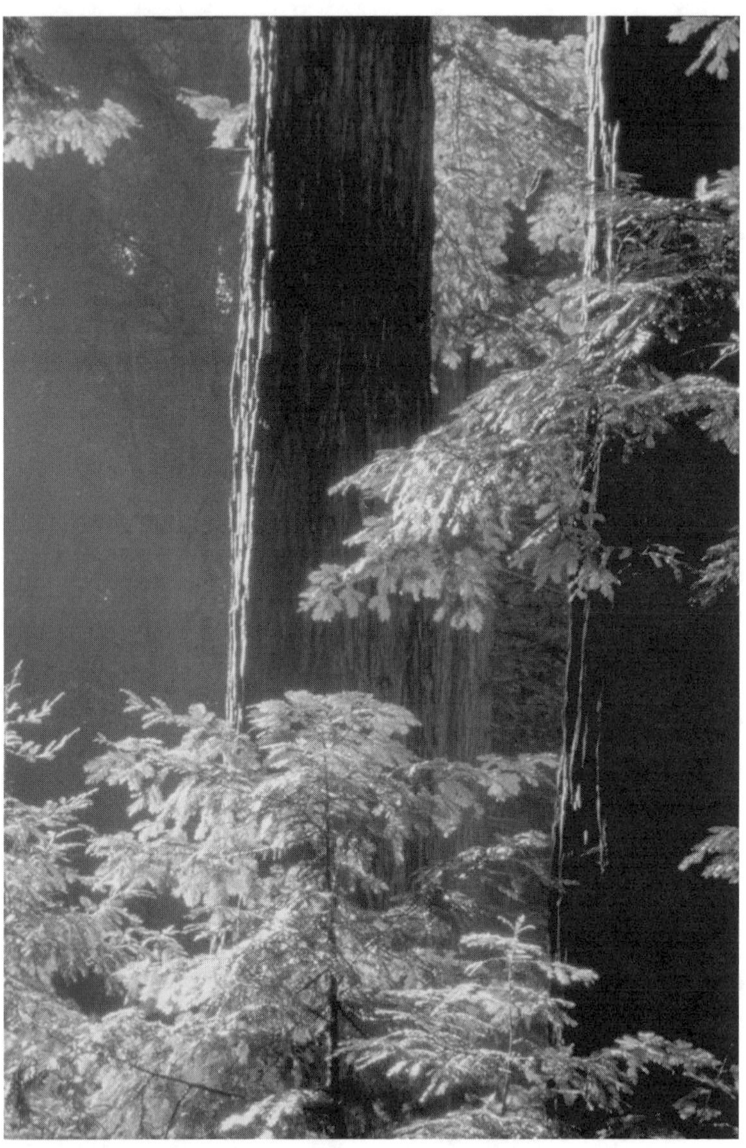

Second-growth redwoods *in Redwood Regional Park have gradually reclaimed hillsides and canyons that were heavily logged in the 19th century.*

entrance; turn left and go 0.5 mile to the farthest parking area, the Canyon Meadow Staging Area.

From State Hwy. 13 southbound, take the Redwood Rd./Carson St. exit, turn left onto Redwood Rd. and follow the directions above.

There are fees for parking and dogs when the entrance kiosk is attended. The trailhead is on the northwest end of the parking area.

Trail Description

From the parking area, head northwest on the paved **Stream Trail** to a junction▶**1** near the restrooms. Here turn right on a dirt road signed TO CANYON TRAIL, which climbs past the Owl and Quail picnic areas. As lawns yield to wildlands, a dirt road from the parking area merges from the right. Continue climbing, now on the **Canyon Trail**, a well-shaded route beside California bays and coastal scrub, that starts steep but changes to moderate.

After about 0.4 mile of huffing and puffing, gain the ridgetop and join the **East Ridge Trail**, a wide dirt road, by bearing left.▶**2** The route follows a rolling course along the initially viewless ridgeline, passes the Redwood Trail, right, and climbs to a

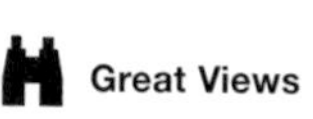

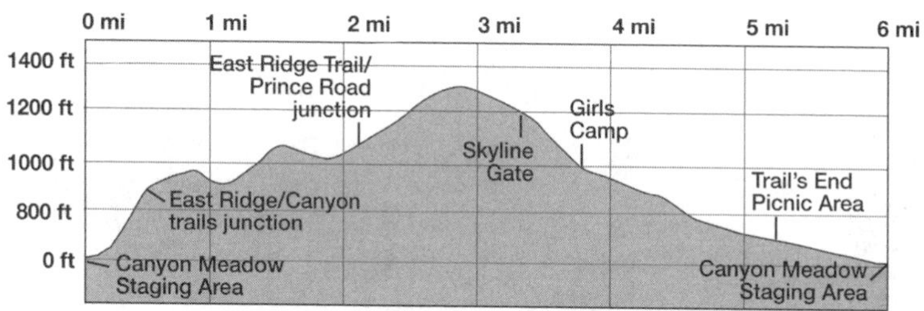

TRAIL 18 Redwood Regional Park: East Ridge Profile

rest bench with views of Mt. Diablo and Redwood Creek.

At about 2.4 miles, Prince Road goes left and downhill. A nearby rest bench provides views of **Redwood Canyon.** Your route stays straight and climbs, soon reaching a fork with the Phillips Loop, left. Here you bear right and continue climbing. Now heading through a corridor of pine, eucalyptus, and madrone, the route passes a junction with the Eucalyptus Trail, left, and begins to bend west.

With the **Skyline Gate parking area** in view, you pass the Phillips Loop, left, and the East Bay Skyline/Bay Area Ridge Trail, right. Nearby are toilets, a rest bench, and a phone. Ahead is a junction with the Stream and West Ridge trails, where water is available.**▶3**

Stream

Turn left on the **Stream Trail** and descend moderately—first through scrub and then through an oak–bay forest—to **Girls Camp**, a grassy meadow with a shelter and picnic tables shaded by plum and walnut trees.**▶4** Now on a gentle descent beside **Redwood Creek**, you pass the Eucalyptus Trail, left. Here the vegetation changes dramatically, and you now walk in a shady forest of magnificent redwoods growing straight and tall, towering overhead. A moderate descent soon brings you to a rest bench and a junction with the Tres Sendas Trail, right. In fall, thousands of breeding ladybugs cluster on the

OPTIONS

More Redwood Regional Park Trails

The **Stream Trail** is closed to bicycles from Skyline Gate to the Trail's End picnic area, but the **West Ridge Trail** is open to bicycles all the way from Skyline Gate to just below Canyon Meadow, making an 8.2-mile round trip on bicycle possible. For hikers, a shadier, more strenuous loop of 7.7 miles can be made using the **Stream, French,** and **Orchard trails.** The West Ridge Trail is part of the Bay Area Ridge Trail/East Bay Skyline Trail between Tilden and Chabot Regional Parks.

foliage near this junction, with others flying through the air, creating a fascinating spectacle.

You continue straight on the Stream Trail through deep forest, crossing several bridges over Redwood Creek. After a junction with Prince Road, left, you emerge briefly into an open area, then reenter the redwood forest. Past the Mill Site group camp, you cross Redwood Creek on a rustic bridge to a T-junction with the Mill Trail, where you stay left on the Stream Trail, now a dirt road.

As you enjoy your level walk on the Stream Trail, you pass several more picnic areas and junctions with the Fern and Chown trails, both right. You reach pavement at the **Trail's End picnic area,** ►5 and, after another 0.5 mile or so, leave the forest near the Fern Dell picnic area and shelter. Where the Bridle Trail goes right, you stay left on the paved Stream Trail, signed TO CANYON MEADOW, on a bridge over Redwood Creek. The Stream Trail curves past a children's play area and the **Orchard picnic area,** and then, after a final shady grove, closes the loop at the restrooms. From here, go straight and retrace your route to the parking area.►6

MILESTONES

►1	0.0	Take paved Stream Trail northwest, then right on Canyon Trail
►2	0.4	Left on East Ridge Trail
►3	3.3	Skyline Gate; go left on Stream Trail
►4	3.7	Girls Camp
►5	5.2	Stream Trail becomes paved near Trail's End picnic area
►6	6.0	Junction with Canyon Trail, left; go straight to parking area

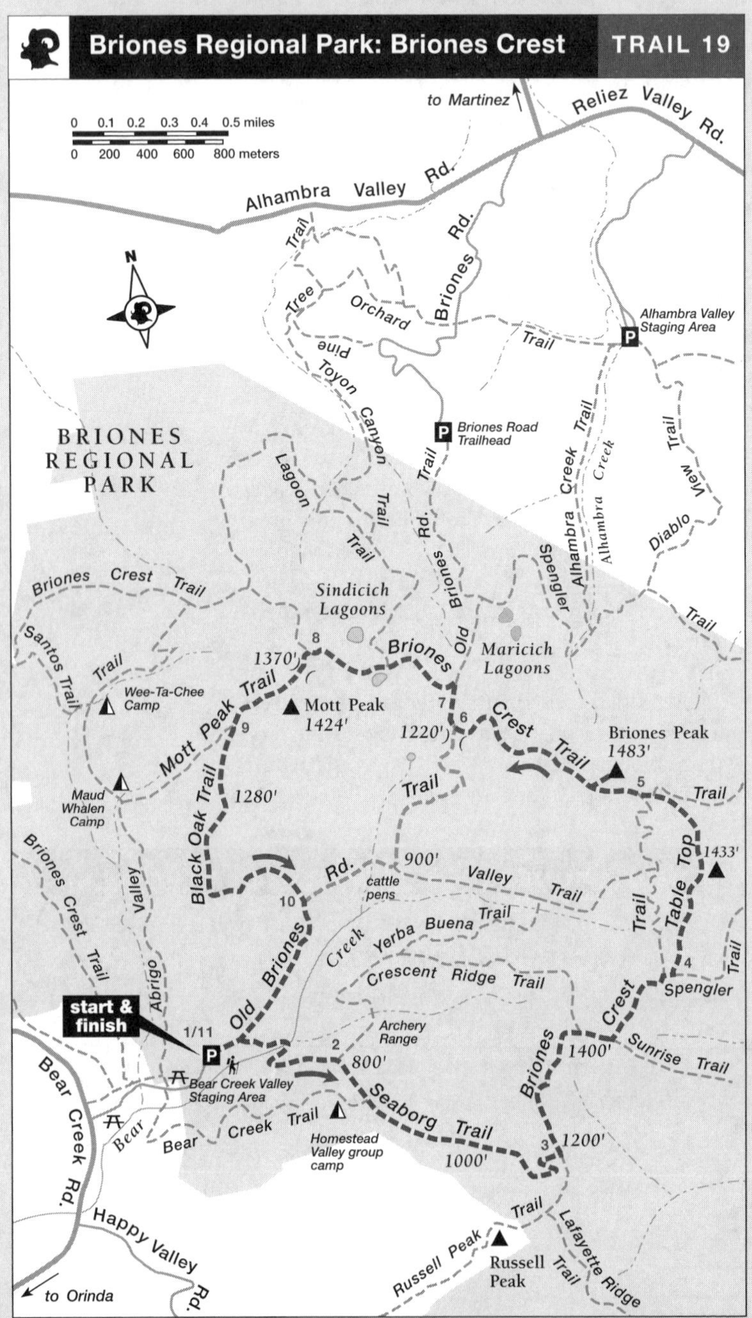
Briones Regional Park: Briones Crest
TRAIL 19
to Martinez
Reliez Valley Rd.
Alhambra Valley Rd.
0 0.1 0.2 0.3 0.4 0.5 miles
0 200 400 600 800 meters
N
BRIONES REGIONAL PARK
Alhambra Valley Staging Area
Briones Road Trailhead
Sindicich Lagoons
Maricich Lagoons
Mott Peak 1424'
Briones Peak 1483'
Wee-Ta-Chee Camp
Maud Whalen Camp
start & finish
Bear Creek Valley Staging Area
Homestead Valley group camp
Archery Range
cattle pens
Russell Peak
Briones Crest Trail
Mott Peak Trail
Black Oak Trail
Old Briones Rd.
Seaborg Trail
Table Top Trail
Spengler Trail
Sunrise Trail
Crescent Ridge Trail
Yerba Buena Trail
Valley Trail
Abrigo Valley Trail
Santos Trail
Lagoon Trail
Toyon Canyon Trail
Pine Tree Trail
Orchard Trail
Alhambra Creek Trail
Diablo View Trail
Bear Creek Trail
Russell Peak Trail
Lafayette Ridge Trail
Bear Creek Rd.
Happy Valley Rd.
to Orinda
Briones Rd.
1370'
1220'
1280'
900'
800'
1000'
1200'
1400'
1433'

Briones Regional Park: Briones Crest

This rambling loop offers a great introduction to the southwest half of this expansive park, an area of rolling hills, high ridges, and forested canyons. The rewards for climbing along the Briones Crest include spring wildflowers and 360-degree views.

TRAIL USE
Hike, Run, Bike, Dogs Allowed

LENGTH
6.8 miles, 4–6 hours

VERTICAL FEET
±1300'

DIFFICULTY
– 1 2 3 **4** 5 +

TRAIL TYPE
Loop

SURFACE TYPE
Dirt, Paved

FEATURES
Fee
Lake
Summit
Wildflowers
Birds
Great Views
Photo Opportunity

FACILITIES
None

Best Time

Best access is in spring and fall; trails may be muddy in wet weather.

Finding the Trail

From State Hwy. 24 in Orinda, take the Orinda Exit and go northwest 2.2 miles on Camino Pablo to Bear Creek Rd. Turn right and go 4.5 miles to the park's Bear Creek Valley entrance. Turn right, and after 0.3 mile reach the entrance kiosk; continue 0.1 mile to the last parking area. The park charges fees for parking and dogs.

The trailhead is at the end of the park entrance road, just past the last parking area.

Trail Description

Passing a trail post bearing the emblem of the **Ivan Dickson Memorial Loop,**▸1 you go through a gate and follow a paved road—the continuation of the park entrance road—east through a brushy area, soon reaching a fork and the end of pavement.▸2 Here the Old Briones Road Trail, once the main route between Orinda and Martinez, heads left, and the **Seaborg Trail,** your route, goes right. You

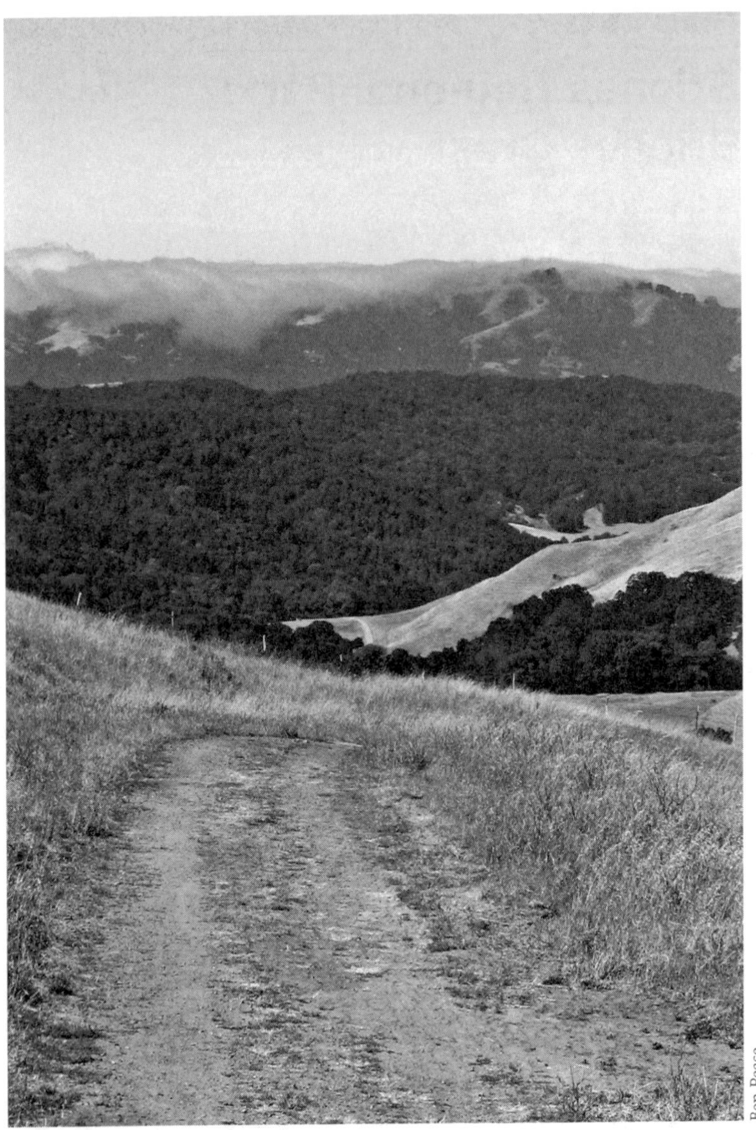

Ben Pease

View of fog *settling in over the Berkeley Hills from Briones Crest*

HISTORY

Dedicated Hiker

Part of this scenic loop follows a route named for Ivan Dickson, a dedicated member of the Berkeley Hiking Club and park enthusiast who, upon his death in 1993 at age 95, left a surprise bequest of $500,000 to EBRPD.

cross **Bear Creek,** then climb past a cattle gate and into the open. Reaching a junction with the Crescent Ridge Trail, which goes straight, you turn right and continue on the Seaborg Trail. After about 0.8 mile, you pass the Bear Creek Trail and **Homestead Valley group camp**, where there are picnic tables, water, and toilets.

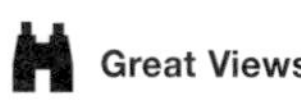

The route reenters forest and climbs moderately. Breaking into the open again and sweeping uphill on several sharp bends, you pass through a gate and reach the **Briones Crest Trail.▶3** Turning left, you follow the rolling ridgetop through a wooded area. The view east is of Walnut Creek and Mt. Diablo, beautifully set off by a foreground of rolling hills.

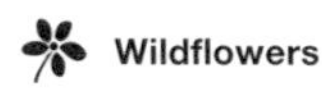

Now you pass the Crescent Ridge Trail, left. Continuing straight, the trail stays in the open, on top of the world. When you reach a fork with the

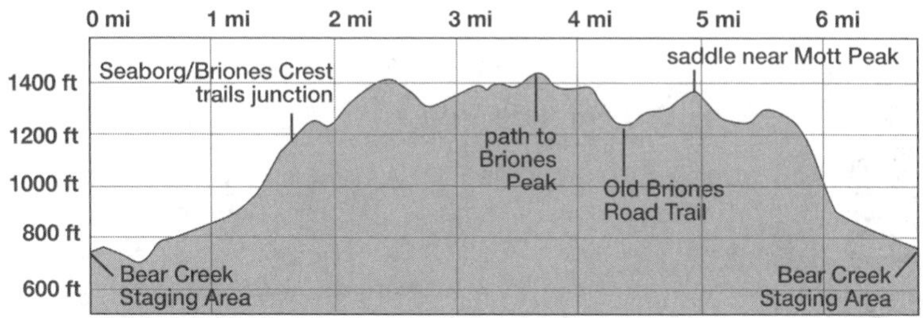

TRAIL 19 Briones Regional Park: Briones Crest Elevation Profile

Sunrise Trail, right, bear left and descend past several cattle gates through a lush wildflower meadow.

At the next junction, where the Briones Crest Trail veers left,►4 go straight on a connector to the Table Top and Spengler trails. Soon the Spengler Trail makes a hard right, and you continue straight on the **Table Top Trail,** heading for the high ground around Briones Peak. A short, steep climb soon levels out. The great views are marred only by the large cable-television facility ahead.

Great Views

Photo Opportunity

When you come to a cattle gate and the next junction, leave the Table Top Trail, which descends right, and continue straight on a short connector to merge with the Briones Crest Trail,►5 joining from the left. Beyond a small grove of oaks, just before the route begins to descend, you come upon an unsigned path, right, which leads to the summit of **Briones Peak** (1483'), where a rest bench and terrific views await. Martinez, Benicia, the Carquinez Strait, and Suisun Bay, home to the mothball fleet of World War II ships, are all in view.

Sindicich Lagoons are a breeding ground for thousands of California newts, which migrate here in early spring from hiding places in nearby forests.

After a well-deserved break, return to the main route, turn right, and continue northwest over rolling terrain to a T-junction with **Old Briones Road Trail.**►6 Here you turn right. For 200 yards, the Briones Crest Trail and Old Briones Road Trail are the same, then you follow the **Briones Crest Trail** as it splits left.►7

OPTIONS

Loop via Old Briones Road

This option shaves 1 mile and 170 feet of elevation gain and loss from the described route. For this shorter option, turn left on the **Old Briones Rd. Trail,**►6 which descends moderately to the valley of Bear Creek. Passing the Valley Trail, left, bear right past the cattle pens and go about 0.4 mile to a junction where the **Black Oak Trail** joins from the right.►10 From here, follow the described route to the parking area.

The Briones Crest Trail climbs from the saddle past one of the **Sindicich Lagoons,** left, to a junction with the **Mott Peak Trail,**▶**8** a wide dirt road. Here turn left and cross a high saddle just north of Mott Peak. At the next junction,▶**9** the Mott Peak Trail descends right; you continue straight on the **Black Oak Trail,** following a roller-coaster ride over a hilltop with a final vista of Briones Crest and then descending steeply to the valley floor.

At a T-junction with Old Briones Road Trail,▶**10** turn right, crossing a tributary of Bear Creek. After passing through a cattle gate, you arrive at the junction with the Seaborg Trail. Bear right, now on pavement, and retrace your route to the parking area.▶**11**

MILESTONES

▶1	0.0	Take paved road east
▶2	0.2	Right on Seaborg Trail
▶3	1.7	Left on Briones Crest Trail
▶4	2.7	Straight on connector, straight on Table Top Trail
▶5	3.4	Table Top Trail goes right, straight on connector to merge with Briones Crest Trail; trail to Briones Peak ahead on right
▶6	4.2	Right at T-junction with Old Briones Rd. Trail
▶7	4.3	Left to stay on Briones Crest Trail
▶8	4.8	Left on Mott Peak Trail
▶9	5.2	Straight on Black Oak Trail
▶10	6.1	Right at T-junction with Old Briones Rd. Trail
▶11	6.8	Back at parking area

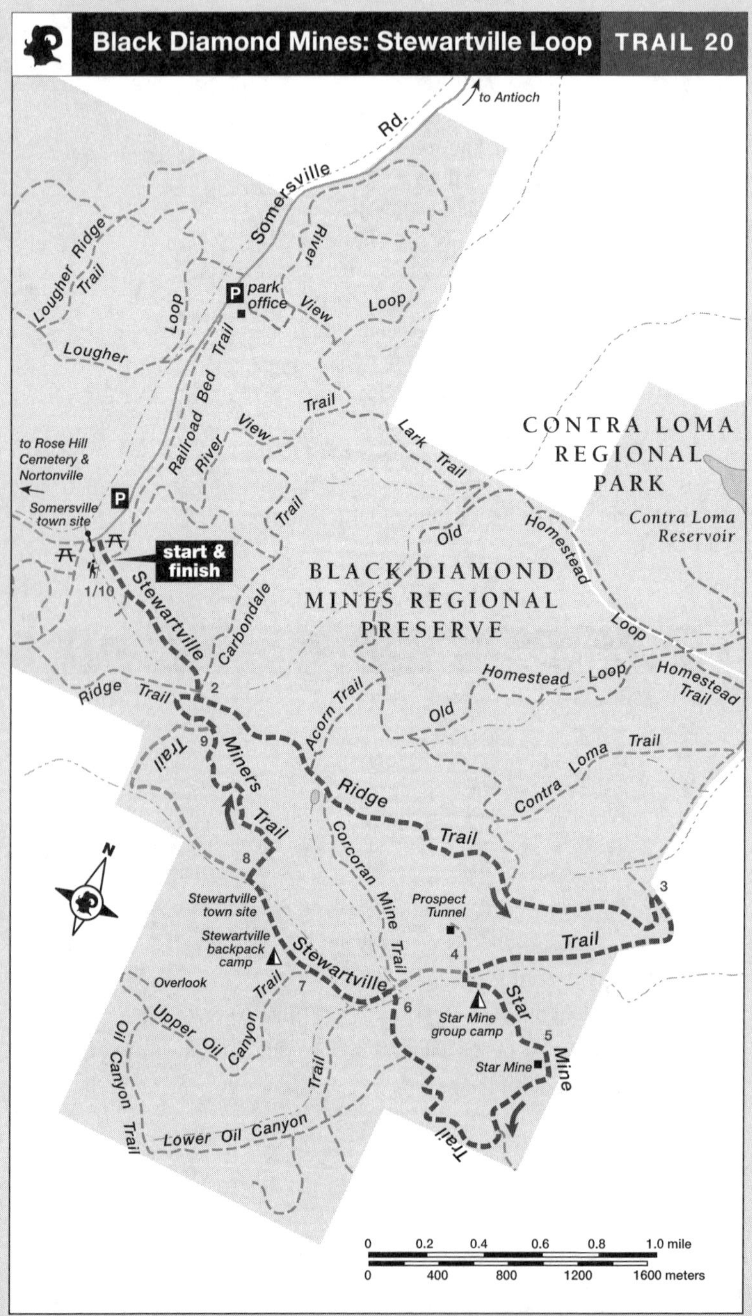
Black Diamond Mines: Stewartville Loop
TRAIL 20
to Antioch
Somersville Rd.
Lougher Ridge Trail
River View Loop
park office
Loop
Lougher
Railroad Bed Trail
River View Trail
Lark Trail
CONTRA LOMA REGIONAL PARK
Contra Loma Reservoir
to Rose Hill Cemetery & Nortonville
Somersville town site
start & finish
1/10
Stewartville
Carbondale
Old Homestead
BLACK DIAMOND MINES REGIONAL PRESERVE
Loop
Homestead Loop
Homestead Trail
Ridge Trail
2
Acorn Trail
Old
Trail
9
Miners Trail
Ridge Trail
Contra Loma Trail
Corcoran Mine Trail
8
3
Stewartville town site
Stewartville backpack camp
Prospect Tunnel
4
Trail
Stewartville
Overlook
7
6
Star Mine
Star Mine group camp
5
Star Mine
Upper Oil Canyon Trail
Oil Canyon Trail
Lower Oil Canyon Trail
Trail
N
0 0.2 0.4 0.6 0.8 1.0 mile
0 400 800 1200 1600 meters

Black Diamond Mines Regional Preserve: Stewartville Loop

This loop from Nortonville to Stewartville, two long-vanished mining towns, is like a trip back in time. Where eager miners pried coal loose from deep underground with clanging picks and shovels, only mine tailings and tunnels remain today. Other echoes of the Old West are grassy valleys dotted with grazing cows and sweeping vistas from high ridgetops.

TRAIL USE
Hike, Run, Bike, Dogs Allowed

LENGTH
7.6 miles, 4–6 hours

VERTICAL FEET
±1900'

DIFFICULTY
– 1 2 3 **4** 5 +

TRAIL TYPE
Loop

SURFACE TYPE
Dirt, Paved

FEATURES
Fee
Mountain
Wildflowers
Birds
Historic
Geologic Interest
Secluded
Camping

FACILITIES
Restrooms
Picnic Tables
Water

Best Time

Fall through spring, but trails may be extremely muddy in wet weather.

Finding the Trail

From State Hwy. 4 in Antioch, take the Somersville Rd. exit and go south, staying in the left lane as you approach and pass Buchanan Rd. At 1.5 miles, follow Somersville Rd. as it continues straight, where the main road, here called James Donlon Blvd., bends sharply left. At 2.6 miles from State Hwy. 4, you reach the entrance kiosk, park office, and emergency telephone; continue another 0.9 mile to a large parking area, right, with an overflow area, left.

Trail Description

From the south end of the parking area,▶1 you pass a gate and continue uphill on the **Nortonville Trail**, a paved road, for about 200 feet to a level area and

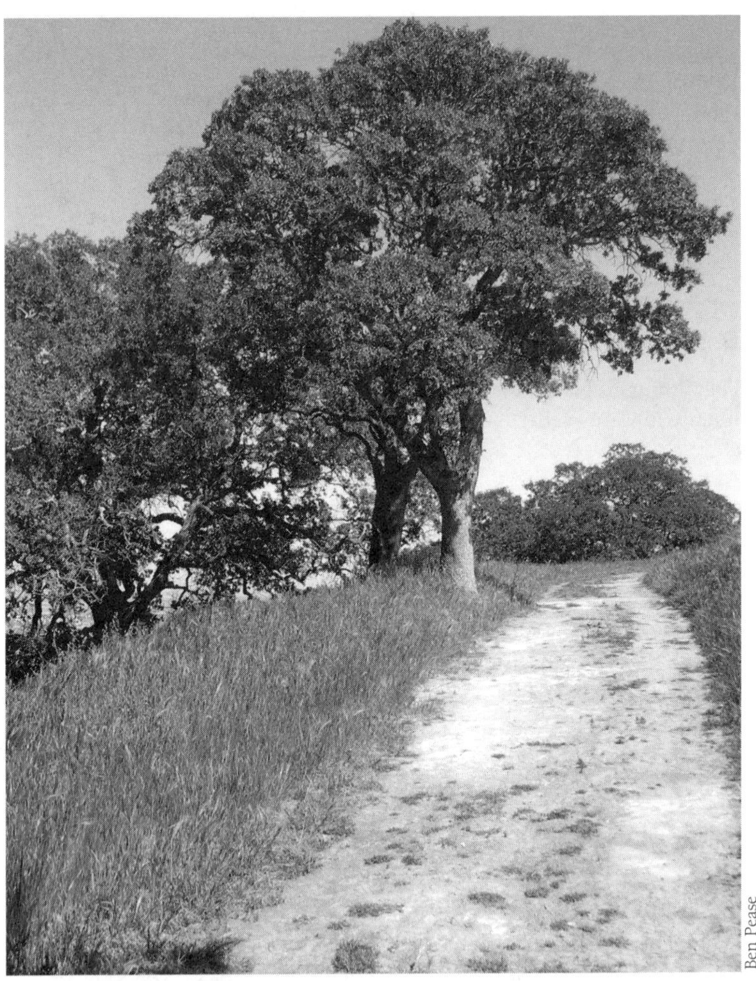

Ben Pease

The Stewartville Ridge Trail *follows a grassy ridge dotted with stately oak groves.*

then a junction, left, with the **Stewartville Trail,** a dirt road. Turn left and begin walking uphill on a moderate grade that soon levels. Once through a cattle gate, you pass the Railroad Bed Trail, left. About 150 yards ahead, the Pittsburg Mine Trail, part of the Somersville History Hike, branches right. Nearby are stands of nonnative black locust trees, which bloom fragrantly in spring, and a pile of gray mine tailings, the residue of years of backbreaking labor.

Continue straight on the Stewartville Trail, climbing southeast to an obvious notch in the skyline, where there are fine views of Mt. Diablo and the Stewartville Valley. As you crest a ridge, you come to a junction with the **Ridge Trail,** right, and the Carbondale Trail, left. Continue straight, now on the Ridge Trail, through a cattle gate. About 75 feet beyond the gate, you turn left at a T-junction to stay on the Ridge Trail.►2 Here you turn left and head uphill on a moderate and then steep grade, soon arriving at another ridgetop.

You turn east and follow the narrow ridgetop, alternating between its north and south sides. The north side features a blue-oak woodland, whereas the south side is open grassland. Just past a pond you come to a junction with the Corcoran Mine

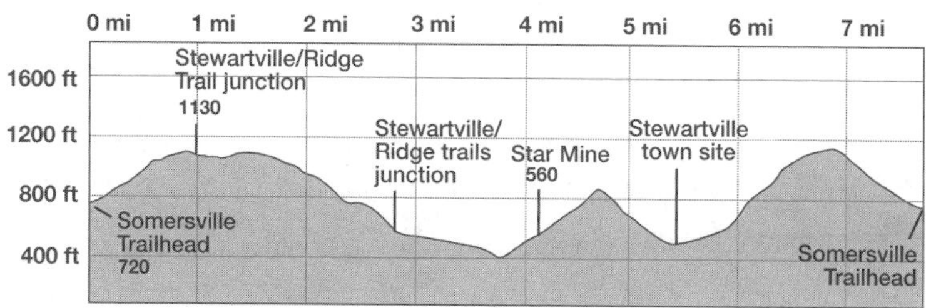

TRAIL 20 Black Diamond Mines: Stewartville Loop Profile

Trail. Here you stay on the Ridge Trail by bearing left. The encroaching subdivisions near Contra Loma Reservoir show why protecting open space in the Bay Area is essential.

You continue straight on the Ridge Trail and make a moderate and then steep descent to the Stewartville Trail,▶3 a level, dirt-and-gravel road with sections of broken pavement. You turn right and follow this road as it swings right, rounding the end of the ridge you just descended and emerging into a broad valley.

Almost a mile from the last junction, you come to a four-way junction, marked by a trail post.▶4 The Prospect Tunnel Trail branches right, but you turn left onto the **Star Mine Trail.** (Bicyclists should stay straight on the Stewartville Trail about 0.4 mile to a second junction with the Star Mine Trail,▶6 and there rejoin the described route.)

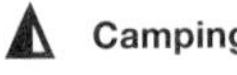
Camping

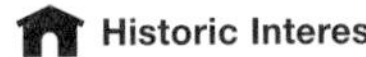
Historic Interest

The dirt-and-gravel road crosses the creek and climbs past **Star Mine group camp** (picnic tables, shelter, and toilet), then climbs on a moderate grade over a ridge and down into an adjacent valley. To the right of the road, look for the gated tunnel of **Star Mine,**▶5 one of the last coal mines in the area to shut down.

The road turns southwest, climbs through a rocky canyon that includes a sandstone quarry, and levels out in a pine forest. You bear right at a fork, staying on the Star Mine Trail, which now climbs steeply. Soon you reach one of the star attractions of this route, in addition to the mines—a manzanita

HISTORY

Rose Hill Cemetery

Nortonville's **Rose Hill Cemetery** is the last resting place for some of the miners, their wives, and children who came here in the 1860s to mine coal—"black diamonds." The cemetery is a short climb from the parking area on the **Nortonville Trail.**

forest. Two kinds of this hardy, fire-adapted shrub grow here: common manzanita, with green leaves that are shiny, smooth, and attach to the branch with a stem; and Mt. Diablo manzanita, with gray, feltlike leaves that clasp the branch and attach without a stem. Common manzanita, as its name suggests, is found in many parts of California, but the Mt. Diablo variety is restricted to its namesake mountain and this preserve.

Soon the road ends; you turn right and descend on a single track, closed to bicycles and horses. Losing elevation via switchbacks, the Star Mine Trail reaches a broad valley. Here you pass through a wooden gate in a barbed-wire fence and, in about 75 feet, reach a fork in the trail, where you bear right (the path to the left shortcuts through the grass to the Lower Oil Canyon Trail). Your route skirts the edge of the valley, circles a possibly wet area, and climbs an embankment to meet the **Stewartville Trail.**►6

Turn left on this dirt road and go past a windmill, a cattle pen, and the Lower Oil Canyon Trail, which departs left. About 0.2 mile ahead, you pass the Upper Oil Canyon Trail and the **Stewartville backpack camp,** where a toilet is available. Camping here is by reservation; call (510) 636-1684.

The Stewartville Trail narrows and dips into a shaded wash, which may be flooded in winter. Now you reach a valley marked with mine tailings on the right.►7 This is the site of **Stewartville,** one of five mining towns that thrived in this area between the

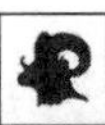

OPTIONS

Prospect Tunnel

►4 Up a short side trail, the **Prospect Tunnel** is a restored mining tunnel you can explore with a flashlight.

1860s and the turn of the century. At a junction, turn sharply right on the **Miners Trail,**▶**8** a single track closed to bicycles and horses, and climb gently north. (Bicyclists continue west on the Stewartville Trail and rejoin the route about 0.9 mile ahead, at the junction with the Miners Trail.) An old railroad grade runs east—west here, across your route. Continue uphill, steeply now, past more mine tailings.

After crossing a small wooden bridge, you join the **Stewartville Trail** at the elbow of a sharp switchback.▶**9** Bear right and continue to climb on a moderate grade. After making a switchback right, you pass a rest bench and reach a flat area where the Stewartville and Ridge trails meet. Turn left, go through the gate, and retrace your route to the parking area.▶**10**

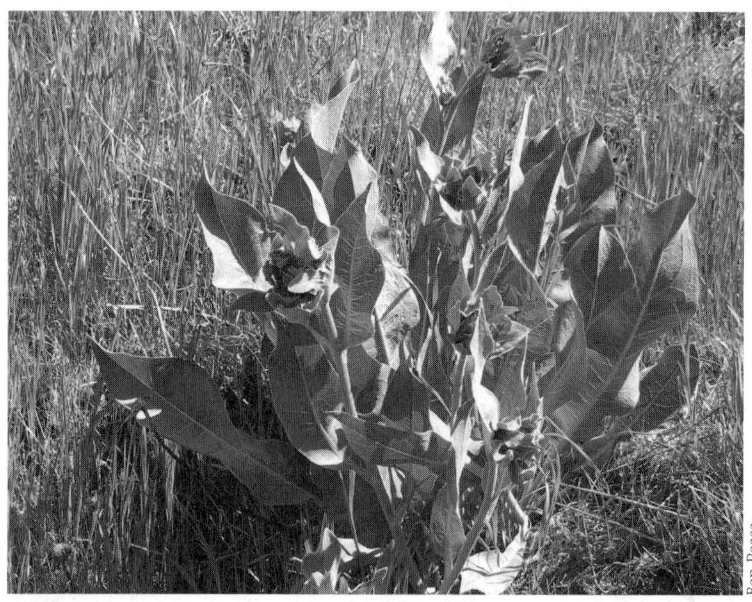

Ben Pease

Mule ears *bear a passing resemblance to their namesake.*

MILESTONES

▶1 0.0 Take Nortonville Trail south, then left on Stewartville Trail
▶2 0.7 Left at T-junction on Ridge Trail
▶3 2.8 Right on Stewartville Trail
▶4 3.7 Hikers turn left on Star Mine Trail
▶5 4.2 Pass Star Mine
▶6 5.3 Hikers turn left on Stewartville Trail
▶7 5.5 Backpack camp and Stewartville town site
▶8 6.0 Right on Miners Trail
▶9 6.5 Right on Stewartville Trail
▶10 7.6 Back at parking area

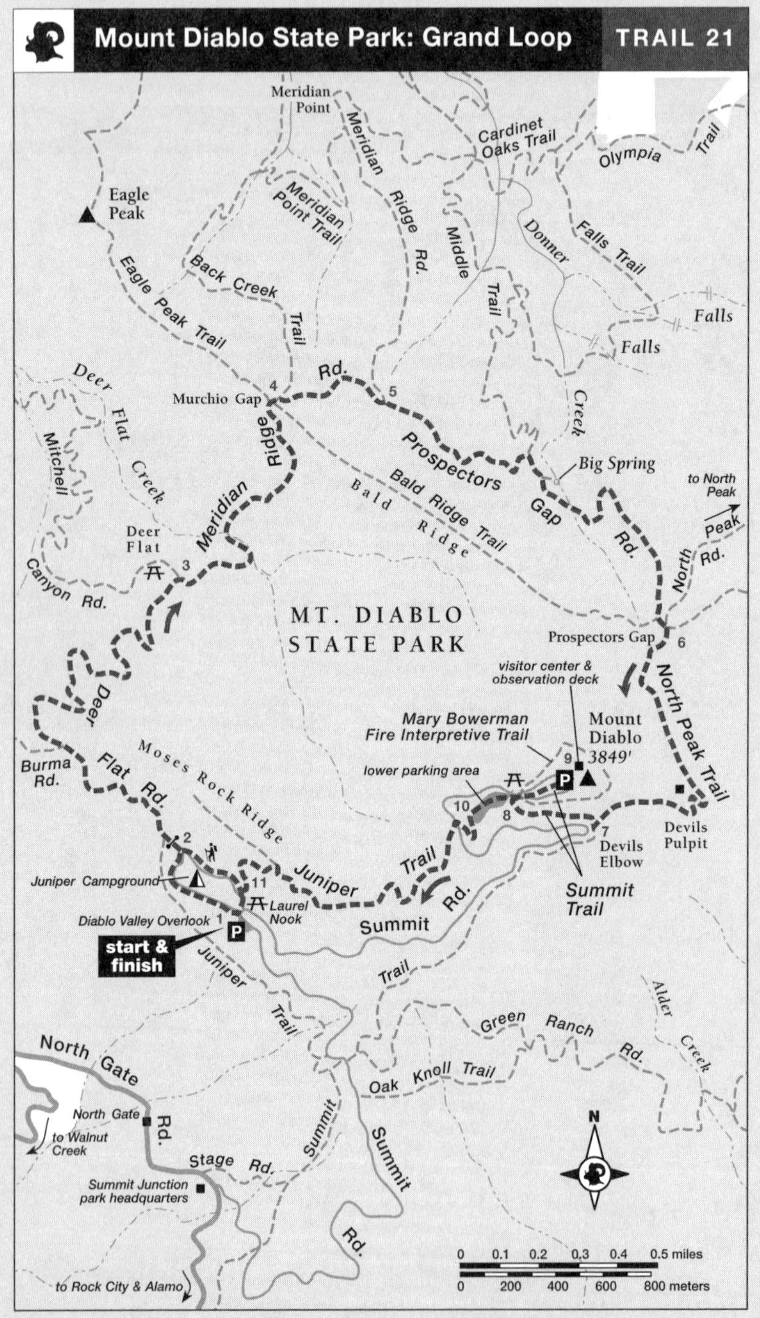
Mount Diablo State Park: Grand Loop
TRAIL 21
Meridian Point
Meridian Ridge Rd.
Cardinet Oaks Trail
Olympia Trail
Eagle Peak
Meridian Point Trail
Middle Trail
Donner Creek
Falls Trail
Back Creek Trail
Eagle Peak Trail
Falls
Falls
Deer Flat Creek
Murchio Gap
Rd.
Prospectors Gap Rd.
Mitchell Canyon Rd.
Meridian Ridge Rd.
Bald Ridge Trail
Bald Ridge
Big Spring
to North Peak
North Peak Rd.
Deer Flat
MT. DIABLO STATE PARK
Prospectors Gap
visitor center & observation deck
Deer Flat Rd.
North Peak Trail
Mary Bowerman Fire Interpretive Trail
Mount Diablo 3849′
Burma Rd.
Moses Rock Ridge
lower parking area
Devils Pulpit
Devils Elbow
Juniper Trail
Juniper Campground
Summit Trail
Laurel Nook
Diablo Valley Overlook
Summit Rd.
start & finish
Juniper Trail
Trail
Alder Creek
Green Ranch Rd.
North Gate Rd.
Oak Knoll Trail
North Gate
to Walnut Creek
Summit Trail
Summit Rd.
Stage Rd.
Summit Junction park headquarters
N
0 0.1 0.2 0.3 0.4 0.5 miles
0 200 400 600 800 meters
to Rock City & Alamo

Mount Diablo State Park: Grand Loop

A complete circle around Mt. Diablo, the East Bay's tallest peak, plus a trip to the summit, make this one of the region's premier hikes, and a great way to learn more about the trees, shrubs, and wildflowers that struggle for survival on the rugged mountain's upper reaches. This strenuous route uses Deer Flat, Meridian Ridge, and Prospectors Gap roads, and the North Peak, Summit, and Juniper trails.

TRAIL USE
Hike, Run, Bike

LENGTH
6.5 miles, 4–5 hours

VERTICAL FEET
±2200'

DIFFICULTY
– 1 2 3 4 **5** +

TRAIL TYPE
Loop

SURFACE TYPE
Dirt, Paved

FEATURES
Fee
Mountain
Summit
Wildflowers
Birds
Historic
Great Views
Photo Opportunity
Steep
Camping

FACILITIES
Visitor Center
Picnic Tables
Water
Restrooms

Best Time

Fall through spring, but trails may be muddy in wet weather.

Finding the Trail

From Interstate 680 in Danville, take the Diablo Rd./Danville exit and follow Diablo Rd. 3 miles east to Mt. Diablo Scenic Blvd. Turn left onto Mt. Diablo Scenic Blvd., which soon becomes South Gate Rd., and go 3.7 miles to the South Gate entrance station. Continue on South Gate Rd. another 3.2 miles to Park Headquarters and a junction with North Gate and Summit roads. Turn right onto Summit Rd. and go 2.3 miles to Diablo Valley Overlook, a large parking area at a sharp bend in the road, just left of the entrance to Juniper Campground and the Laurel Nook group picnic area. The trailhead is on the north end of Diablo Valley Overlook.

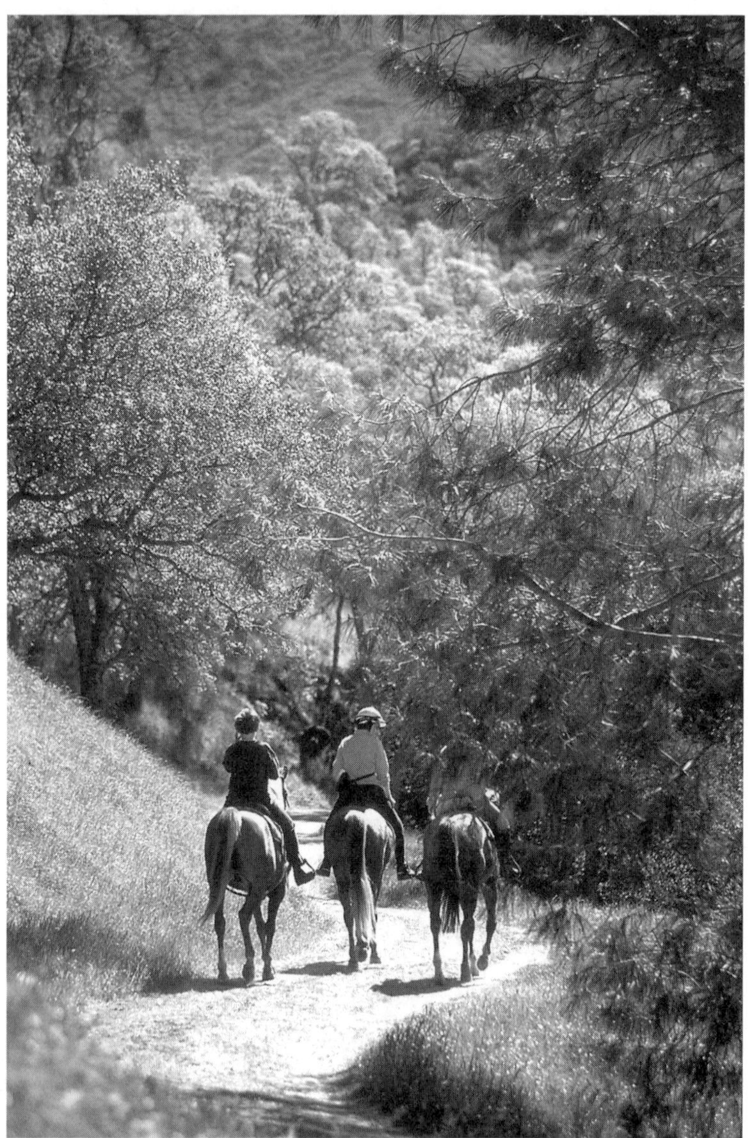

Equestrians *ride on Mt. Diablo.*

Trail Description

From the north end of the parking area,►1 follow either of two paved roads downhill into the **Juniper Campground.** From the point where they join,►2 near the restrooms and Campsite 23, continue walking northwest, now on **Deer Flat Road** (a dirt road also named Mitchell Canyon Road). At a gate, the Juniper Trail descends left. The road descends moderately across a grassy hillside that slopes precipitously to the wooded valleys far below. Looking west on a clear day you have expansive views across Pine Canyon to the hills of Oakland and Berkeley and distant Mt. Tamalpais.

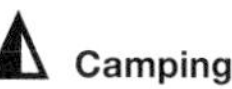

On a clear day, the view west from Mitchell Canyon Rd. takes in the Diablo foothills, the East Bay hills, Mt. Tamalpais, and the Golden Gate.

Passing Burma Road, left, you continue straight and then bear right as the road descends via well-graded but in places steep S-bends, giving you a look at Mt. Diablo's 3849-foot summit, your goal. The road levels in a little valley named **Deer Flat,** one of the prettiest spots on Mt. Diablo, especially in fall when bigleaf maple, California wild grape, and poison oak add touches of color to the scene. Soon you come to a junction►3 where Mitchell Canyon Road goes left. (You can turn left down this road about 150 yards to find a pleasant, tree-shaded picnic area with a watering trough for horses.)

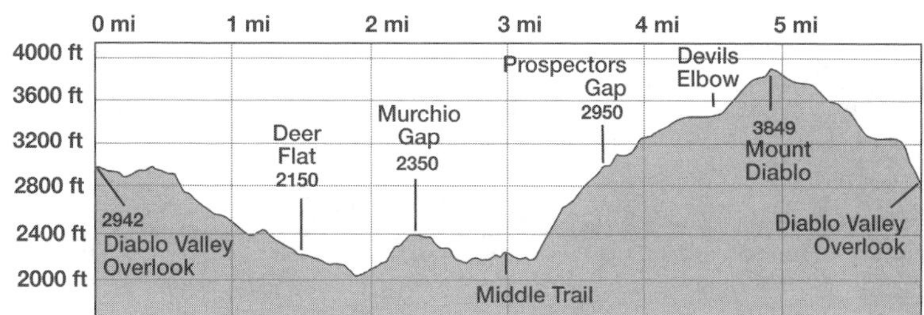

TRAIL 21 Mount Diablo State Park: Grand Loop Profile

At the junction, turn right on **Meridian Ridge Road,** which descends on a gentle grade, crosses a gravelly creek bed, begins a relentless ascent in the open, and brings you to **Murchio Gap,**▶4 between Bald Ridge and Eagle Peak. This important junction has many trails. Clockwise from the left as you face north, they are the Eagle Peak Trail, Back Creek Trail, Meridian Ridge Road, and the Bald Ridge Trail.

From Murchio Gap, follow Meridian Ridge Road east and gently downhill. You are treated to fine vistas of the Clayton Valley and Black Diamond Mines Regional Park. At a junction,▶5 Meridian Ridge Road turns left, but you go straight on **Prospectors Gap Road.** On a rocky nose you pass a junction with the Middle Trail, left, then come within earshot of **Donner Creek** and walk by a spur trail to Big Springs. Now begins a long, extremely steep climb—perhaps the steepest in this guide—up the rocky flank of **North Peak.**

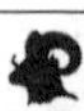 **Steep**

The grade eases slightly just before **Prospectors Gap,** a saddle between North Peak and Mt. Diablo's summit.▶6 At the saddle, the Bald Ridge Trail enters right, Prospectors Gap Road drops steeply in front of you, and North Peak Road heads left to North Peak. Your route is the **North Peak Trail,** right, one of the few single-track trails in the park open to bicycles and horses.

OPTIONS

Variations on the Grand Loop

The **Bald Ridge Trail** is an alternate route from Murchio Gap to Prospectors Gap. It is only a little less steep than the Meridian Ridge and Prospectors Gap roads, and nearly as strenuous.

Bicyclists can ride this loop all the way to Devils Elbow, then ride paved **Summit Rd.** up to the summit and back to the Diablo Valley Overlook. (Be alert for cars.)

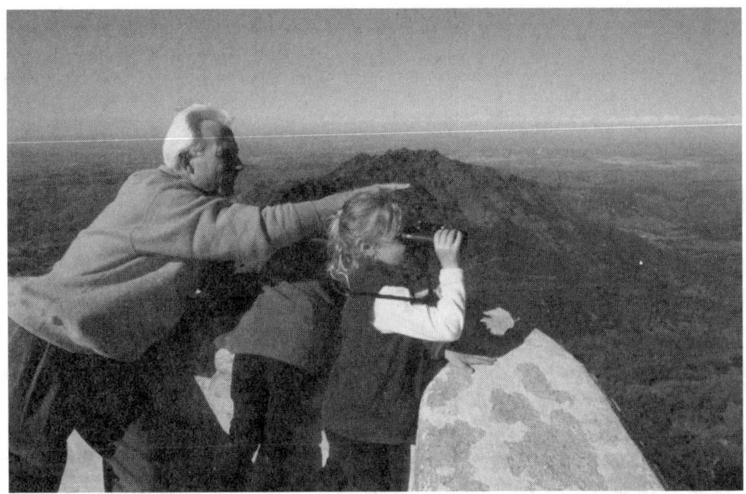

The view *from Mt. Diablo's summit is one of the Bay Area's best.*

Climb steeply across an open, rocky hillside, then settle into a rolling, moderate ascent beside mossy outcrops and a forest of California bay. Switchbacks near craggy **Devils Pulpit** reveal a stunning 180-degree view of the west Delta, the Central Valley, Livermore, Pleasanton, the Sunol/Ohlone Wilderness, and Mission Peak. Now the trail turns west toward **Devils Elbow,** a sharp bend in Summit Road. Above are the Summit Museum and communication towers on Mt. Diablo's summit.

Stop a moment in Deer Flat, one of the prettiest spots on Mt. Diablo.

As you reach pavement at Devils Elbow,►7 turn sharply right and begin climbing the **Summit Trail,** which rises through chaparral to emerge at the summit's lower parking area.►8 To reach **Mt. Diablo's 3849-foot summit** from the lower parking area, turn right and follow signs for the 0.2-mile continuation of the Summit Trail, which runs between the two paved roads that link the parking area with the summit.►9

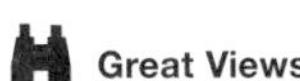

After resting and enjoying the scenery, retrace your route to the big lower parking area,►10 then

OPTIONS

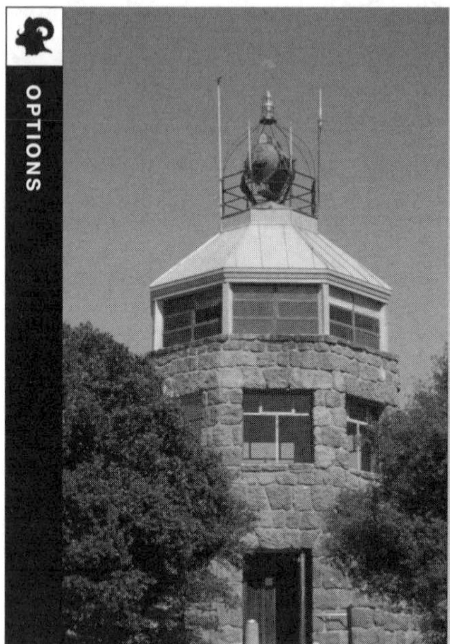

Summit Museum

The stone building at the summit (left) houses the **Mt. Diablo Interpretive Association visitor center,** which has information on the mountain's geology, flora, and fauna. You can climb to the observation deck for spectacular 360-degree views. Restrooms and water are available. For more information about the museum, which is open Wednesday–Sunday, call (925) 837-6119 or visit www.mdia.org/museum.htm.

continue west across pavement to the parking area's west end and a trail post marking the **Juniper Trail.** This single track makes a steep, rugged descent on loose dirt, rocks, and railroad ties to Summit Road. Cross the road carefully, turn right, and walk uphill about 90 feet to a trail post, left, marking the continuation of the Juniper Trail.

You drop via a series of switchbacks and then continue to descend along the crest of a broad ridge, with a sea of chaparral on both sides of the trail. As the route flattens out at a saddle, you come to a junction with a trail to Moses Rock Ridge. A trail post with an arrow pointing left directs you down the Juniper Trail, which descends through groves of bay and juniper to the **Laurel Nook group picnic area** beside the Diablo Valley Overlook.►11

MILESTONES

- ▶1 0.0 Go northwest on paved road through Juniper Campground
- ▶2 0.3 Straight on Deer Flat Rd.
- ▶3 1.4 Deer Flat; right on Meridian Ridge Rd.
- ▶4 2.2 Murchio Gap; angle right to stay on Meridian Ridge Rd.
- ▶5 2.4 Straight on Prospectors Gap Rd.
- ▶6 3.5 Prospectors Gap; right on North Peak Trail
- ▶7 4.6 Devils Elbow; right on Summit Trail
- ▶8 4.8 Lower parking area; right on paved road, then uphill on continuation of Summit Trail
- ▶9 5.0 Mt. Diablo summit
- ▶10 5.3 Go to west end of lower parking area and descend Juniper Trail
- ▶11 6.5 Back to Diablo Valley Overlook

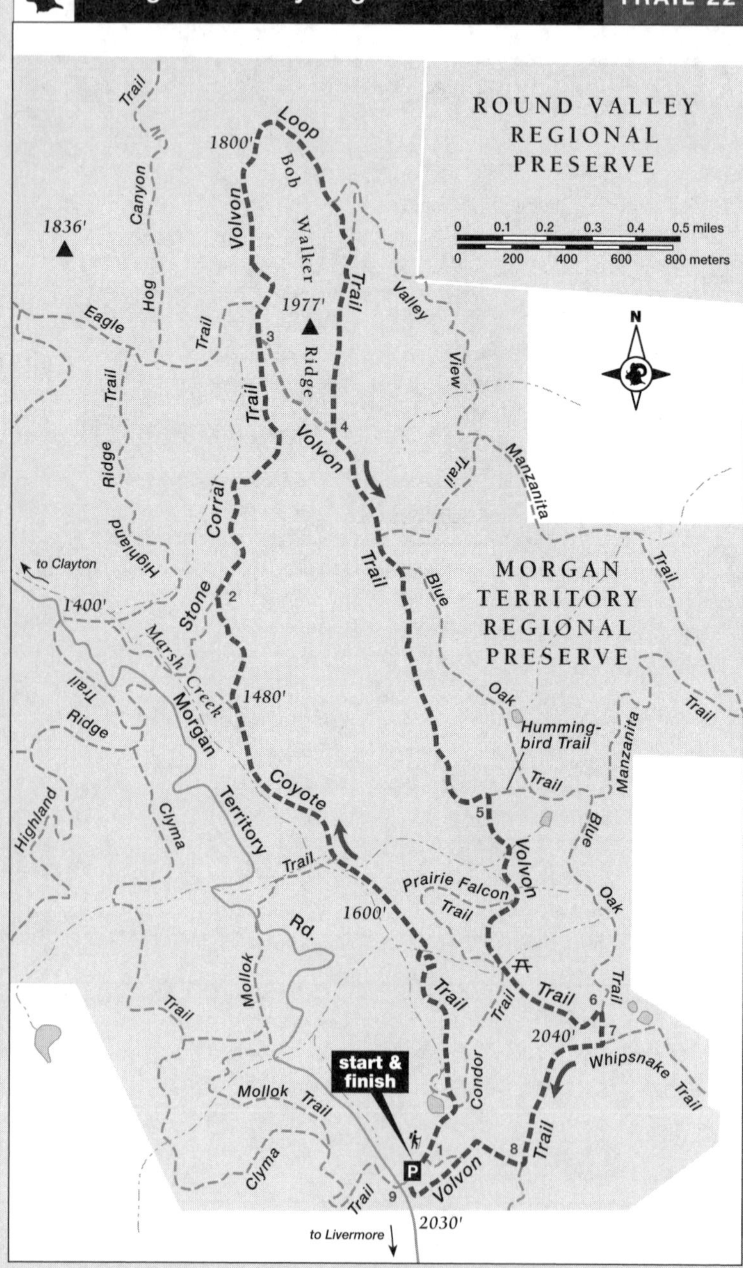
Morgan Territory Regional Preserve
TRAIL 22
ROUND VALLEY
REGIONAL
PRESERVE
MORGAN
TERRITORY
REGIONAL
PRESERVE
0.5 miles
800 meters
N
Volvon Loop
Bob Walker Ridge Trail
Volvon Trail
Coyote Trail
Stone Corral Trail
Highland Ridge Trail
Hog Canyon Trail
Eagle Trail
Valley View Trail
Manzanita Trail
Blue Oak Trail
Hummingbird Trail
Prairie Falcon Trail
Condor Trail
Whipsnake Trail
Mollok Trail
Clyma Trail
Marsh Creek
Morgan Territory Rd.
to Clayton
to Livermore
start & finish
1800'
1836'
1977'
1400'
1480'
1600'
2040'
2030'

Morgan Territory Regional Preserve: Bob Walker Ridge

This is one of the most remote and scenic parks in the East Bay, perched at 2000 feet on the southeastern edge of Mt. Diablo State Park, within sight of Livermore, Altamont Pass, and the Central Valley. Seclusion and wilderness make hiking here a special experience. This loop takes full advantage of these attributes, dropping into a deep canyon, then climbing lofty Bob Walker Ridge for views of the Livermore and Central valleys and Altamont Pass.

Bob Walker was a photographer and environmentalist who helped the East Bay Regional Park District build public support for land acquisitions in Morgan Territory Regional Preserve and Pleasanton Ridge Regional Park, from 1984 until his death in 1993.

TRAIL USE
Hike, Run, Bike, Dogs Allowed

LENGTH
5.9 miles, 4 hours

VERTICAL FEET
±1050'

DIFFICULTY
– 1 2 3 **4** 5 +

TRAIL TYPE
Loop

SURFACE TYPE
Dirt

FEATURES
Canyon
Autumn Colors
Birds
Great Views
Secluded

FACILITIES
Restrooms
Picnic Tables
Water

Best Time

Spring and fall. This is a region of extremes: hot in summer, cold in winter, and potentially windy all year.

Finding the Trail

From Interstate 580 in Livermore, take the North Livermore exit and go north on North Livermore Ave., and then west on its continuation, Manning Rd. At 4.4 miles from the interstate, just after a sharp bend to the west, you turn right onto Morgan Territory Rd., and go 6.3 miles to the Volvon Staging Area, right. (Use caution: After 0.7 mile, Morgan Territory Rd. becomes a one-lane paved road with turnouts.)

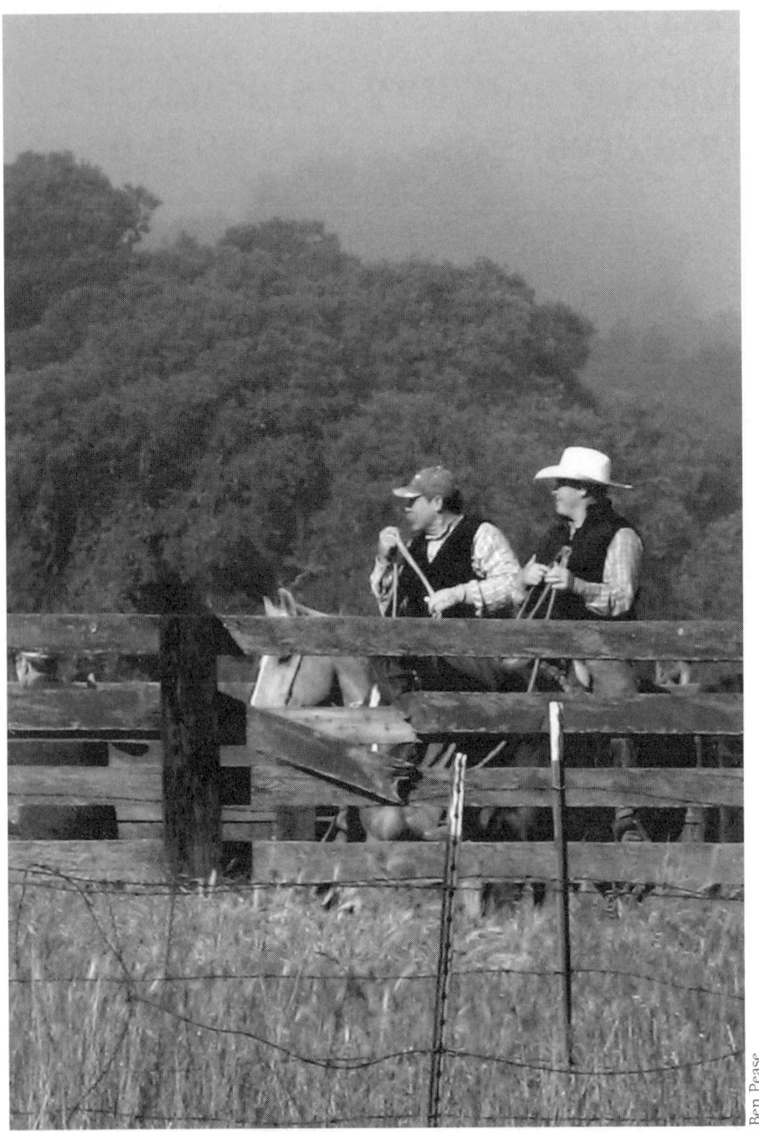

Ben Pease

Cowboys *at Morgan Territory Regional Preserve*

From Marsh Creek Rd. in Clayton, turn right onto Morgan Territory Rd. and go southeast 9.4 miles to the Volvon Staging Area, left.

The trailhead is on the northeast edge of the parking area.

Trail Description

From the trailhead, where the Volvon Trail, a multiuse dirt road ascends right, you descend left►1 on the single-track **Coyote Trail.** Reaching a stock pond, bear left past the Condor Trail. Beyond the pond, the trail, initially indistinct, descends through a narrow, rocky canyon. This is rugged terrain, colorful in fall, with a distinct wilderness feel. In the canyon, you pass a junction with the Mollok Trail, left, at about 0.8 mile.

The Coyote Trail descends gently another 0.3 mile along wooded **Marsh Creek,** then veers right and ascends through a low notch. Passing through a gate, you angle left on the edge of a large, open valley, soon reaching an indistinct fork. Bear right, in places following just a matted path in the grass. Climbing across a grassy hillside, you reach a T-junction with the **Stone Corral Trail,** a dirt road.►2 Here turn right and climb north on a gentle and then moderate grade through oak savanna. About 0.7 mile ahead, you meet the **Volvon Trail,** merging sharply from the right.

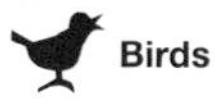

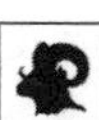

OPTIONS

Bicycling Bob Walker Ridge

Bicyclists and equestrians can visit **Bob Walker Ridge** by riding the 2.5-mile Volvon Trail as an out-and-back trip. Bear left on the Volvon Trail►4 for 0.3 mile to a junction with the Stone Corral Trail,►3 then continue around and retrace your route on the Volvon Trail.

Continue straight a few steps to a second T-junction, where you go right on the Volvon Loop Trail.▶3 The road bends sharply right at the north end of **Bob Walker Ridge**, presenting a vista that stretches east to the Central Valley and, on a clear day, the Sierra Nevada. Now heading southeast through a blue oak woodland, you pass on your left the first of two connections to the Valley View Trail, about 0.1 mile apart. Just ahead on the right is a good place for a picnic, with rocks to sit on.

After about 0.5 mile, you reach a notch in the ridge where a trail enters sharply from the right, but you stay straight, now on the **Volvon Trail.▶4** Soon you pass the Valley View and Blue Oak trails, both going left. Another 0.6 mile or so along the ridge brings you to a junction.▶5 Here the Hummingbird Trail goes straight, but you turn sharply right to stay on the Volvon Trail. Soon you pass two junctions, about 0.2 mile apart, with the Prairie Falcon Trail, right. Just beyond the second of these you pass the Condor Trail, also right.

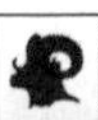

The Volvon Trail climbs to its second junction with the Blue Oak Trail.▶6 Here follow the Volvon Trail as it swings sharply right, and in about 150 feet you come to a T-junction where the Whipsnake Trail, a dirt-and-gravel road, goes left.▶7 Turn right here to stay on the Volvon Trail and begin an easy descent through open grassland. When you reach a fork signed TO PARK STAGING AREA,▶8 bear right and

HISTORY

Trail Names

Morgan Territory's trail names are based on Native American history and tradition: Coyote is a mythic personality in Indian legends, and the Volvon were one of the East Bay groups that resisted the Spanish mission system.

follow the gently rolling road until you can see the parking area, below and right. Bear left at the next fork and switchback moderately down to the parking area.►9

MILESTONES

►1	0.0	Left on Coyote Trail
►2	1.6	Right at T-junction on Stone Corral Trail
►3	2.3	Right at T-junction on Volvon Loop Trail
►4	3.5	Straight on Volvon Trail
►5	4.5	Right at junction with Hummingbird Trail to stay on Volvon Trail
►6	5.2	Second junction with Blue Oak Trail; stay on Volvon Trail by veering right
►7	5.3	Right again at T-junction with Whipsnake Trail, a dirt-and-gravel road
►8	5.5	Right at fork to stay on Volvon Trail
►9	5.9	Left on single-track trail; back at parking area

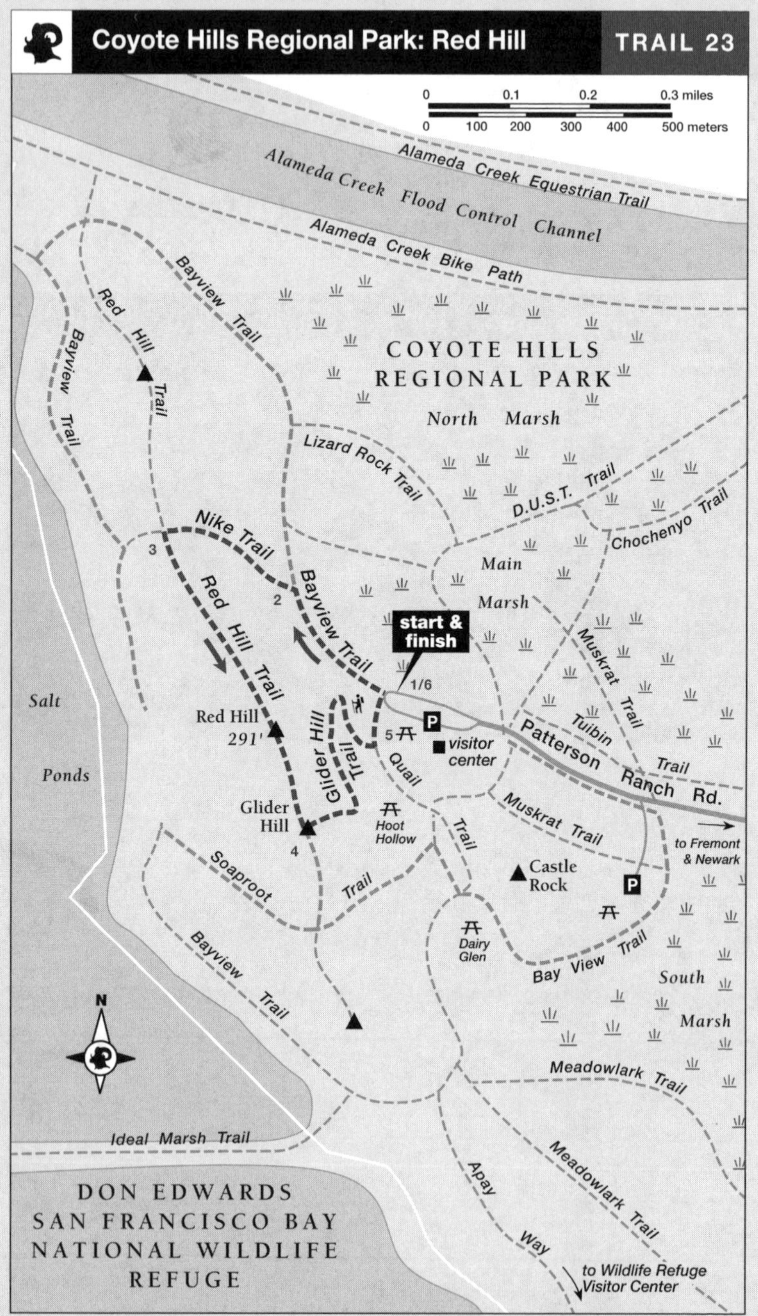
Coyote Hills Regional Park: Red Hill
TRAIL 23
0 0.1 0.2 0.3 miles
0 100 200 300 400 500 meters
Alameda Creek Equestrian Trail
Alameda Creek Flood Control Channel
Alameda Creek Bike Path
COYOTE HILLS REGIONAL PARK
North Marsh
Bayview Trail
Red Hill Trail
Lizard Rock Trail
D.U.S.T. Trail
Chochenyo Trail
Nike Trail
Main Marsh
start & finish
Muskrat Trail
Tuibin Trail
Patterson Ranch Rd.
Salt Ponds
Red Hill 291'
Glider Hill Trail
visitor center
Quail Trail
Glider Hill
Hoot Hollow
Muskrat Trail
to Fremont & Newark
Castle Rock
Soaproot Trail
Dairy Glen
Bay View Trail
South Marsh
Meadowlark Trail
Ideal Marsh Trail
Apay Way
to Wildlife Refuge Visitor Center
DON EDWARDS SAN FRANCISCO BAY NATIONAL WILDLIFE REFUGE
N

Coyote Hills Regional Park: Red Hill

This short loop over the Coyote Hills offers more scenery per calorie than any other hike in the East Bay, with 360-degree views extending from Mt. Tamalpais to Mission Peak and the Santa Cruz Mountains. The extensive brackish marsh and shimmering salt ponds surrounding the hills are habitat for waterfowl and shorebirds.

TRAIL USE
Hike, Run, Bike, Child Friendly, Dogs Allowed
LENGTH
1.0 mile, 1 hour
VERTICAL FEET
±350'
DIFFICULTY
– 1 **2** 3 4 5 +
TRAIL TYPE
Loop
SURFACE TYPE
Dirt

FEATURES
Fee
Lake
Summit
Wildflowers
Birds
Great Views
Photo Opportunity

FACILITIES
Visitor Center
Restrooms
Picnic Tables
Water

Best Time

This route is enjoyable all year.

Finding the Trail

From State Hwy. 84 at the east end of the Dumbarton Bridge in Fremont, take the Thornton Ave./Paseo Padre Pkwy. exit, and go north 1.1 miles on Paseo Padre Pkwy. to Patterson Ranch Rd. Turn left and go 0.5 mile to the entrance kiosk. Another 1.0 mile brings you to the parking area for the visitor center. The park charges fees for parking and dogs. The trailhead is on the west end of parking area, at its entrance.

Trail Description

From the west end of the parking area►**1** head northwest on the paved **Bayview Trail**, passing the Quail Trail, a dirt road, left. On your right is brackish Main Marsh, a haven for birds, including herons, egrets, ducks, and shorebirds. When you reach the **Nike Trail**, about 0.1 mile from the trailhead, turn left►**2** and start a moderate climb. (The Nike Trail

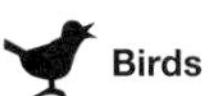

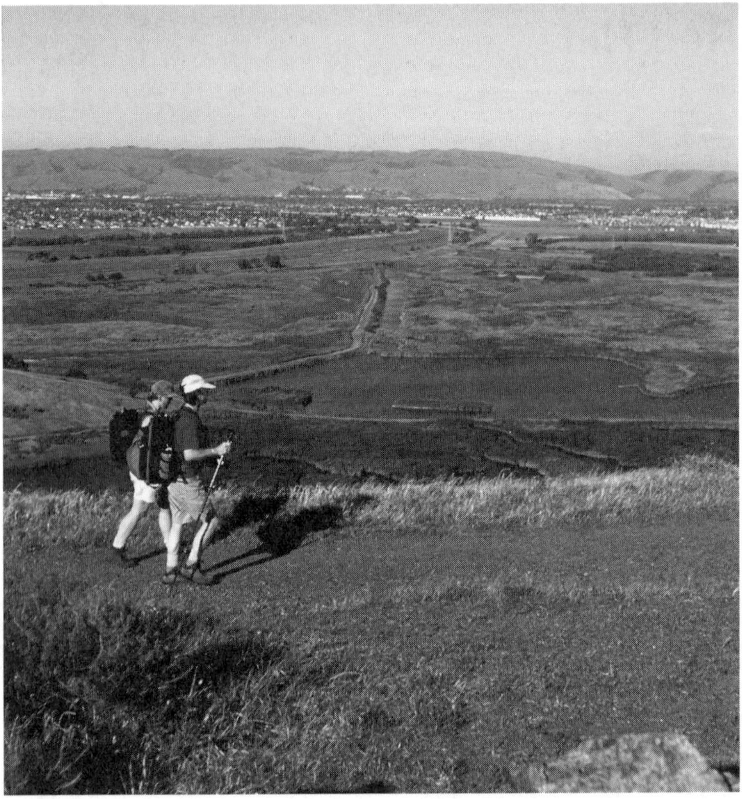

Hikers on Red Hill *overlook the Main Marsh, with the East Bay hills and Fremont on the distant horizon.*

is named for the missiles located nearby during the Cold War, not for the athletic apparel company.)

Turning left at a four-way junction on the **Red Hill Trail,▶3** a dirt road, continue your ascent over open terrain. After a short, steep pitch just below the summit of **Red Hill,** you gain the summit itself. To the northwest is the faint outline of San Francisco, with the dark hulk of Mt. Tamalpais looming behind. Oakland is also in view, beyond Hayward, San Leandro, and Alameda. To the south, the vista extends past the Dumbarton Bridge and the Don Edwards San Francisco Bay National Wildlife Refuge, all the way to the Santa Cruz Mountains.

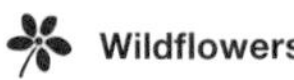

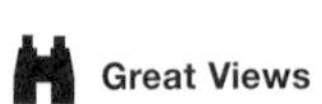

OPTIONS

Bicycle Route

Bicyclists continue straight from atop Glider Hill on the **Red Hill Trail,** descending steeply to a T-junction with the **Soaproot Trail.** From here you can go either left or right. The shorter return is to turn left and ride about 0.3 mile to the **Bayview Trail,** then turn left about 0.4 mile to **Patterson Ranch Rd.** From there, turn left on the road (or on the Bayview Trail, on the road's north side) about 0.3 mile to parking area, closing the loop. A longer return is to turn right on the **Soaproot Trail** about 0.3 mile, then turn right on the **Bayview Trail.** Circle clockwise around the north end of the Coyote Hills about 1.7 miles to the parking area.

After crossing the level summit, you descend steeply to a saddle, then reach the top of **Glider Hill,**►4 where the views equal those from Red Hill. The open, grassy summit even has a convenient picnic table. From here, hikers turn left and descend on the hiking-only **Glider Hill Trail.** In a few hundred feet, the trail drops left off the ridge and descends easily across the east slope of the Coyote Hills, through coastal scrub and grassland. The trail switchbacks south to a junction with the **Quail Trail**►5, a wide, gravel road. Turn left on the Quail Trail and soon meet the **Bayview Trail,** closing the loop. Now turn right and retrace your route to the parking area.►6

The Coyote Hills visitor center features excellent exhibits on native Ohlone people, birds, animals, and history, plus a small store. The building was a Nike barracks during the Cold War.

MILESTONES

►1	0.0	Take paved Bayview Trail east
►2	0.1	Left on Nike Trail
►3	0.4	Left on Red Hill Trail
►4	0.8	Left on Glider Hill Trail
►5	0.9	Left on Quail Trail
►6	1.0	Back at parking area

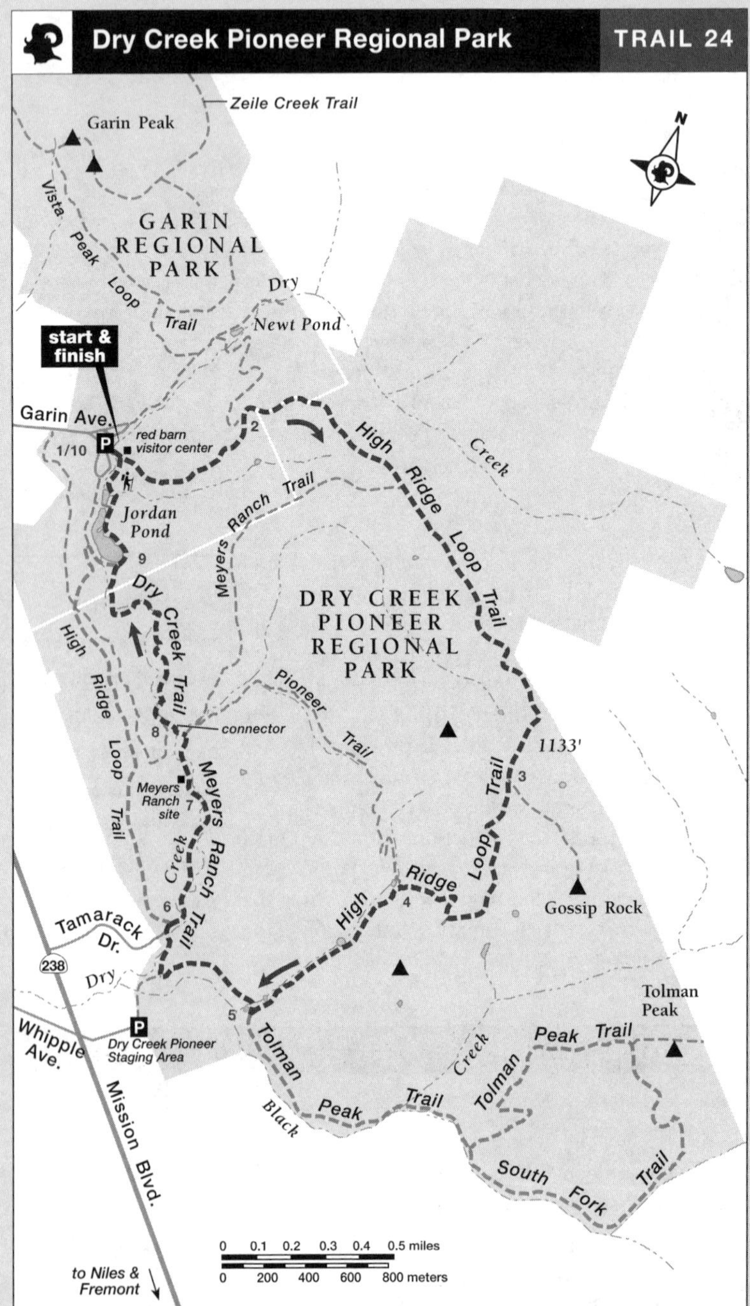

Dry Creek Pioneer Regional Park
TRAIL 24
Zeile Creek Trail
Garin Peak
N
Vista Peak Loop Trail
GARIN REGIONAL PARK
Dry
Newt Pond
start & finish
Garin Ave.
1/10
P
red barn visitor center
2
High Ridge Loop Trail
Creek
Meyers Ranch Trail
Jordan Pond
9
Dry Creek Trail
DRY CREEK PIONEER REGIONAL PARK
High Ridge Loop Trail
Pioneer Trail
8
connector
1133'
3
Meyers Ranch site
7
Meyers Ranch Trail
Creek
Ridge
High
4
Gossip Rock
6
Tamarack Dr.
238
Dry
5
Tolman Peak
P
Dry Creek Pioneer Staging Area
Whipple Ave.
Tolman Peak Trail
Creek
Tolman
Peak Trail
Black
Mission Blvd.
South Fork Trail
0 0.1 0.2 0.3 0.4 0.5 miles
0 200 400 600 800 meters
to Niles & Fremont

Dry Creek Pioneer Regional Park: High Ridge Loop

This route explores a regional-park gem—an oasis in the middle of one of the East Bay's most heavily industrial and residential areas. Scenery, views, and variety of habitat combine to make hiking these ridges more than just a challenging workout. An optional ascent of Tolman Peak will reward those wanting a longer route.

TRAIL USE
Hike, Run, Bike, Dogs Allowed

LENGTH
5.7 miles, 3–4 hours

VERTICAL FEET
±1100'

DIFFICULTY
– 1 2 3 **4** 5 +

TRAIL TYPE
Loop

SURFACE TYPE
Dirt

FEATURES
Fee
Lake
Summit
Birds
Wildlife
Great Views
Secluded

FACILITIES
Visitor Center
Restrooms
Picnic Tables
Water
Phone

Best Time

Spring and fall, but trails may be muddy in wet weather.

Finding the Trail

From Interstate 580 eastbound in Castro Valley, take the Hayward/State Hwy. 238 exit and follow signs for Hayward. From the first traffic light, continue straight, now on Foothill Blvd., for 1.7 miles to Mission Blvd., staying in the left lanes as you approach Mission Blvd. Bear left onto Mission Blvd. and go 3.5 miles to Garin Ave. Turn left and go 0.9 mile uphill to the entrance kiosk. At the kiosk bear right and proceed to parking areas; park in the lowest area if space is available.

From I-580 westbound in Castro Valley, take the Strobridge exit and go 0.2 mile to the first stop sign. Turn right, go 0.1 mile to Castro Valley Blvd., and turn left. Follow Castro Valley Blvd. 0.5 mile to Foothill Blvd., turn left, and follow the directions above. The park charges fees for parking and dogs when the entrance kiosk is attended.

To find the trailhead, go to the northeast corner of the lower parking area, turn east and cross a creek on a wooden bridge, then continue straight on a path into a picnic area. The route starts at the visitor center, a big red barn about 100 yards north of the wooden bridge.

Trail Description

From just south of the visitor center, follow a dirt road heading east across a large meadow to a metal gate. When you come to a four-way junction with a gravel road,▶1 continue straight and begin climbing the **High Ridge Loop Trail,** a dirt road with a grassy gulch on the right. At about 0.5 mile the grade eases briefly, and the Newt Pond Trail enters on your left.▶2 Soon the route levels, turns southeast, and then passes a junction, at about 1.1 miles, with the Meyers Ranch Trail, right. Ground squirrels abound in the open pastures.

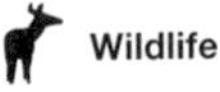
Wildlife

Near the start of the climb, perhaps only the distant blue blur of the Santa Cruz Mountains were visible above a strip of San Francisco Bay. But as you continue, a grand scene is revealed—San Francisco Bay National Wildlife Refuge, Coyote Hills, the Dumbarton and San Mateo bridges, Fremont, Newark, and Union City. On a clear day even Mt. Tamalpais, Mt. Diablo, and Loma Prieta may present themselves for inspection.

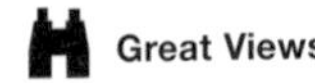
Great Views

A short climb earns your first view of Mission Peak, to the southeast, and the southern end of San Francisco Bay. Ahead is a junction with the Gossip Rock Trail, which goes left.▶3 There is a rest bench

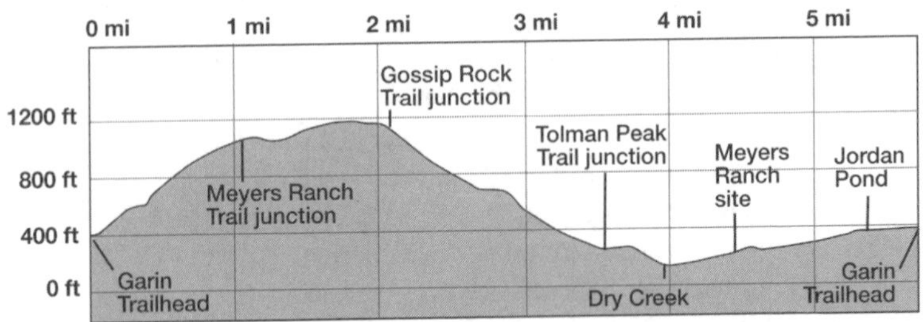

TRAIL 24 Dry Creek Pioneer Regional Park: High Ridge Loop Profile

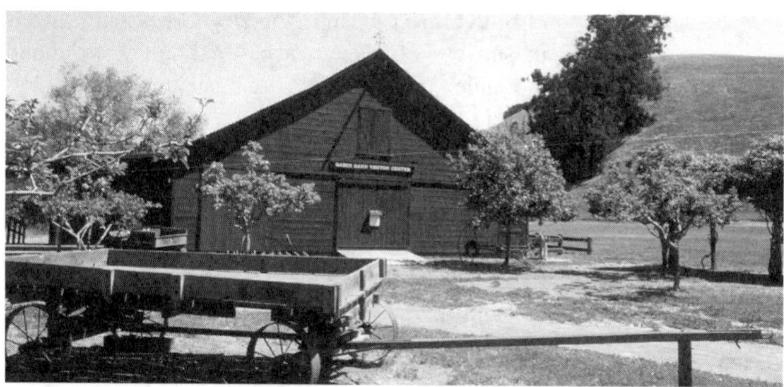

Garin/Dry Creek visitor center, *in a restored barn, has displays of antique farm equipment and information about Hayward's ranching and farming history.*

here, but on a hot day you may want to walk the short distance to **Gossip Rock** and enjoy the shade of the large California bay trees there.

Leaving the junction and going straight, you descend moderately through open grassland, flanked by wooded canyons. About 0.5 mile past the Gossip Rock Trail, bear sharply right at a junction with an unnamed road and continue downhill, now steeply. Scrubland soon gives way to a shady oak woodland. In a lovely valley, the Pioneer Trail departs right, and your route continues straight.▶4 The trail emerges from the woods and reaches a T-junction near a stock pond.▶5 Here the Tolman Peak Trail (see sidebar on page 176) goes left, but your route, the **High Ridge Loop Trail**, turns right.

Climbing on a gentle grade, the road crosses a grassy slope with a view west, then descends. Where the May Trail descends left to the Dry Creek Pioneer Staging Area, you bear sharply right. After crossing Dry Creek, you reach a four-way junction.▶6 Left is a gate leading to Tamarack Drive. Ahead and slightly left, the High Ridge Loop Trail ascends a high, open ridge (bicyclists angle left up this dirt road about 1 mile, then veer right as it descends to Jordan Pond; turn right to cross the dam and rejoin the hiking route).

Hikers bear right on the **Meyers Ranch Trail.** The dirt road descends gently, then crosses a series of bridges over meandering **Dry Creek,** and ducks in and out of trees in a pastoral valley. In about 0.5 mile, you come to an open area signed for Meyers Ranch;►7 look for rusted, antique farm equipment lying in the grass to your right. Although no buildings remain, planted poplars and fruit trees show this was once a homestead.

After leaving the Meyers Ranch site, find a single track on your left signed DRY CREEK TRAIL. Hikers descend this narrow connector, which is closed to

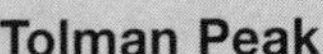

OPTIONS

Tolman Peak

The side trip to Tolman Peak adds 3.9 miles and an elevation gain and loss of 800 feet to the trip. Turning left on the **Tolman Peak Trail,►5** a dirt-and-gravel road, you pass a stock pond and amble through Black Creek Valley. Beyond a cattle pen, left, eucalyptus at an old ranch site provide a shady resting place. Beyond a gate, the road crosses a creek on a small bridge and then twice crosses the rocky creek bed itself. Soon the Tolman Peak Trail turns left, but you continue straight on the dirt road you have been following, now called the **South Fork Trail**. The road continues up the canyon another 0.5 mile or so to a bench at the regional-park boundary. Bicyclists, and hikers seeking just a creekside saunter, should turn back here and retrace your route through Black Creek Valley to the High Ridge Loop Trail, for a 2.8-mile side trip.

Energetic hikers turn left on the **South Fork Trail**, now a single track, and climb across a steep hillside. Once out of the forest, the trail may be hard to spot: Look for a line of matted grass. A bench affording a grand view of San Francisco Bay and the regional park's nearby canyons marks the trail's high point. Gossip Rock, which you passed earlier, is to the north. Just past the bench is a T-junction with the **Tolman Peak Trail**, a faint path that leads right and uphill to Tolman Peak. (The 0.2-mile side trip to the very summit is fun but does not gain you any better views.)

As you wind downhill on a moderate and then steep grade, you follow a small creek to close the short loop at a junction with the **South Fork Trail.** From here, turn right and retrace your route through Black Creek Valley to the junction with the **High Ridge Loop Trail.►5**

bikes, and cross Dry Creek on a narrow footbridge (an alternate equestrian trail fords the creek to the right of the bridge). Several hundred feet past the bridge is a T-junction with the **Dry Creek Trail.**▶8 Here you turn right, toward Jordan Pond and the visitor center.

Your route now winds through a shady area and crosses the creek on another wooden bridge. After traversing a low ridge, you come to a grove of bay trees. Here one branch of the trail leads straight to a horse crossing at the creek, but you turn left and cross the creek on a wooden bridge.

Once across the creek, turn right and, at a big rock, join the path coming from the horse crossing. Ahead the trail forks again: right for horses, straight for hikers. One last bridge takes you over the creek, and soon, heading straight, you ascend a paved section of trail and reach a T-junction at **Jordan Pond.**▶9

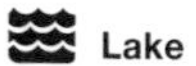

Here the High Ridge Loop Trail goes left, but you turn right and begin circling the pond on a dirt road, through an area of picnic tables and fire grates. Past the upstream end of the pond, you come to a fork in the route: bear right through the picnic area to return to the visitor center, then turn left to the parking area.▶10

MILESTONES

▶1	0.0	Start southeast, through gate, up High Ridge Loop Trail
▶2	0.5	Newt Pond Trail on left
▶3	2.1	Trail to Gossip Rock on left
▶4	2.9	Straight at T-junction with Pioneer Trail
▶5	3.5	Right at T-junction to stay on High Ridge Loop Trail
▶6	4.0	Right on Meyers Ranch Trail
▶7	4.5	Meyers Ranch
▶8	4.7	Right at T-junction with Dry Creek Trail
▶9	5.4	Jordan Pond; right at T-junction, then right at fork
▶10	5.7	Back at visitor center

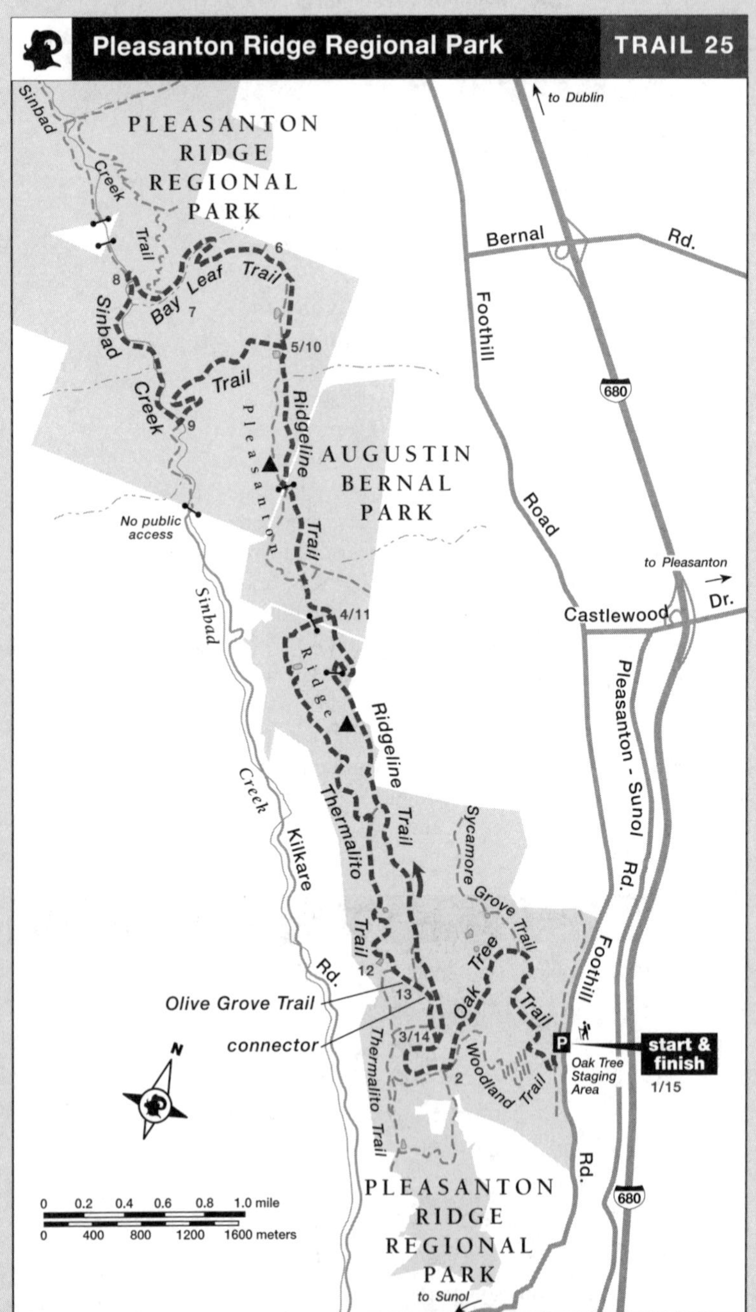
Pleasanton Ridge Regional Park
TRAIL 25
PLEASANTON RIDGE REGIONAL PARK
to Dublin
Bernal
Rd.
Foothill
680
Sinbad Creek Trail
Bay Leaf Trail
Sinbad Creek Trail
Ridgeline Trail
Pleasanton Ridge
AUGUSTIN BERNAL PARK
Road
No public access
to Pleasanton
Castlewood
Dr.
Pleasanton - Sunol Rd.
Sinbad Creek
Kilkare Rd.
Ridgeline Trail
Thermalito Trail
Sycamore Grove Trail
Oak Tree Trail
Foothill Rd.
Olive Grove Trail
connector
Woodland Trail
Thermalito Trail
Oak Tree Staging Area
start & finish
1/15
2
3/14
4/11
5/10
6
7
8
9
12
13
N
0 0.2 0.4 0.6 0.8 1.0 mile
0 400 800 1200 1600 meters
PLEASANTON RIDGE REGIONAL PARK
to Sunol

Pleasanton Ridge Regional Park

The hike along Pleasanton Ridge, although one of the longest and most challenging in this guide, is also one of the most rewarding (several shorter options are also enjoyable). Outstanding views extend from Pleasanton, San Ramon, and Mt. Diablo to Sunol Valley, the Sunol/Ohlone Wilderness, and Mission Peak. Bird and plant life flourish in this relatively undeveloped park. The varied terrain includes dense woodland, open grassland, and even a restored olive orchard.

TRAIL USE
Hike, Run, Bike, Dogs Allowed

LENGTH
12.3 miles, 6–8 hours

VERTICAL FEET
±3000'

DIFFICULTY
– 1 2 3 4 **5** +

TRAIL TYPE
Loop

SURFACE TYPE
Dirt

FEATURES
Stream
Canyon
Summit
Wildflowers
Birds
Great Views
Photo Opportunity
Secluded

FACILITIES
Restrooms
Picnic Tables
Water

Best Time

Fall through spring, but trails may be muddy in wet weather.

Finding the Trail

From Interstate 680 in Pleasanton, take the Sunol Blvd./Castlewood Dr. exit and go southwest on Castlewood Dr., staying straight where Pleasanton–Sunol Rd. bends left. After 0.3 mile, you reach Foothill Rd.; turn left and go south 1.6 miles on Foothill Rd. to the Oak Tree Staging Area, right. The trailhead is on the west side of the first parking area.

Trail Description

From the parking area, follow a dirt road west through a cattle gate, then bear left at a junction▶1 and begin climbing moderately on the **Oak Tree Trail**, also a dirt road. Continue past the hiking-only Woodland Trail, left.

The route ascends on a winding, open course through open grassland dotted with valley oaks.

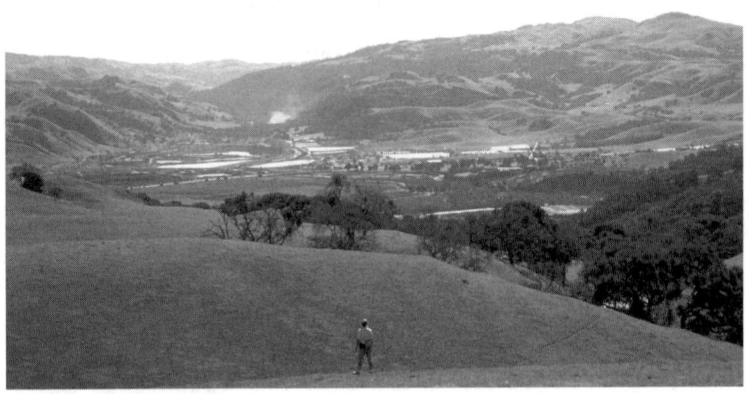

The view south from Pleasanton Ridge *includes Mission and Monument Peaks (right).*

Midway through a broad 180-degree bend, you pass a junction with the Sycamore Grove Trail, right. As the road climbs south, an unsigned single track parallels it below and left.

At about 1.3 miles, you emerge from a wooded area and reach a five-way junction near a barbed-wire fence.►**2** Here, the Woodland Trail joins on the left, and an unnamed dirt road follows the fence left and right. Your route, the Oak Tree Trail, turns right and goes through an opening in the fence. About 30 feet beyond the fence is a junction. Here you leave the Oak Tree Trail, which goes left, and join the **Ridgeline Trail** by angling right.

The Ridgeline Trail makes a 180-degree bend to gain the ridgetop. Soon you pass a connector to the Olive Grove Trail, which branches left. Follow the

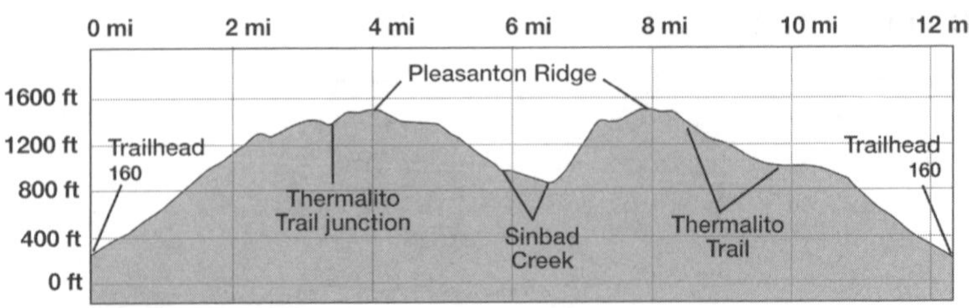

TRAIL 25 Pleasanton Ridge Regional Park Profile

Ridgeline Trail by bearing right, heading generally northwest, and climbing moderately past the first of two stately **olive groves.** The groves here were planted between about 1890 and the 1920s, but there is no record of who planted them. Just beyond the grove are a drinking faucet, a watering trough for animals, and another fork, where you continue straight. Rising steeply over rocky ground, your route eventually levels and comes into the open.

Where there are oaks in the East Bay, you are likely to find acorn woodpeckers.

Pause often to enjoy the view, which extends from Mt. Diablo south to Mission and Monument peaks. San Antonio Reservoir, with the Sunol/Ohlone Wilderness behind it, is southeast; and forested Sunol Ridge, topped by a single communication tower, rises above Kilkare Canyon and Sinbad Creek to the west. Now you pass a junction▶**3** with the Olive Grove Trail merging sharply from the left. Along the ridgetop, you climb over several high points, the first of which is just ahead. There is a picnic table atop one of these rounded summits. Soon you descend to a saddle and a fork. Your route bends right and climbs steeply to the summit of a grassy hill.

Continuing on the Ridgeline Trail, you climb steeply over several more hills. Finally, the route leaves the ridgetop, veering right and downhill through a cattle gate, then descends over steep and rocky ground. Traversing north through dense forest, you soon enter Pleasanton's **Augustin Bernal Park.** Now out of dense forest, you drop to an oak-shaded saddle and a junction, left, with the Thermalito Trail, your eventual return route.▶**4** A few steps left along the trail are drinking water and a trough for animals.

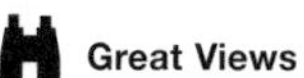

Continue straight on the Ridgeline Trail, sauntering moderately uphill through an oak savanna. Soon, an equestrian-only trail crosses your route, and then the Valley View Trail merges from the right. Ahead about 0.3 mile is a gate marking the boundary between the city and regional parks. Just beyond the gate is a fork. Bear right and enjoy a mostly level stroll through a beautiful oak savanna. After about 0.4 mile, the left branch of the previous fork rejoins, and now the Ridgeline Trail begins to climb.

As the route breaks into the open, you pass a pond, left, and a junction with the Sinbad Creek Trail, also left, part of your return route.►5 For now, continue straight, passing another small pond. At a junction near the park boundary, you go straight on the **Bay Leaf Trail,►6** then bend left and begin to descend. Soon the route turns sharply right and drops into a ravine on a moderate grade.

Now the route crosses two creeks that flow under the road through culverts. After an open section, you pass a junction right, with the single-track Sinbad Creek Trail.►7 Your route follows the road, now also named the **Sinbad Creek Trail**, downhill. You soon reach **Sinbad Creek** at the bottom of Kilkare Canyon.►8 Step across the creek on rocks and, at a T-junction with a dirt road, turn left. After a pleasant, 0.7-mile streamside stroll, you arrive at a T-junction in a clearing.►9 Here you turn left, recross the creek, and begin climbing steeply out of the canyon on the Sinbad Creek Trail, a dirt road.

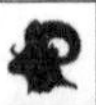 **Stream**

Cresting the ridge, you soon come to a T-junction with the **Ridgeline Trail.►10** Turn right on the Ridgeline Trail and retrace your route to the junction of the Ridgeline and Thermalito trails. When you reach that junction,►11 turn right on the **Thermalito Trail**, a dirt road.

OPTIONS

Shorter Trips

For a different shorter loop, another good turnaround point is the **Ridgeline/Sinbad Creek trail** junction,►5/10, which reduces your total trip distance to 9.3 miles. But first, continue right on an unsigned path to a rest bench overlooking the I-680 corridor and Pleasanton. Then return to the junction and start back on the Ridgeline Trail.

Another option is, when you're in Augustin Bernal Park, to turn left on the **Thermalito Trail►4** and follow the route description from►11. This route reduces your trip distance to about 7 miles.

Now the route roller coasters over rocky ground, passing a picturesque pond, to a T-junction, where you stay right on the Thermalito Trail. Out in the open now, the road descends past a stock pond to a small ravine, which may hold water during wet weather. Crossing to the other side of the ravine, the route climbs slightly, bringing you to another pond, right, and a junction.►**12** Leaving the Thermalito Trail as it turns right, you continue straight on a connector to the **Olive Grove Trail.** Walking east about 100 yards, you get on the Olive Grove Trail by going straight. At the next junction, where the Olive Grove Trail swings right, go straight on a connector to the Ridgeline Trail.►**13** At the junction with the Ridgeline Trail,►**14** bear right and retrace your route to the parking area.►**15**

MILESTONES

►1	0.0	Take dirt road west to junction and start up the Oak Tree Trail
►2	1.3	Right at five-way junction to stay on Oak Tree Trail, then right on Ridgeline Trail
►3	1.9	Olive Grove Trail merges from left
►4	3.4	Thermalito Trail on left; go straight to stay on Ridgeline Trail
►5	4.5	Sinbad Creek Trail on left; go straight
►6	4.9	Straight on Bay Leaf Trail
►7	5.7	Straight on Sinbad Creek Trail (dirt road)
►8	5.8	Cross Sinbad Creek, then left at T-junction to stay on Sinbad Creek Trail
►9	6.5	Left at T-junction, cross creek to stay on Sinbad Creek Trail
►10	7.4	Right at T-junction with Ridgeline Trail
►11	8.5	Right on Thermalito Trail
►12	10.5	Straight on connector to Olive Grove Trail; straight on Olive Grove Trail
►13	10.7	Straight on connector to Ridgeline Trail
►14	10.8	Right on Ridgeline Trail, then follow Oak Tree Trail
►15	12.3	Back at parking area

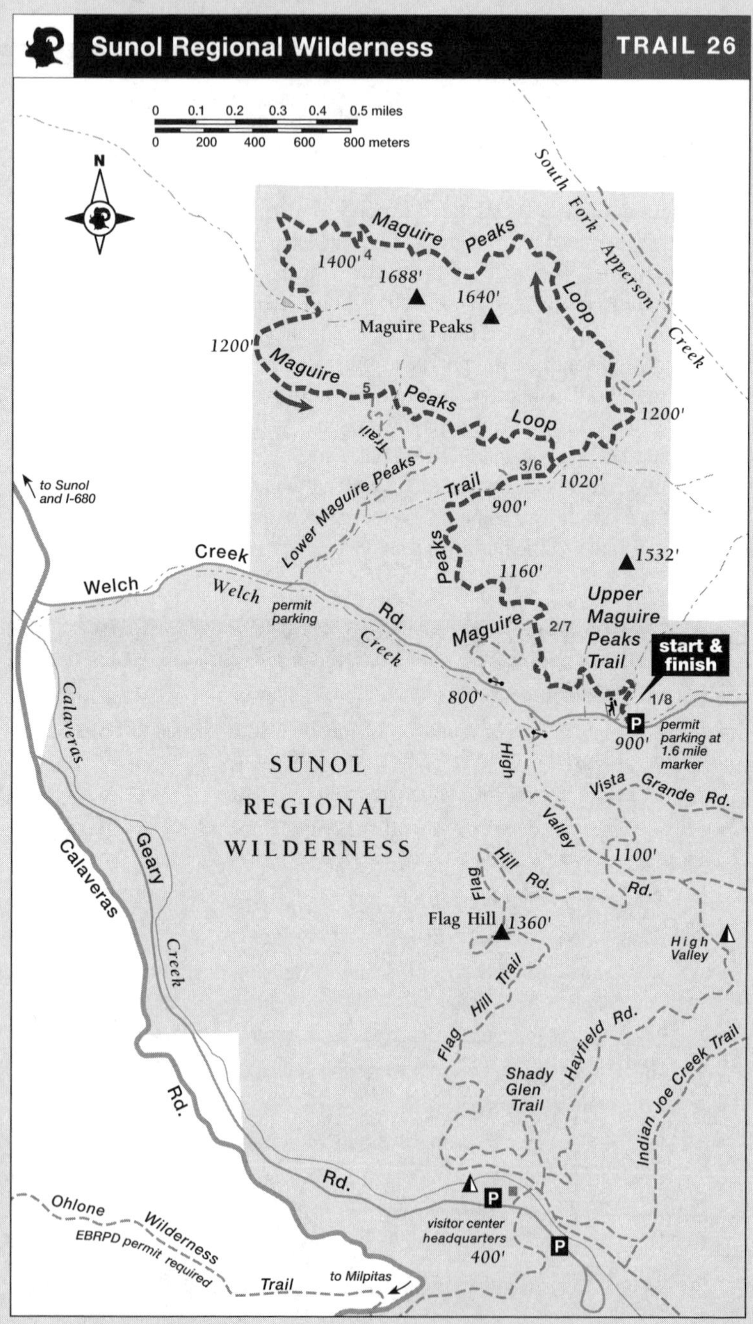

Sunol Regional Wilderness
TRAIL 26
0 0.1 0.2 0.3 0.4 0.5 miles
0 200 400 600 800 meters
N
South Fork Apperson Creek
Maguire Peaks Loop
1400'
4
1688'
1640'
Maguire Peaks
1200'
5
1200'
Lower Maguire Peaks Trail
3/6
1020'
900'
Maguire Peaks Trail
1160'
1532'
Upper Maguire Peaks Trail
2/7
start & finish
1/8
to Sunol and I-680
Welch Creek
Welch Creek Rd.
permit parking
800'
900'
permit parking at 1.6 mile marker
SUNOL REGIONAL WILDERNESS
High Valley Rd.
Vista Grande Rd.
1100'
Flag Hill Rd.
Flag Hill
1360'
High Valley
Flag Hill Trail
Hayfield Rd.
Shady Glen Trail
Indian Joe Creek Trail
Calaveras
Calaveras Rd.
Geary Rd.
Creek
visitor center headquarters
400'
Ohlone Wilderness Trail
EBRPD permit required
to Milpitas

Sunol Regional Wilderness: Maguire Peaks

This circuit of Maguire Peaks explores a hidden corner of Sunol Regional Wilderness, divided by Welch Creek Road from the main part of the park. The scenery is beautiful and serene, and the vistas from several vantage points are superb. Literally to top it off, you can make an ascent of Maguire Peaks west summit (1688'), a mountain climb in miniature.

TRAIL USE
Hike, Run, Bike, Dogs Allowed

LENGTH
5.9 miles, 4 hours

VERTICAL FEET
±1400'

DIFFICULTY
– 1 2 3 **4** 5 +

TRAIL TYPE
Loop

SURFACE TYPE
Dirt

FEATURES
Permit Required
Canyon
Summit
Wildflowers
Birds
Great Views
Secluded

FACILITIES
None

Best Time

All year, but trails may be extremely muddy in wet weather.

Finding the Trail

To park on Welch Creek Rd., you must have either a parking permit, available at the Sunol visitor center on Geary Rd., or a Regional Parks Foundation membership card—whichever you have, be sure to leave it on your dashboard when you park.

From Interstate 680 southbound in Scotts Corner, take the Calaveras Rd. exit, and at a stop sign turn left onto Paloma Rd. Go back under I-680, stay in the left lane, and at the next stop sign continue straight, now on Calaveras Rd. Go south 3.9 miles to Welch Rd., a winding, one-lane road. Turn left and go to the 1.6 mile marker, where two turnouts have space for about 6 to 8 cars total. The trailhead is on the north side of small parking area.

From I-680 northbound in Scotts Corner, take the Calaveras Rd. exit, bear right onto Calaveras Rd., then follow directions above.

OPTIONS

Biking Maguire Peaks

For a 9.3-mile route, bicyclists should start from the Sunol visitor center and pedal up the **Hayfield** and **High Valley Trails** to reach Welch Creek Rd. Turn left, go about 0.3 mile, and then turn right on the **Maguire Peaks Trail**, a dirt road. Climb about 0.3 mile to the intersection with Upper Maguire Peaks Trail,►2 then follow the described route.

Sunol Wilderness is one of the best places in the Bay Area to see yellow-billed magpies—large black-and-white birds with long tails, which are usually found in flocks.

To reach the Sunol visitor center, proceed past Welch Creek Rd. another 0.3 mile, turn left on Geary Rd., and go 1.8 miles to the entrance kiosk. Then continue 0.1 mile to the visitor center parking area, left. The area charges fees for parking and dogs.

Trail Description

From the parking area on Welch Creek Road,►1 walk north down a small embankment and cross Welch Creek on rocks, finding a trail post and the **Upper Maguire Peaks Trail**, a single track heading north. About 50 feet past the trail post, you step across a little tributary of Welch Creek and then follow its left-hand bank upstream on a level grade. About 100 yards from the trailhead, bear left at fork marked by a trail post and begin to climb across a steep, oak-shaded hillside on a generally northwest course.

Soon the trail climbs to a clearing, where you have a beautiful view north to Maguire Peaks—two rocky summits behind a foreground of rolling, grassy hills studded with oaks. For a short distance ahead, the route becomes indistinct: Follow metal trail posts and descend to a T-junction with the **Maguire Peaks Trail,** near the side of an old homestead.►2

Turn right and follow the dirt road, which soon bends sharply left and climbs moderately across a grassy slope. As you turn a corner and head north, enjoy another view of Maguire Peaks, then descend moderately through an oak woodland.

Reaching the bottom of a shady canyon, the route crosses a tributary of Welch Creek flowing through a culvert, and then climbs straight past an unnamed side road, left. Leaving the dense forest behind and entering oak savanna, you pass a junction with the Maguire Peaks Loop.►3 Here you continue straight, still on an ascending dirt road, and after another 0.3 mile reach a junction, marked by a metal trail post with an arrow pointing left.

Turn left, now on the **Maguire Peaks Loop**, with Mt. Diablo just visible over hills to the north. The route, a dirt road, bends north and then swings northwest to skirt the end of a ridge topped by the easternmost of the two **Maguire Peaks**, left.

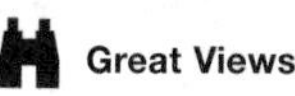

Circling around the north side of Maguire Peaks on a mostly level course, you reach an open area where the view extends northwest to Pleasanton and Sunol ridges. Soon the route begins a moderate climb, aiming for a flat spot in a ridge extending northwest from the west peak. The trail now turns left and briefly follows the ridgetop southeast, toward Maguire Peaks. Just before the route turns right and begins to descend, you arrive at a bench.►4

The taller of the two Maguire Peaks is the west peak (1688'), its grassy summit guarded by a rock rampart.

To climb the 1688-foot west peak, find an unsigned path beside the bench, angling southeast up a steep hillside. After you gain the main ridge, staying well to the right of a severe drop-off, the grade eases.

OPTIONS

Wet-Weather Access

During wet weather, the **Upper Maguire Peaks Trail** may be almost impassably muddy. As an alternate, walk from the parking area about 0.3 mile back (westward) on Welch Rd. to the Maguire Peaks trailhead, on the north side of the road (be alert for cars). Ascend **Maguire Peaks Trail** for about 0.3 mile to the Upper Maguire Peaks Trail junction►2, then follow the described route.

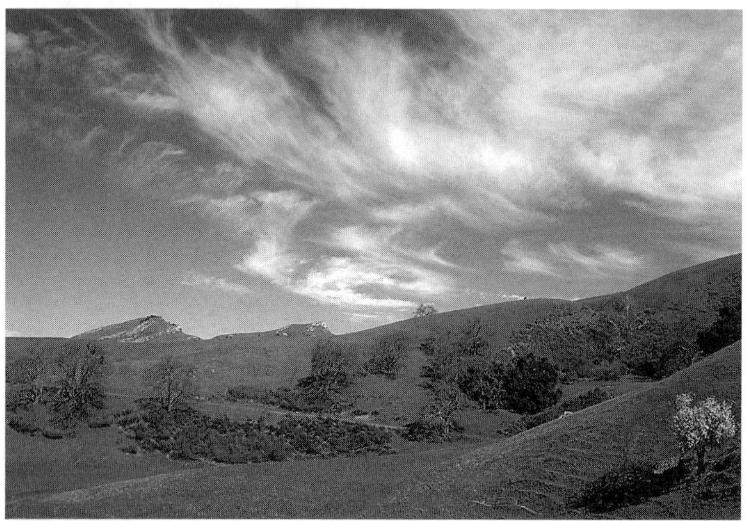

Maguire Peaks *are a prominent landmark on the north edge of Sunol Regional Wilderness.*

Soon you cross a rocky area, then tackle the final pitch up a grassy slope to the summit. A path leads across the summit to a 360-degree viewpoint.

Back on the Maguire Peaks Loop►4, you follow a winding course downhill, soon reaching level ground. Heading generally west, the route comes to the end of a long ridge, then bends around it to the south, crossing a culvert that drains a marshy area with a stock pond on the right. Now you pass a junction with the Lower Maguire Peaks Trail, right.►5 From here the Maguire Peaks Loop rises and falls gently to its junction with the **Maguire Peaks Trail.**►6 Turn right, then turn left at the junction near the old homestead,►7 and retrace your route to the parking area.►8

MILESTONES

▶1	0.0	Cross Welch Creek, north on Upper Maguire Peaks Trail, then bear left at fork
▶2	0.6	Right at T-junction with Maguire Peaks Trail
▶3	1.4	Straight on Maguire Peaks Loop
▶4	2.3	Unsigned path going southeast to west peak (out-and-back side trip)
▶5	3.8	Lower Maguire Peaks Trail on right; straight to stay on Maguire Peaks Loop
▶6	4.5	Right on Maguire Peak Trail
▶7	5.3	Straight on Upper Peaks Trail
▶8	5.9	Back at parking area

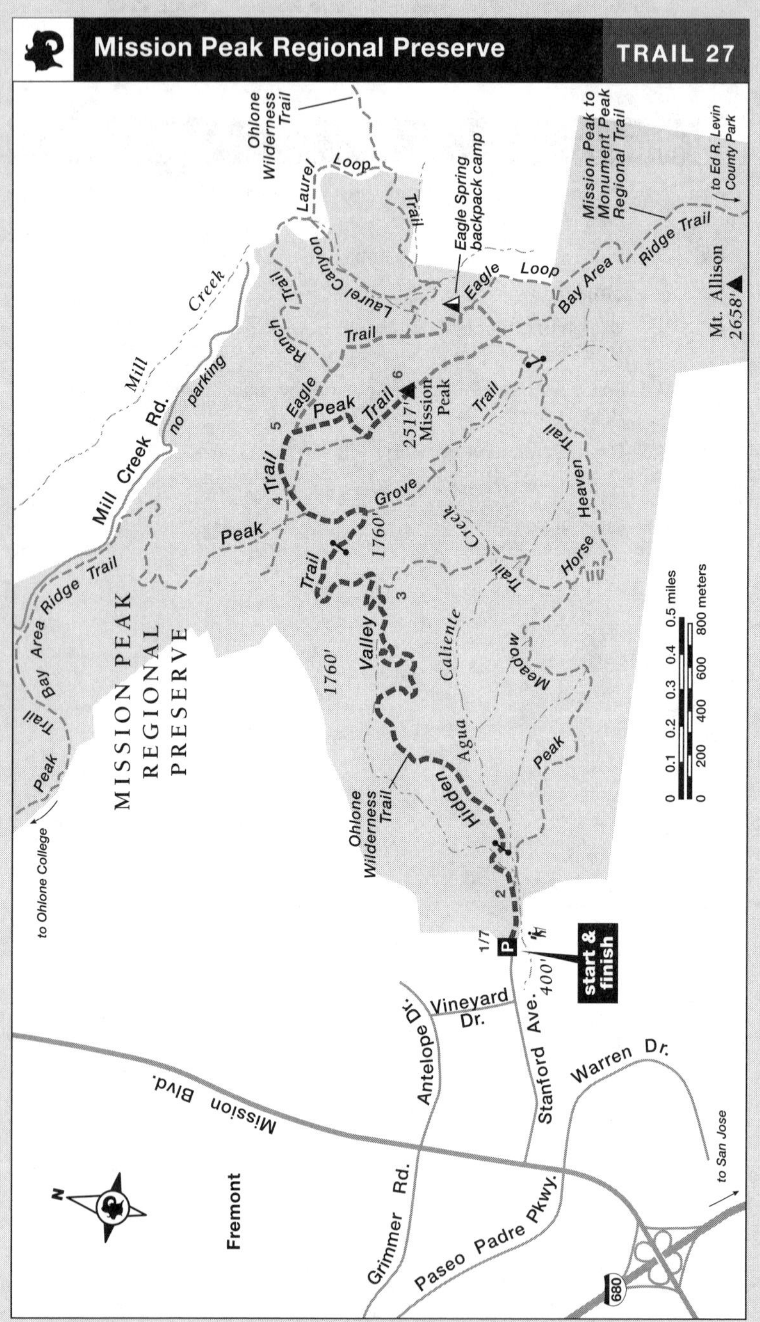
Mission Peak Regional Preserve
TRAIL 27
MISSION PEAK REGIONAL PRESERVE
Ohlone Wilderness Trail
Laurel Loop
Trail
Eagle Spring backpack camp
Mission Peak to Monument Peak Regional Trail
to Ed R. Levin County Park
Mill Creek
Mill Creek Rd.
no parking
Laurel Canyon
Ranch Trail
Eagle Trail
Eagle Loop
Bay Area Ridge Trail
Mt. Allison 2658'
Peak Trail
Eagle Peak Trail
2517' Mission Peak
Trail
Horse Heaven Trail
Peak Grove Trail
Creek
1760'
Valley Trail
Caliente
Meadow
Agua
Hidden Valley
Peak
Ohlone Wilderness Trail
Peak Trail
Bay Area Ridge Trail
to Ohlone College
0.5 miles
800 meters
start & finish
400'
Vineyard Dr.
Antelope Dr.
Stanford Ave.
Warren Dr.
Mission Blvd.
Fremont
Grimmer Rd.
Paseo Padre Pkwy.
680
to San Jose

Mission Peak Regional Preserve: Mission Peak

A steady climb of more than 2,000 feet in just over 3 miles brings you to one of the East Bay's most dramatic summits, offering views of the entire Bay Area. Not a hike for hot weather, try Mission Peak just after a winter or spring storm, when the air is clear and the hills green. Even on a warm day, however, take extra clothes and a wind shell—the mountain environment can quickly turn hostile.

TRAIL USE
Hike, Run, Bike, Dogs Allowed

LENGTH
6.3 miles, 4 hours

VERTICAL FEET
±2250'

DIFFICULTY
– 1 2 3 4 **5** +

TRAIL TYPE
Out & Back

SURFACE TYPE
Dirt

FEATURES
Mountain
Birds
Great Views
Steep

FACILITIES
Restrooms
Water

Best Time

Fall through spring; pick a clear day with good visibility.

Finding the Trail

From Interstate 880 in Fremont, take the Mission Blvd./Warren Ave. exit and go northeast on Mission Blvd. 1.8 miles to Stanford Ave. Turn right and go 0.6 mile to a parking area at the end of Stanford Ave.

From Interstate 680 in Fremont, take the Mission Blvd./Warms Springs District exit and follow signs for Mission Blvd. eastbound. Once on Mission Blvd., follow it for 0.6 mile to Stanford Ave. Turn right and go 0.6 mile to the parking area at the end of Stanford Ave.

Trail Description

From the east side of the parking area,►1 the **Hidden Valley Trail**, a dirt road, heads uphill toward Mission Peak. After about 200 yards, stay left

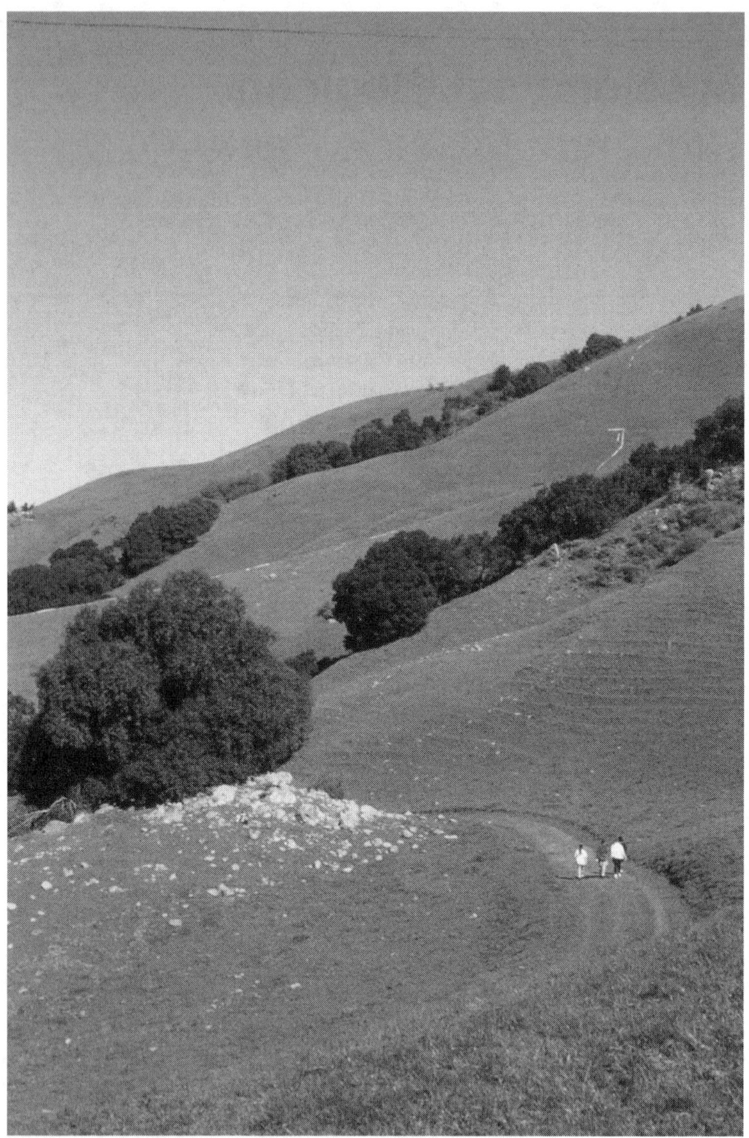

Hidden Valley Trail *ascends the west slope of Mission Peak.*

at the first fork, a unsigned junction with the Peak Meadow Trail.▶2 The road curves around several low knolls and passes through a gate. Please stay on the main road and observe all AREA CLOSED: NO ENTRY signs.

After about 0.3 mile, you reach an unsigned fork. Bear left and begin a gentle climb which soon becomes moderate. Just beyond a gate, the right-hand branch of the fork rejoins, but it diverges at the base of a rocky hill; here you again bear left.

Rising across grassy slopes, your route passes a wooded area, then bends south and continues to climb—and climb. You come to a short, steep section and then pass a junction with the Peak Meadow Trail, right.▶3 Here, 1.5 miles from the trailhead, you have already climbed 1,000 feet! Now the road begins the series of switchbacks that will carry you to the summit. Ahead, the terrain around you becomes more rugged.

If the day you've chosen is especially clear, you may be thrilled, when you crest the ridge, to see a line of snow-capped peaks in the distance—the Sierra Nevada—rising behind Livermore and Altamont Pass.

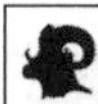

OPTIONS

Eagle Trail Descent

For hikers, a longer (another 0.7 mile) but easier descent from the summit is to follow the **Peak Trail** south 0.3 mile to a junction with the Horse Heaven Trail. Turn left and soon reach a junction with the **Eagle Loop Trail**, a dirt road. After a little more than 0.1 mile, stay left on the **Eagle Trail**. After 0.3 mile, you come to **Eagle Spring backpack camp**, which has four tent sites (available by reservation only; call 510-636-1684) with picnic tables, a toilet, and untreated water.

Now the Eagle Trail ambles north across rolling grassland, with the steep east face of Mission Peak looming left. Where the Laurel Canyon and Ranch trails go right, stay straight. At about 0.6 mile from the backpack camp the **Peak Trail**,▶5 enters left. Continue straight on the Peak Trail, then turn left onto the **Hidden Valley Trail** ▶4 at the next junction, and retrace your route to the parking area.

Just below a band of cliffs you come to a T-junction with the Grove Trail. To the southeast are old ranch buildings used by East Bay Regional Park District rangers, and looming above them is Mt. Allison, bristling with communication towers. Your route, now a gravel road, turns left and—surprise!—climbs steeply toward the skyline ridge. Respite arrives, just as you crest the ridge, in the form of a broad, flat area.

Steep

Where the gravel road branches left, you bear right on a dirt road, soon getting your first view today of Mt. Diablo and Pleasanton Ridge. Continue straight to the next junction, where you go straight on the **Peak Trail,** a dirt road.►4 Ahead, to the east, the land drops away to the Alameda Creek drainage, then rises up on the other side to form the highlands of the Sunol/Ohlone Wilderness.

Soon you reach a fork in the road.►5 Left is the Eagle Trail (part of the Ohlone Wilderness Regional/Bay Area Ridge Trails), but you angle right to stay on the Peak Trail and begin a gentle climb that soon turns steep, bringing you to the end of the road and a hitching post for horses and bikes. From here, join one of the several dirt paths that head southeast and steeply uphill to the summit of **Mission Peak.**►6

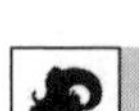
Summit

OPTIONS

Regional Trails from Mission Peak

The 28-mile **Ohlone Wilderness Regional Trail** passes through some of the East Bay's most scenic and remote territory. It starts at the Stanford Ave. parking area and follows your route up the west side of Mission Peak. From here it continues east to Sunol Wilderness, the Ohlone Wilderness, and Del Valle Regional Park near Livermore. The emblem for this trail, which you may see on trail posts here, is a white oak leaf in a red disk.

The **Bay Area Ridge Trail**, which runs north to Mission College and south to Ed R. Levin County Park, is also East Bay Regional Park District's **Mission Peak-to-Monument Peak Regional Trail.**

When you have finished enjoying this exhilarating and hard-won perch, retrace your route to the parking area.►7

Some of the most notable landmarks visible from Mission Peak include Mt. Hamilton's Lick Observatory (4209'); Rose Peak (3817') in the Ohlone Wilderness; Flag Hill, behind the visitor center in Sunol Wilderness; Moffett Field in Mountain View; Mt. Tamalpais; San Francisco; and Coyote Hills Regional Park.

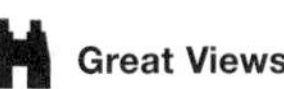

MILESTONES

►1	0.0	Take Hidden Valley Trail east
►2	0.1	Left at unsigned junction with Peak Meadow Trail
►3	1.5	Straight at junction with Peak Meadow Trail
►4	2.5	Right at four-way junction with Peak Trail
►5	2.7	Right at fork with Eagle Trail to stay on Peak Trail
►6	3.15	Mission Peak summit
►7	6.3	Retrace to parking area

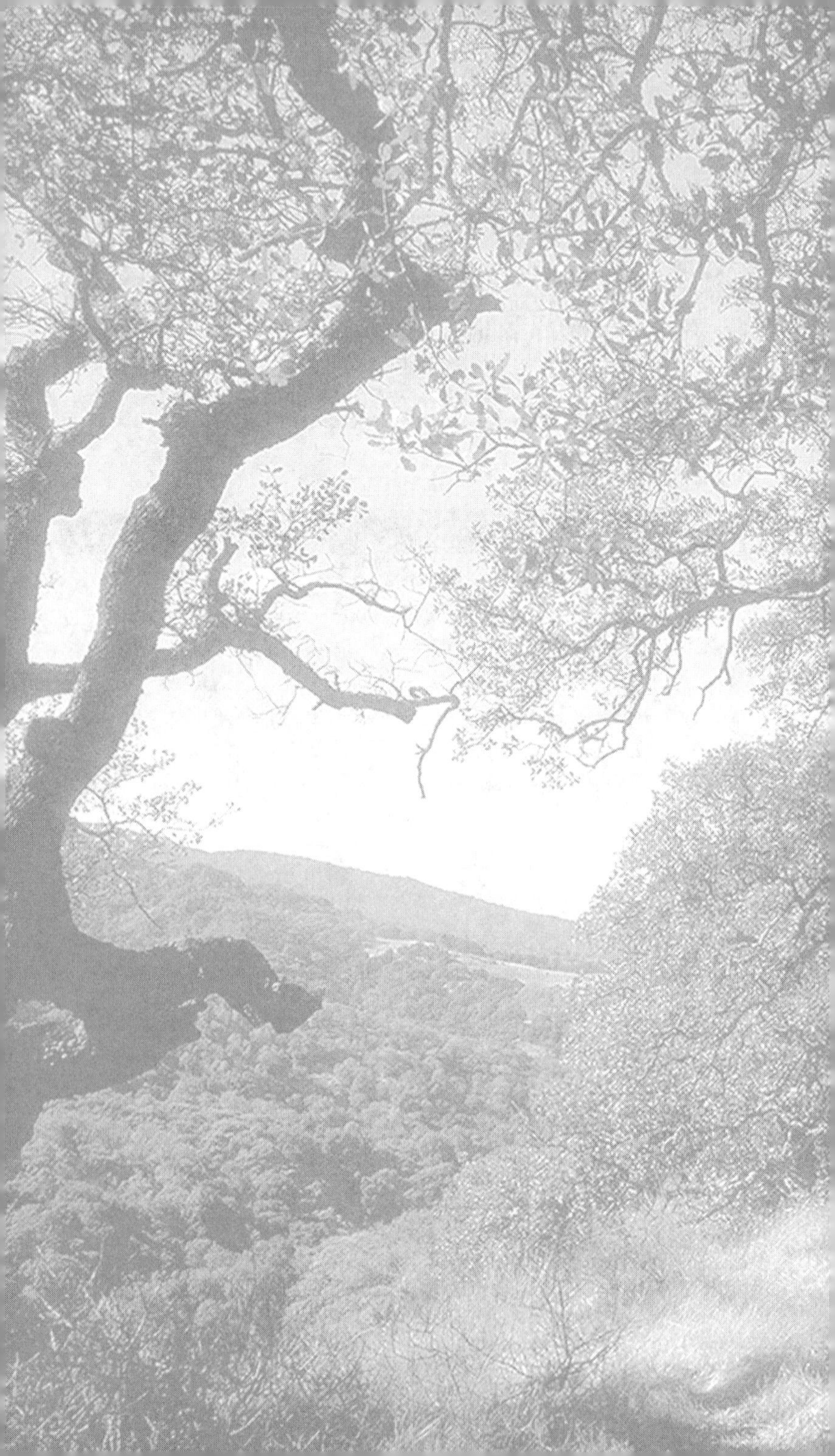

CHAPTER 3

South Bay

28. Ed R. Levin County Park
29. Joseph D. Grant County Park
30. Henry W. Coe State Park
31. Almaden Quicksilver County Park
32. Sierra Azul Open Space Preserve: Limekiln–Priest Rock Loop
33. Fremont Older Open Space Preserve

South Bay

The South Bay is home to Silicon Valley and San Jose, California's third-largest city. But the South Bay also includes some of the Bay Area's wildest and most biologically diverse terrain. To the west of the broad, relatively flat **Santa Clara Valley** rise the Santa Cruz Mountains, where redwood and Douglas-fir forests mingle with oak groves and dry chaparral. To the east the grassy foothills soar to the pine-clad ridges of the Diablo Range, which extend in ever drier stages to the Central Valley.

Winter rains turn the South Bay hills verdant green, and when cold winter storms arrive, the road to the University of California's Lick Observatory atop 4213-foot Mt. Hamilton may be closed by snow. But summer temperatures are often among the warmest in the Bay Area, and wildfires are not uncommon.

Santa Clara Valley, the backbone of the South Bay, was settled by immigrants drawn by its fertile soil Known as the "Valley of Heart's Delight," the orchards and farms here provided an abundant harvest of fruits, nuts, vegetables, and grain. Loggers made camps in the rugged Santa Cruz Mountains and began cutting the seemingly endless stands of coast redwoods. After World War II, technology and computer chips became the new basis of the South Bay's economy, and suburbs and industrial parks began to dominate the landscape. You may see the remnants of orchards in Fremont Older Open Space Preserve and on the way to Mt. Hamilton.

Although the South Bay lay far from the Sierra Nevada gold fields, mining also left its mark on the landscape. On the site of today's Almaden Quicksilver County Park, the New Almaden Mines operated from 1845 into the 1970s. Local cinnabar ore was refined into mercury, which was used in the extraction of gold and silver from their ores.

The South Bay has a growing network of county parks. Several, including Joseph D. Grant and Almaden Quicksilver, are quite large. On the west edge of San Jose, Midpeninsula Regional Open Space District's Sierra Azul is a vast work-in-progress which will someday provide access to 3806-foot Loma Prieta and 3486-foot Mt. Umunhum. Also here is Northern California's largest state park, Henry W. Coe, a vast tract in the remote country east of Morgan Hill.

See Appendix 2 for agency contact information (page 314) and Appendix 6 for maps (page 321).

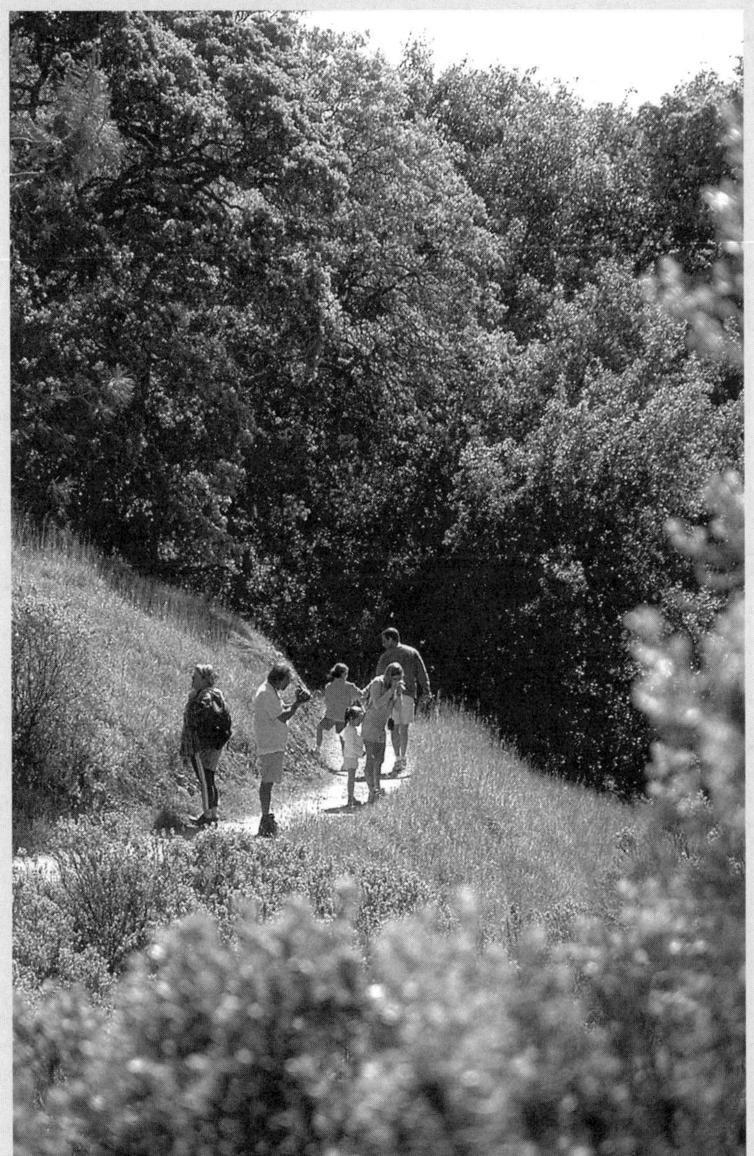

Hikers amble along the Corral Trail *in Henry W. Coe State Park (Trail 30).*

OVERVIEW MAP

South Bay

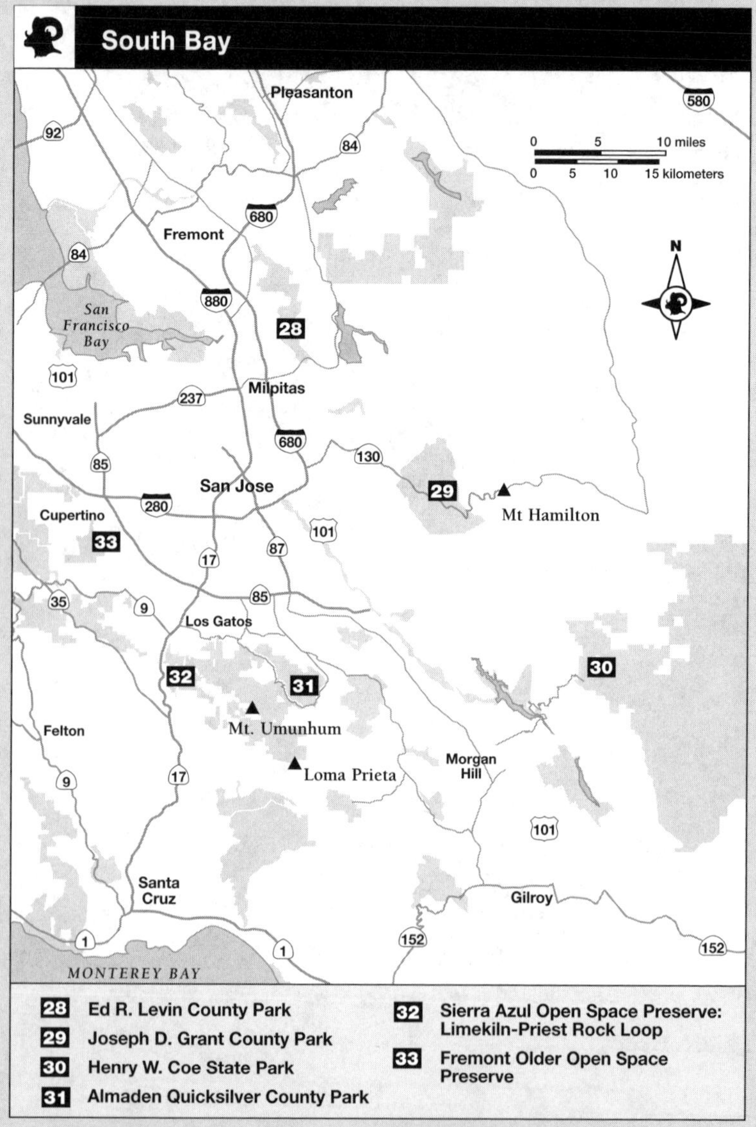

TRAIL FEATURE TABLE

South Bay

TRAIL	Difficulty	Length	Type	USES & ACCESS	TERRAIN	FLORA & FAUNA	OTHER
28	5	7.8	Loop	Hiking, Running, Fee	River or Stream, Canyon, Summit	Birds, Wildlife	Great Views, Steep
29	5	9.8	Loop	Hiking, Running, Biking	Summit	Birds	Great Views, Secluded, Camping
30	4	6.3	Loop	Hiking, Running, Fee	River or Stream, Canyon	Wildflowers, Birds, Wildlife	Historic, Secluded, Camping
31	5	7.0	Loop	Hiking, Running, Dogs Allowed	River or Stream, Canyon, Summit	Birds	Historic, Geologic Interest, Great Views, Secluded, Steep
32	3	5.2	Loop	Hiking, Running, Biking, Dogs Allowed	River or Stream, Canyon	Autumn Colors, Wildflowers, Birds	Historic, Great Views, Secluded
33	3	3.1	Loop	Hiking, Running, Biking, Child Friendly, Dogs Allowed	Canyon, Summit	Wildflowers, Birds	Great Views

USES & ACCESS
- Hiking
- Running
- Biking
- Child Friendly
- Dogs Allowed
- $ Fee
- Permit Required

TYPE
- Loop
- Out & Back
- Point to Point

DIFFICULTY
-1 2 3 4 5 +
less more

TERRAIN
- River or Stream
- Waterfall
- Lake or Shore
- Canyon
- Mountain
- Summit

FLORA & FAUNA
- Autumn Colors
- Wildflowers
- Birds
- Wildlife

OTHER
- Historic
- Geologic Interest
- Great Views
- Photo Opportunity
- Secluded
- Cool & Shady
- Camping
- Steep

1 *Bicyclists use described alternate trails or trailheads*

South Bay

TRAIL 28

Hike, Run
7.8 miles, Loop
Difficulty: 1 2 3 4 **5**

Explore the high ground on the border of Alameda and Santa Clara counties for great views and the chance to spot hawks, falcons, and even golden eagles. Open grasslands dominate here, with occasional shady, creek-filled canyons.

TRAIL 29

Hike, Run, Bike
9.8 miles, Loop
Difficulty: 1 2 3 4 **5**

Following a rolling, ridgetop course to Antler Point, you enjoy views of nearby Mt. Hamilton and the distant Santa Cruz Mountains. Returning, the trail dips to Deer Camp and a marshy meadow, then resumes its quest of high places.

TRAIL 30

Hike, Run
6.3 miles, Loop
Difficulty: 1 2 3 **4** 5

This loop to Frog Lake and Middle Ridge samples only a small corner of Northern California's largest state park, but may whet your appetite for exploring this magnificent area's rugged canyons, oak-studded ridges, and skyscraping slopes.

TRAIL 31

Hike, Run,
Dogs Allowed
7.0 miles, Loop
Difficulty: 1 2 3 4 **5**

Travel back in time on this strenuous route through one of the Bay Area's most famous mining areas, where cinnabar ore was mined and converted into mercury in fiery brick furnaces. Today, oak woodlands, grasslands, and chaparral are the main attractions of this rugged and remote park.

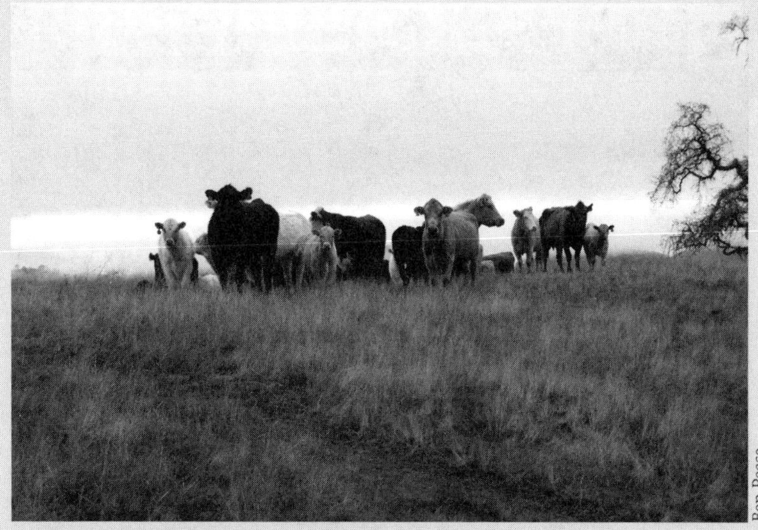
Ben Pease

A herd of cows *at Joseph Grant County Park (Trail 29)*

Sierra Azul Open Space Preserve: Limekiln–Priest Rock Loop 227

TRAIL 32

Hike, Run, Bike, Dogs Allowed
5.2 miles, Loop
Difficulty: 1 2 **3** 4 5

This loop visits the northwest corner of Sierra Azul, Midpeninsula Regional Open Space District's largest, most remote preserve. Much of the journey is over serpentine soil, which gives rise to a fascinating community of shrubs and wildflowers. Early blooming shrubs, such as manzanita and currant, may add splashes of unexpected color as early as December, and bright red toyon berries attract numerous species of hungry songbirds.

Fremont Older Open Space Preserve 233

TRAIL 33

Hike, Run, Bike, Child Friendly, Dogs Allowed
3.1 miles, Loop
Difficulty: 1 2 **3** 4 5

Varied terrain and superb views from Hunters Point make this route a favorite among South Bay hikers. In spring, the grasslands come alive with wildflowers, and the Seven Springs Trail offers shady respite on a warm day. Remnants of walnut and apricot orchards hearken back to Santa Clara Valley's heyday as an agricultural paradise.

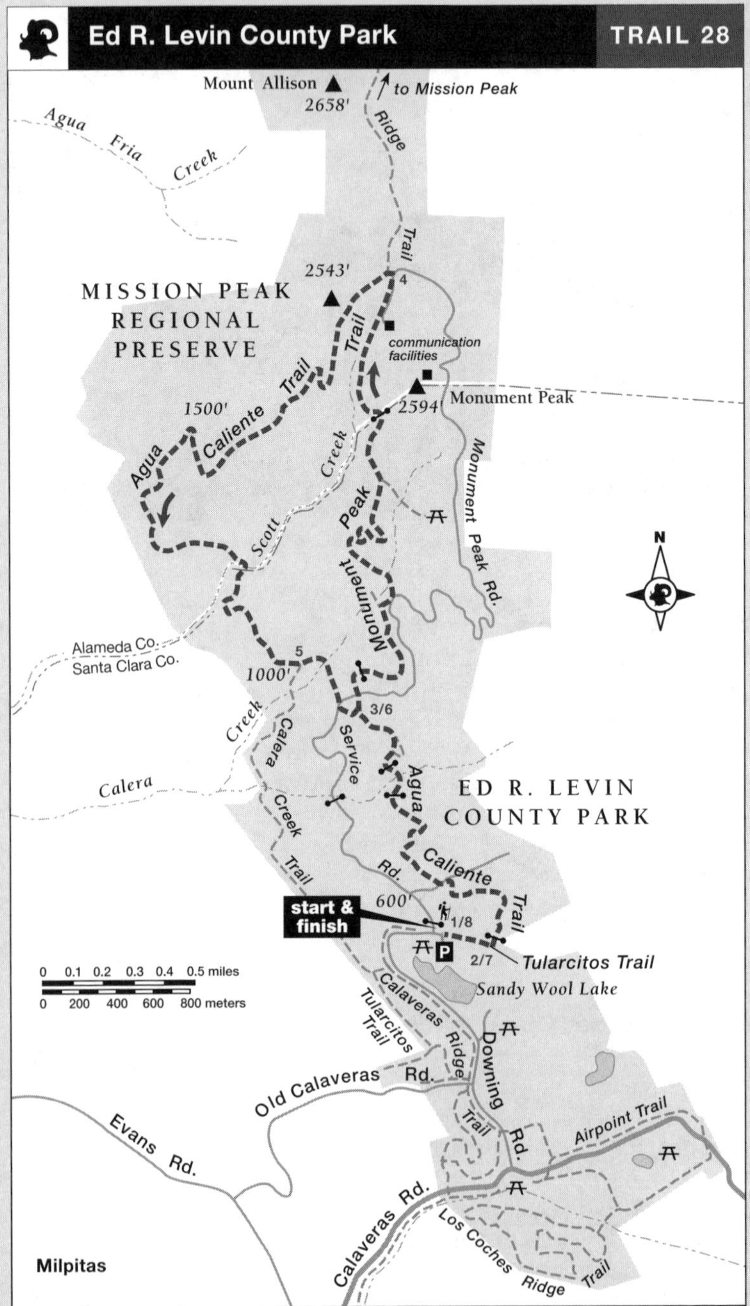
Ed R. Levin County Park
TRAIL 28
Mount Allison
2658'
to Mission Peak
Agua Fria Creek
Ridge Trail
2543'
MISSION PEAK REGIONAL PRESERVE
Trail
communication facilities
Monument Peak
2594'
1500'
Agua Caliente Trail
Scott Creek
Monument Peak Trail
Monument Peak Rd.
N
Alameda Co.
Santa Clara Co.
5
1000'
3/6
Creek
Calera
Service Rd.
Agua Caliente Trail
ED R. LEVIN COUNTY PARK
Calera
Creek Trail
600'
start & finish
1/8
2/7
Tularcitos Trail
Sandy Wool Lake
0 0.1 0.2 0.3 0.4 0.5 miles
0 200 400 600 800 meters
Calaveras Ridge
Tularcitos Trail
Downing Rd.
Old Calaveras Rd.
Trail
Airpoint Trail
Evans Rd.
Calaveras Rd.
Los Coches Ridge Trail
Milpitas

Ed R. Levin County Park

Explore the high ground on the border of Alameda and Santa Clara counties via this aerobic route, and you will be rewarded with great views and the chance to spot hawks, falcons, and even golden eagles. Open grasslands dominate here, but you also cross wooded canyons holding Calera and Scott creeks. You may find yourself tracing mini-switchbacks across the steep dirt roads that serve as your trail, but views of Monument Peak and Mt. Hamilton should spur you onward.

TRAIL USE
Hike, Run

LENGTH
7.8 miles, 5–6 hours

VERTICAL FEET
±2800'

DIFFICULTY
– 1 2 3 4 **5** +

TRAIL TYPE
Loop

SURFACE TYPE
Dirt

FEATURES
Fee
Stream
Canyon
Summit
Birds
Wildlife
Great Views
Steep

FACILITIES
Restrooms
Picnic Tables
Water
Phone

Best Time

Fall through spring, but trails may be muddy in wet weather.

Finding the Trail

From Interstate 680 in Milpitas, take the Calaveras Blvd./Milpitas exit and go east 1.9 miles to Downing Rd. Turn left and after 0.5 mile come to an entrance kiosk and self-registration station. Go another 0.9 mile to a paved parking area just north of Sandy Wool Lake. The trailhead is at the end of Downing Rd., about 100 yards northeast of the parking area.►1

Trail Description

Passing an information board, go east on the **Tularcitos Trail,** a dirt road. Skirt a metal gate and climb gently to a junction with a side trail, right, then steeply to meet the **Agua Caliente Trail.**►2 Turn left on this dirt road. There are a number of cattle gates

Look skyward for birds, especially hawks, falcons, kites, and golden eagles.

on this route; make sure you close each one after passing through it.

Your road follows a rolling course, sometimes pitching steeply upward. After passing a hang-glider launch area and a water tank, you cross a service road and then begin a series of switchbacks that climb on a grade alternating between moderate and steep. Now you descend to a wooded ravine that holds a tributary of Calera Creek. Creekside trees include coast live oak, California bay, bigleaf maple, and western sycamore. As you climb from this drainage, an unsigned dirt road departs right and then rejoins.

At a junction with the **Monument Peak Trail,**▶3 you leave the Agua Caliente Trail and veer right. Just ahead, you cross Monument Peak Road, closed to trail users. Here you continue straight, passing a watering trough and an unofficial trail heading downhill and left.

Monument Peak is one of the Bay Area's best places for hang-gliding, under the auspices of the Wings of Rogallo hang-gliding club.

Now the trail ascends steeply though a gate and beside a wooded gulch. Monument Peak Road, uphill, is visible from time to time. Ignore a prominent cow path branching left; instead, turn right toward a large rock outcrop above the trail.

Now the trail comes to **Calera Creek,** which you may have to step across on rocks. North of the creek, the trail finds level ground, and you begin to see the communication towers atop **Monument Peak** (2594'), which is uphill and right. Soon the trail swings right and begins a steep, winding ascent.

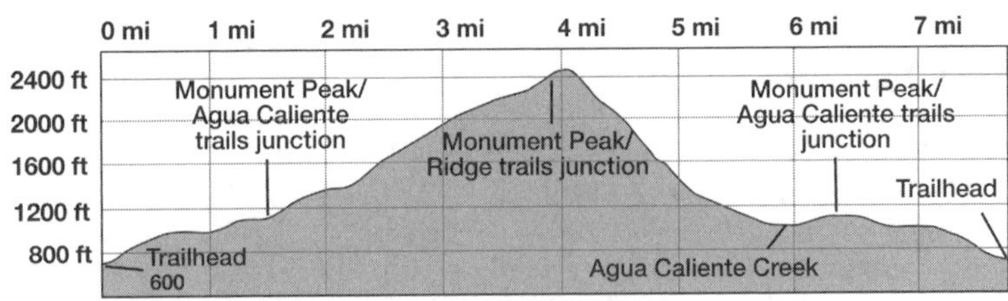

TRAIL 28 Ed R. Levin County Park Profile

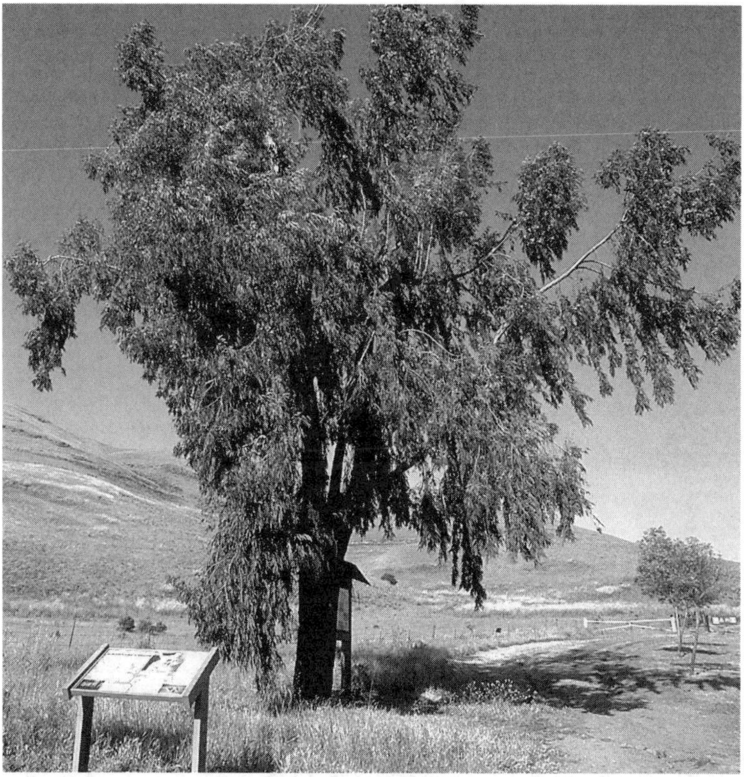

A eucalyptus tree *and signs mark the start of the Tularcitos Trail.*

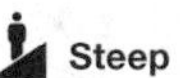
Steep

Climb past a junction with the Sierra Trail, right. Just southwest of Monument Peak, you leave Santa Clara County and enter the East Bay Regional Park District's **Mission Peak Regional Preserve** at a gate. Mt. Hamilton, topped with observatory domes, rises to the southeast.

Now, a nearly level walk takes you past the headwaters of Scott Creek. With a communication tower looming overhead, you join a gravel road and head straight for a saddle and a junction.▶**4** Here the gravel road you have been on bends right and enters a restricted area. The road continuing straight

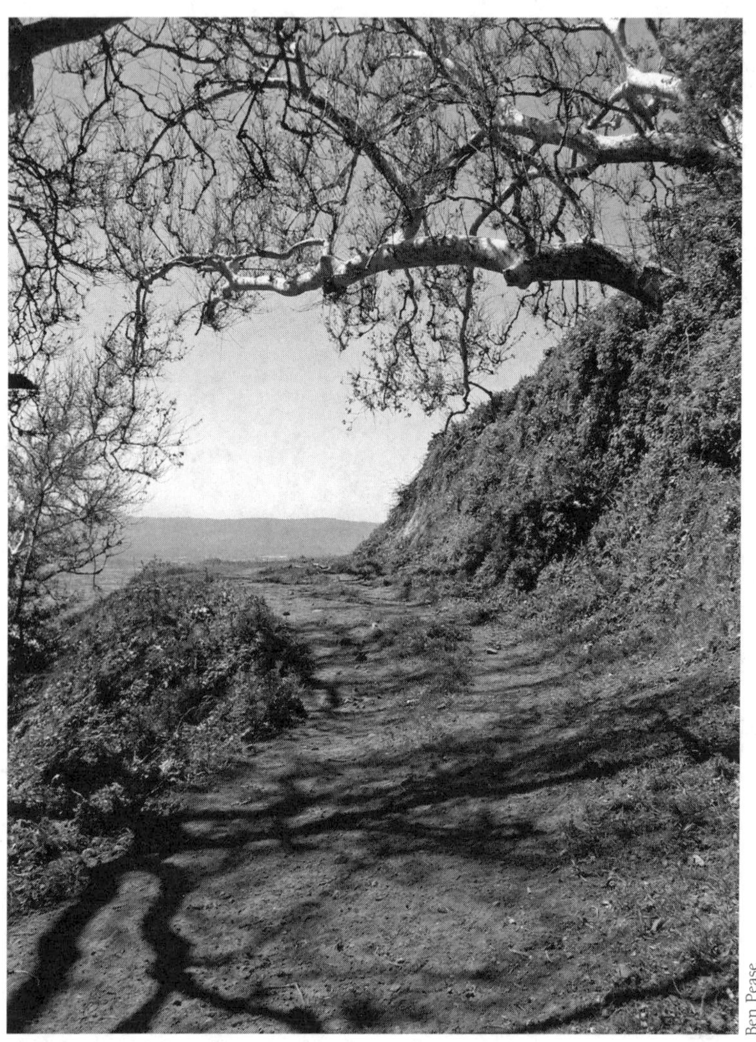

Sycamores *shade the trail near Scott Creek.*

is signed MISSION PEAK TO MONUMENT PEAK REGIONAL TRAIL, and is part of the Bay Area Ridge Trail. You turn sharply left on the **Agua Caliente Trail**, also part of the Bay Area Ridge Trail. This multiuse dirt road climbs gently, soon reaching the route's high point, a grassy summit just 50 feet lower than the summit of Monument Peak. The fine view from here takes in Mission Peak, Mt. Hamilton, Mt. Diablo, and most of the South Bay.

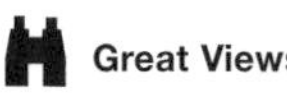

Skirting a communication facility, the road veers left and descends on a grade that shifts between moderate and steep. Eventually the grade eases and you make a winding descent into the wooded canyon holding **Scott Creek.** After crossing the creek, which flows through a culvert, you are faced with a short, steep climb. The road then bends sharply left and descends on a moderate and then steep grade. At a junction with the **Calera Creek Trail,**▶5 right, you stay straight on the **Agua Caliente Trail** to its junction with the **Monument Peak Trail.**▶6 From here, angle right to retrace your route on the **Agua Caliente Trail** to its junction with the **Tularcitos Trail.**▶7 Now turn right and retrace your route to the parking area.▶8

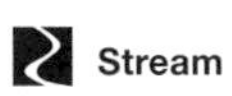

MILESTONES

▶1	0.0	Take Tularcitos Trail east
▶2	0.2	Left on Agua Caliente Trail
▶3	1.5	Right on Monument Peak Trail
▶4	3.9	Left on Agua Caliente Trail, left again at communication facility
▶5	6.0	Junction with Calera Creek Trail; straight to stay on Agua Caliente Trail
▶6	6.3	Junction with Monument Peak Trail; veer right to stay on Agua Caliente Trail and retrace to Tularcitos Trail
▶7	7.6	Right on Tularcitos Trail
▶8	7.8	Back at parking area

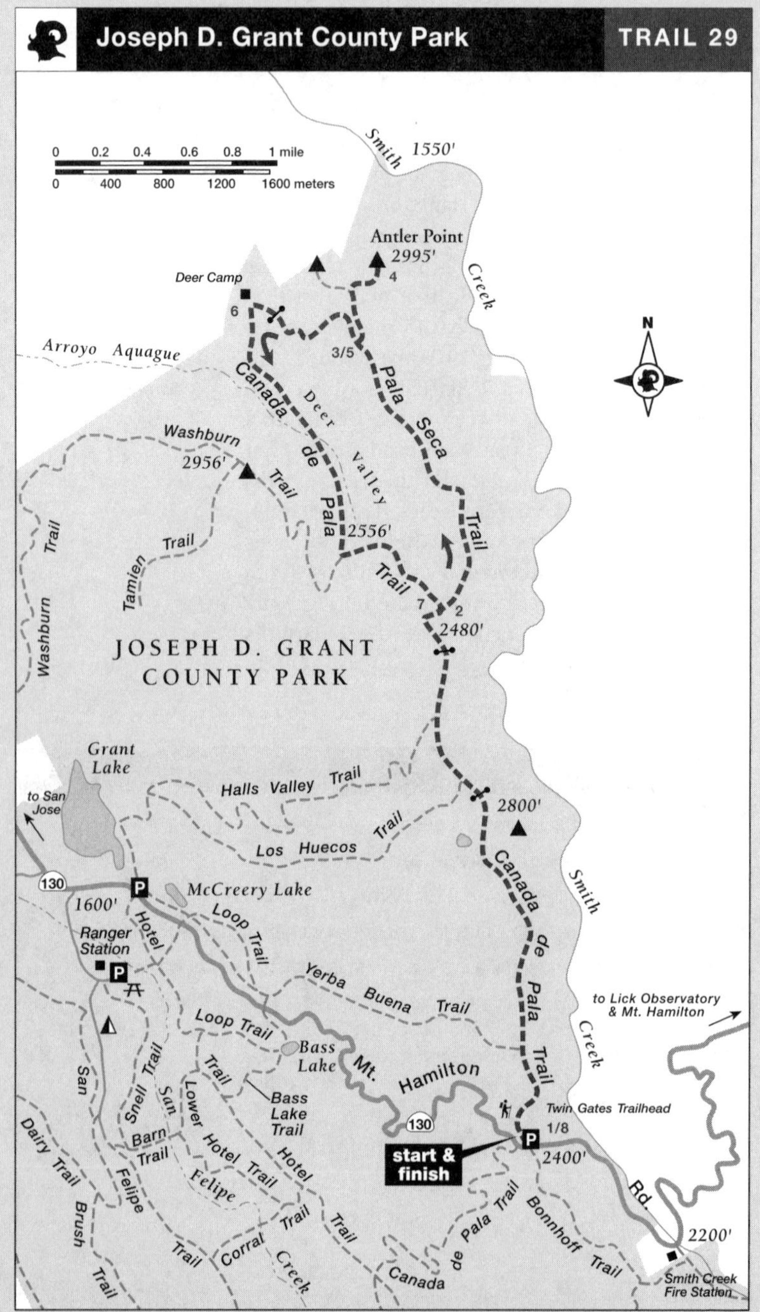
Joseph D. Grant County Park
TRAIL 29
0 0.2 0.4 0.6 0.8 1 mile
0 400 800 1200 1600 meters
Smith
1550'
Antler Point
2995'
Creek
Deer Camp
Arroyo Aquague
3/5
Canada
Deer
Pala
Seca
Washburn
2956'
Trail
de
Valley
Trail
Pala
2556'
Trail
Tamien
Trail
Washburn
2480'
JOSEPH D. GRANT
COUNTY PARK
Grant
Lake
to San
Jose
Halls Valley Trail
2800'
Los Huecos Trail
Canada
Smith
130
1600'
McCreery Lake
Hotel
Loop Trail
de
Ranger
Station
Yerba Buena Trail
Pala
to Lick Observatory
& Mt. Hamilton
Loop Trail
Bass
Lake
Creek
Mt. Hamilton
Trail
San
Snell Trail
San
Trail
Lower
Bass
Lake
Trail
Twin Gates Trailhead
1/8
start &
finish
2400'
Dairy Trail
Barn
Trail
Hotel Trail
Hotel
Felipe
Felipe
Trail
Pala Trail
Bonnhoff
Rd.
2200'
Brush
Trail
Corral
Trail
Creek
Canada
de
Trail
Smith Creek
Fire Station

Joseph D. Grant County Park

Following a mostly rolling, ridgetop course on the Canada de Pala and Pala Seca trails, you enjoy views of the Diablo Range, crowned by nearby Mt. Hamilton, and the distant Santa Cruz Mountains. From Antler Point, the trail dips into lovely Deer Valley but soon resumes its quest of high places. Camping is available in the park's main area. For reservations, phone (408) 355-2201 or reserve online at www.gooutsideandplay.org.

TRAIL USE
Hike, Run, Bike
LENGTH
9.8 miles, 4–6 hours
VERTICAL FEET
±1650'
DIFFICULTY
– 1 2 3 4 **5** +
TRAIL TYPE
Loop
SURFACE TYPE
Dirt

FEATURES
Summit
Birds
Great Views
Secluded
Camping

FACILITIES
Restrooms
Picnic Tables
Water
Phone

Best Time

Fall through spring.

Finding the Trail

From Interstate 680 in San Jose, take the Alum Rock exit, go northeast 2.2 miles to Mt. Hamilton Rd., and turn right. At 7.7 miles you pass the entrance to the park's main area. Continue another 3.4 miles to a paved parking area, left, for the Twin Gates Trailhead. The trailhead is on the west side of the parking area.

Trail Description

From the trailhead,▶1 go through a metal gate and then climb moderately on the **Canada de Pala Trail**, a dirt road. The road bends right and gains the top of a ridge. Mt. Hamilton, a hulking giant topped by 4373-foot Copernicus Peak, rises to your east. The white domes clustered around Mt. Hamilton's

If the Santa Clara Valley is foggy, you may be reveling under clear skies with views of the Santa Cruz Mountains to the west.

summit belong to University of California's Lick Observatory.

Soon the grade eases, and you enjoy a rolling course over mostly open, grassy terrain. At a junction with the Yerba Buena Trail, left, you continue straight, eventually passing a rest bench and a stock pond, both left. After passing through a cattle gate, you descend past a junction, left, with the Los Huecos Trail, a dirt road. Continuing straight and steadily losing elevation, you pass the Halls Valley Trail, left, and then a saddle in the ridge you've been following.

Climbing to a junction where the Canada de Pala Trail►2 bends left, you continue straight, now on the **Pala Seca Trail.** This trail, also a dirt road, climbs moderately and then steeply, still following the crest of a ridge. A rest bench, right, invites you to stay awhile and relish the scenery.

The road levels, curves right, and then begins to descend. Twin summits are just ahead, the right one being **Antler Point.** You reach it via the **Antler Point Trail,** a single track angling right.►3 This trail wanders across a hillside and soon reaches an unsigned fork. You bear right on the less prominent trail and climb gently for 0.2 mile to trail's end.►4 (The left-hand trail also leads to a summit, with a rest bench.) The view northward from Antler Point takes in a rugged ensemble of canyons, ravines, and ridges that make up some of the wildest land in the

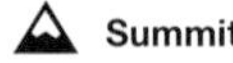

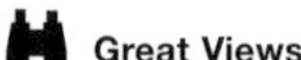

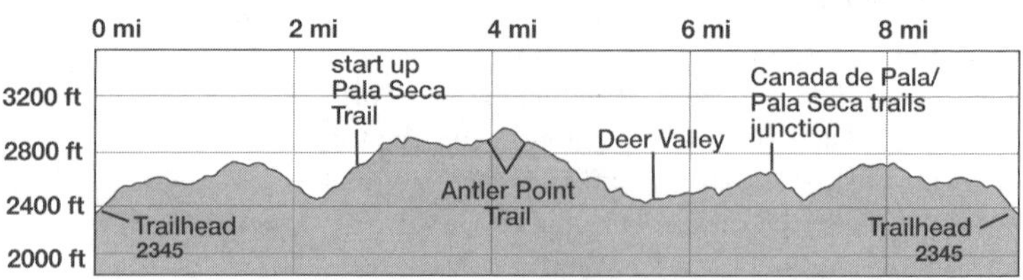

TRAIL 29 Joseph D. Grant County Park Profile

Bay Area. After enjoying this invigorating scene, retrace your route to the **Pala Seca Trail.**►5

Now you make a hard right on the dirt road, pass a rest bench, and begin to descend via S-bends. In places the road is rocky, eroded, and perhaps muddy where a creek trickles across. After losing elevation, you climb on a gentle grade to a barbed-wire fence and a cattle gate. Once through the gate, you pass **Deer Camp,** site of an old hunting cabin that has a picnic table on its shady back porch.►6 Here the Pala Seca Trail ends and blends seamlessly into the **Canada de Pala Trail.** Resuming the descent, you drop steeply into a ravine, then cross a low divide and enter beautiful, wide **Deer Valley.** Soon you are beside a creek that creates a marshy tract of sedges and rushes. A culvert carries the creek under the road and puts it on your left.

A wet meadow, left, marks the head of the creek. An extensive ground squirrel colony is nearby. Now you pass a junction with the Washburn Trail, a dirt road heading right. You continue straight and climb out of the valley at its south end. Soon you reach a cattle gate, and just beyond is the junction with the **Pala Seca Trail.**►7 From here, bear right and retrace your route along the rolling ridge to the parking area.►8

From the Canada de Pala Trail you can see two Bay Area mountain ranges—the Diablo Range and the Santa Cruz Mountains.

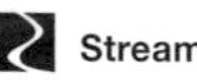

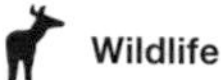

MILESTONES

►1	0.0	Take the Canada de Pala Trail
►2	2.6	Straight on Pala Seca Trail
►3	4.2	Right on trail to Antler Point
►4	4.4	Antler Point; retrace to previous junction
►5	4.6	Right on Pala Seca Trail
►6	5.3	Deer Camp, straight on Canada de Pala Trail
►7	7.2	Right to stay on Canada de Pala Trail, retrace to parking area
►8	9.8	Back at parking area

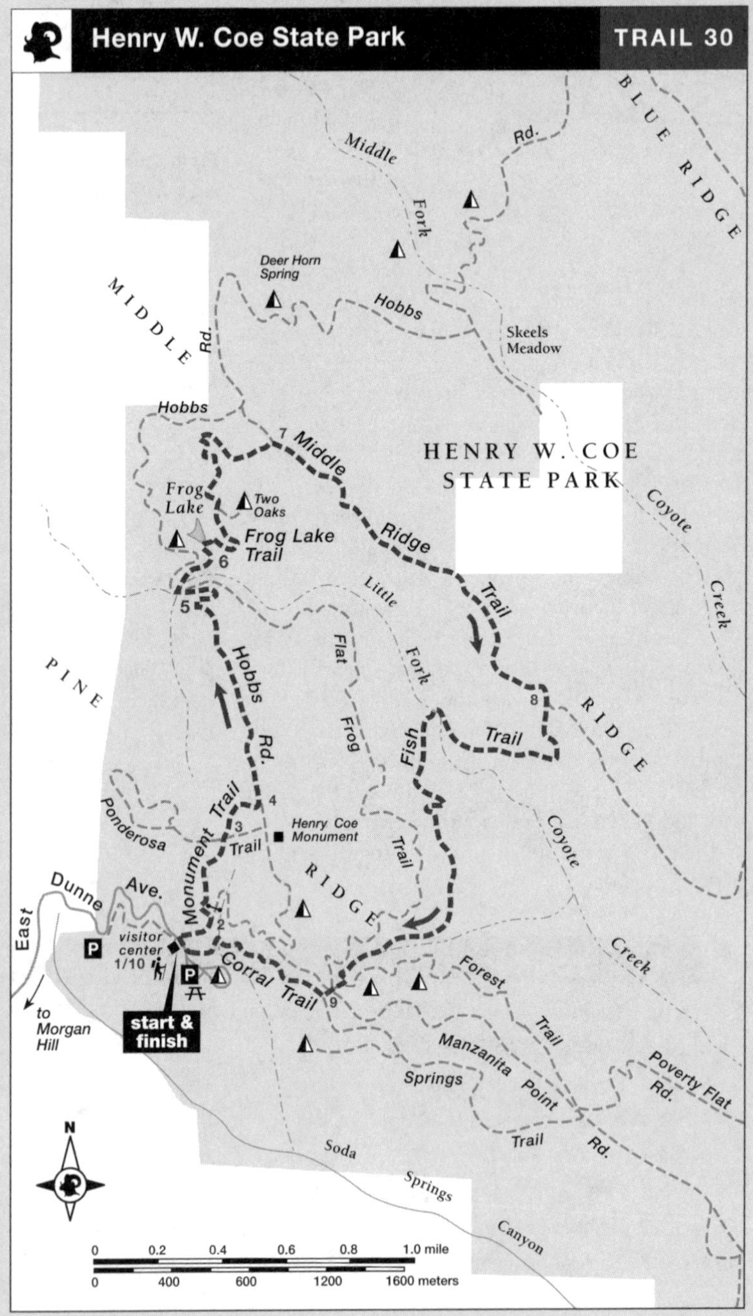
Henry W. Coe State Park
TRAIL 30
HENRY W. COE STATE PARK
BLUE RIDGE
Middle Fork Rd.
Deer Horn Spring
Hobbs
Skeels Meadow
MIDDLE Rd.
Hobbs
7
Middle Ridge Trail
Frog Lake
Two Oaks
Frog Lake Trail
6
5
Coyote Creek
Little Fork
Flat Frog Trail
Hobbs Rd.
PINE
8
Fish Trail
RIDGE
4
3
Monument Trail
Henry Coe Monument
Ponderosa Trail
Coyote Creek
RIDGE
East Dunne Ave.
2
visitor center
1/10
P
P
Corral Trail
9
Forest Trail
to Morgan Hill
start & finish
Manzanita Point Rd.
Springs Trail
Poverty Flat Rd.
Soda Springs Canyon
N
0
0.2
0.4
0.6
0.8
1.0 mile
0
400
600
1200
1600 meters

Henry W. Coe State Park

This loop samples only a small corner of Northern California's largest state park, but it should whet your appetite for further exploration of this magnificent area. From the trailhead you ascend through stands of ponderosa pines, then drop steeply to Little Fork Coyote Creek. On Middle Ridge, you enjoy a long ramble until diverted by the Fish Trail into several canyons. An easy, shady walk completes the circuit. The visitors center is open Friday through Sunday in spring and summer and Saturday and Sunday in fall and winter.

TRAIL USE
Hike, Run

LENGTH
6.3 miles, 3–4 hours

VERTICAL FEET
±1950'

DIFFICULTY
– 1 2 3 **4** 5 +

TRAIL TYPE
Loop

SURFACE TYPE
Dirt, Paved

FEATURES
Fee
Stream
Canyon
Wildflowers
Birds
Wildlife
Historic
Secluded
Camping

FACILITIES
Visitor Center
Picnic Tables
Restrooms
Water
Phone

Best Time

This route is best during spring and fall.

Finding the Trail

From US Hwy. 101 in Morgan Hill, take the E. Dunne Ave./Morgan Hill exit and go northeast on E. Dunne Ave. At 11.7 miles you reach the Coe Ranch entrance and the overflow parking area (a short trail leads from here to the main entrance). At 12.3 miles is the main entrance. There are fees for parking and camping; backpackers must register at the visitor center. The trailhead is several hundred feet back on E. Dunne Ave., at the foot of Manzanita Point Rd.

Trail Description

Climbing moderately from the trailhead▶1 on paved **Manzanita Point Road**, you soon reach a gate and a junction. Here you angle left on the **Monument**

The park's fine stands of ponderosa pines are a rarity in the Bay Area. Usually found in mountains, these stately trees are the most common pine in North America.

Trail, a single track closed to bikes and horses.►2 Switchbacks help you gain elevation to a four-way junction with the Ponderosa Trail.►3 During the climb, you are rewarded with fine southward views. From the junction, the **Henry W. Coe monument** is about 0.1 mile to your right, just across Hobbs Road. Cattle rancher Henry W. "Harry" Coe (1860–1943) lived with his wife, Rhoda Dawson Sutcliffe, at Pine Ridge Ranch, which formed the nucleus of today's state park. In 1953, their daughter, Sada, donated the more than 12,000 acres of ranchland to Santa Clara County, as a memorial to her father. Today, with 87,000 acres under protection, Henry W. Coe is the largest Northern California state park.

Camping

From the four-way junction, continue on the Monument Trail to where it merges with **Hobbs Road,** on which you veer left.►4 Making a long descent on a moderate and then steep grade, you pass the Flat Frog Trail, right, just before **Little Fork Coyote Creek.** Step across the seasonal creek to the next junction, where you turn sharply right on the **Frog Lake Trail,**►5 a single track closed to bikes and horses. After a few tight switchbacks, you meet Hobbs Road at **Frog Lake,**►6 where camping is available. There are 19 designated backcountry campsites in the park; there are also "backpacking zones" where camping is not restricted to designated sites (see Appendix 2, page 314, for more information).

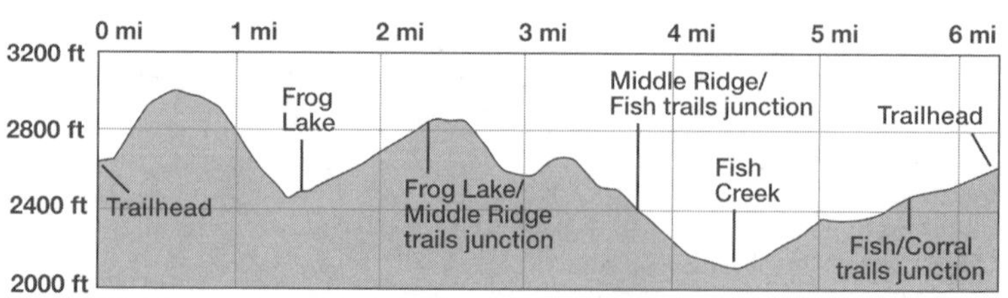

TRAIL 30 Henry W. Coe State Park Profile

Turning right, you cross the earthen dam that made the lake, pass a faint trail that circles the lake, and then start to climb a grassy, oak-shaded hillside by switchbacking right, still on the Frog Lake Trail.

 Camping

Passing a short trail to Two Oaks Camp, right, you wind your way gently uphill to a T-junction with the **Middle Ridge Trail.**▶7 Turning right, you climb gently across an open field and then begin to descend on a moderate grade through stands of gray pine and blue oak. Beyond a saddle, the trail rises steeply, then descends through a corridor of chaparral that includes giant manzanitas.

This park is infested with wild pigs, and you may see evidence beside the trail of their destructive rooting.

At a junction with the **Fish Trail,**▶8 you turn right and leave the ridge you have been following. In places the trail is merely a ledge cut in the hillside, so use caution. A rolling course brings you to **Little Fork Coyote Creek,** which you step across on rocks. Now the trail zigzags uphill and then contours across a hillside that slopes left. After passing a seasonal creek in a mossy, fern-filled ravine, you climb steeply via switchbacks to a saddle. Now a gentle descent over open and then forested ground puts you in a narrow canyon that holds a tributary of Little Fork Coyote Creek, which you follow upstream.

Leaving the canyon, the trail climbs to a broad ridgetop and several junctions with a welter of trails.▶9 First is a four-way junction with the self-guiding Forest Trail, left, and the Flat Frog Trail, right. Then, past an information board, you come to Manzanita Point Road and a short connector trail, just across it. Cross the dirt road, and go straight

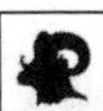

OPTIONS

Ponderosa Trail

From the junction of Monument and Ponderosa trails,▶3 go left on the **Ponderosa Trail** for a gentle, 1.1-mile semiloop through meadows and beneath stately pines overlooking the **Santa Clara Valley.**

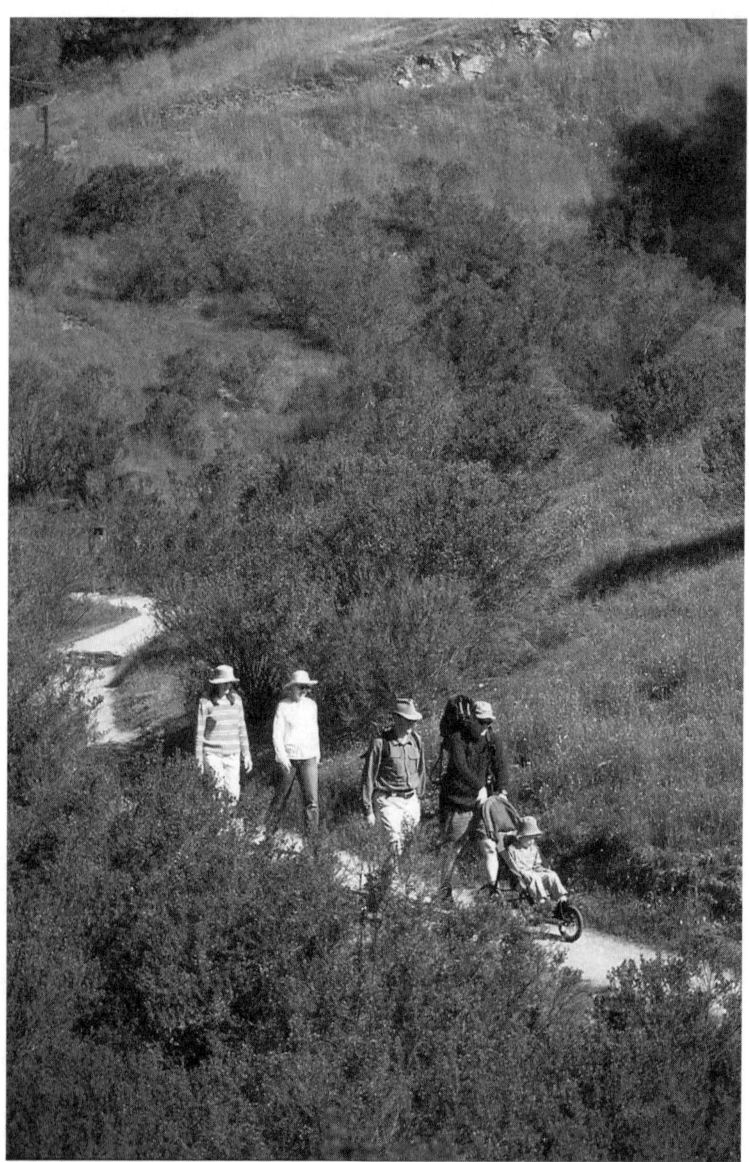

Corral Trail *in Henry Coe State Park*

on the connector trail a few hundred feet to the Corral Trail, on which you turn right. Now you enjoy a level walk across a forested hillside that falls steeply to **Soda Springs Canyon.** The trail ducks into and swings out of ravines cut into the hillside. Climbing on a gentle grade, you reach open ground, curve left, and cross a bridge over a branch of the creek. Just ahead is the parking area and park headquarters.►10

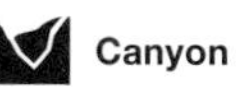

MILESTONES

►1	0.0	Take Manzanita Point Rd. (paved) northeast
►2	0.1	Left on Monument Trail
►3	0.4	Straight at junction with Ponderosa Trail; trail to Coe monument on right
►4	0.6	Left on Hobbs Rd.
►5	1.4	Right on Frog Lake Trail
►6	1.6	Frog Lake; cross dam and climb on Frog Lake Trail
►7	2.4	Right on Middle Ridge Trail
►8	3.8	Right on Fish Trail
►9	5.7	Cross Manzanita Point Rd., then right on Corral Trail
►10	6.3	Back at parking area

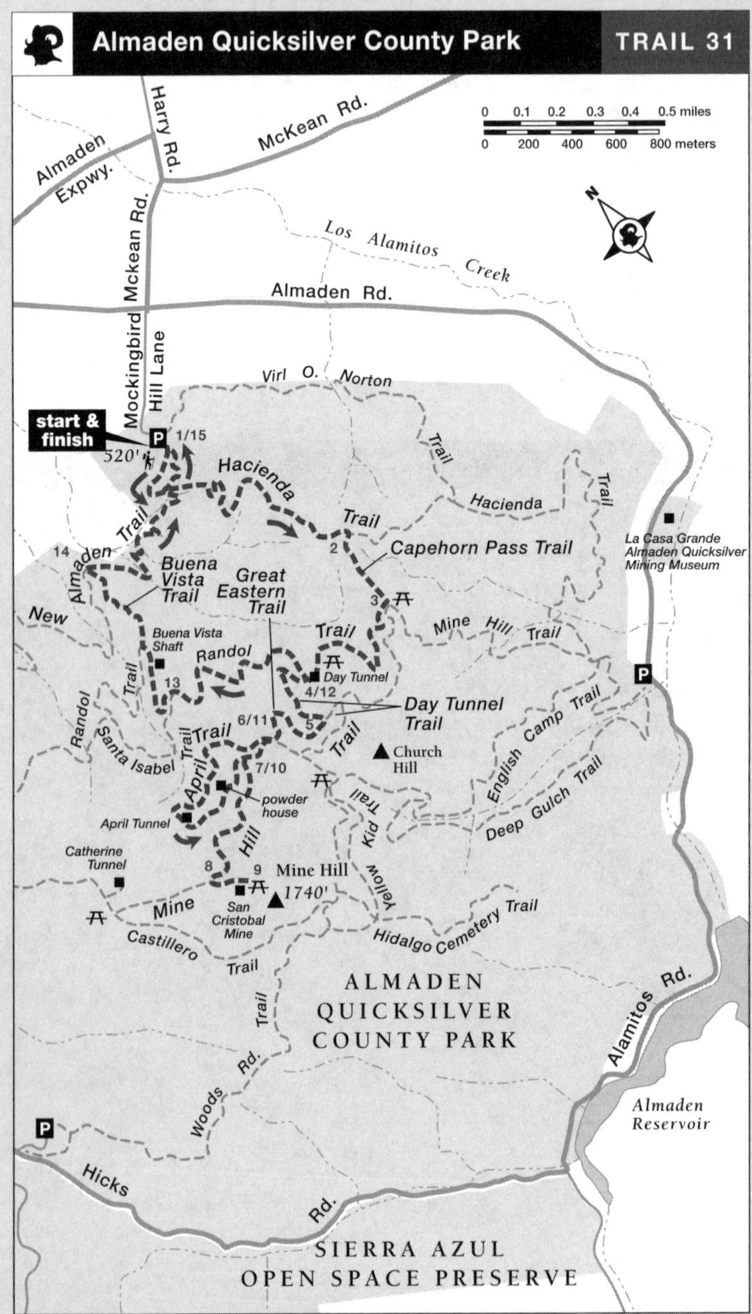
Harry Rd.
McKean Rd.
Almaden Expwy.
0 0.1 0.2 0.3 0.4 0.5 miles
0 200 400 600 800 meters
Mckean Rd.
Los Alamitos Creek
Almaden Rd.
Mockingbird Hill Lane
Virl O. Norton Trail
start & finish
1/15
520'
Hacienda Trail
Hacienda Trail
Capehorn Pass Trail
La Casa Grande Almaden Quicksilver Mining Museum
Almaden Trail
Buena Vista Trail
Great Eastern Trail
New Trail
Mine Hill Trail
Buena Vista Shaft
Randol Trail
Day Tunnel
4/12
Day Tunnel Trail
Randol
Santa Isabel Trail
April Trail
6/11
7/10
Church Hill
powder house
April Tunnel
Kid Trail
English Camp Trail
Deep Gulch Trail
Catherine Tunnel
Mine Hill
1740'
Yellow
Mine
San Cristobal Mine
Castillero Trail
Hidalgo Cemetery Trail
Trail
ALMADEN QUICKSILVER COUNTY PARK
Alamitos Rd.
Almaden Reservoir
Woods Rd.
Hicks Rd.
SIERRA AZUL OPEN SPACE PRESERVE

Almaden Quicksilver County Park

Travel back in time on this strenuous route through one of the Bay Area's most famous mining areas, where cinnabar ore was hauled out of the earth and converted to mercury in fiery brick furnaces. Today, shady oak woodlands, high grasslands, and chaparral are the main attractions of this rugged and remote park. For the South Bay foothills, this trail is relatively shady.

TRAIL USE
Hike, Run, Dogs Allowed

LENGTH
7.0 miles, 4 hours

VERTICAL FEET
±1750'

DIFFICULTY
– 1 2 3 4 **5** +

TRAIL TYPE
Loop

SURFACE TYPE
Dirt

FEATURES
Stream
Canyon
Summit
Birds
Historic
Geologic Interest
Great Views
Secluded
Steep

FACILITIES
Restrooms
Picnic Tables
Water

Best Time

Fall through spring, but trails may be muddy in wet weather.

Finding the Trail

From State Hwy. 85 in San Jose, take the Almaden Expwy. exit and go south 4.4 miles to Almaden Rd. Turn right, go 0.5 mile, then turn right on Mockingbird Hill Ln. and go 0.4 mile to a paved parking area, left. The trailhead is on the south corner of the parking area, near an information board.

Trail Description

From the information board,►1 the New Almaden Trail goes straight, but you go right on the **Hacienda Trail** and begin climbing on a moderate and then steep grade. The forest near the trailhead includes a fine mix of California bay, California buckeye, toyon, and various oaks.

Atop a narrow ridge, you cross the single-track New Almaden Trail. You continue straight on a wide track that rises relentlessly and in places steeply.

Steep

Great Views

Canyon

Mt. Umunhum, to the southwest, was the site of an Air Force station during the Cold War. You can still see the concrete building, used to support a radar system, on its summit.

Finally you reach a flat spot, where a panorama stretches from the San Francisco Bay to Loma Prieta, the two-humped peak bristling with communication towers on the southern skyline.

Crossing one more knoll, your roller-coaster ride subsides at a junction►2 where the Hacienda Trail swings left. You turn right on the **Capehorn Pass Trail** and descend a brushy ridge to a junction with the Randol and Mine Hill trails.►3 Here turn right on the **Randol Trail**, a nearly level dirt road that wanders in and out of wooded canyons.

Piles of red rock beside the trail are mine tailings hauled out of nearby **Day Tunnel**, whose entrance is no longer visible. A picnic area left, sits beside a spring (nonpotable water), shaded by bigleaf maples, willows, and California bay trees. Just beyond the picnic area, the Day Tunnel Trail,►4 veers left. Follow this single track and climb on a mostly moderate grade. At a junction with the **Great Eastern Trail,**►5 turn right and continue uphill on it to a T-junction with the Mine Hill and April trails.►6

Turn right on the **April Trail**, a dirt road that descends gently past the remnants of the **April Tunnel**, which include a wooden trestle and a corrugated metal shed. Looping back toward the Mine Hill Trail, you come to a brick-and-wood replica of a building used to store explosives, called a **powder house.** (The original, built in 1866, was destroyed by the 1989 Loma Prieta earthquake.)

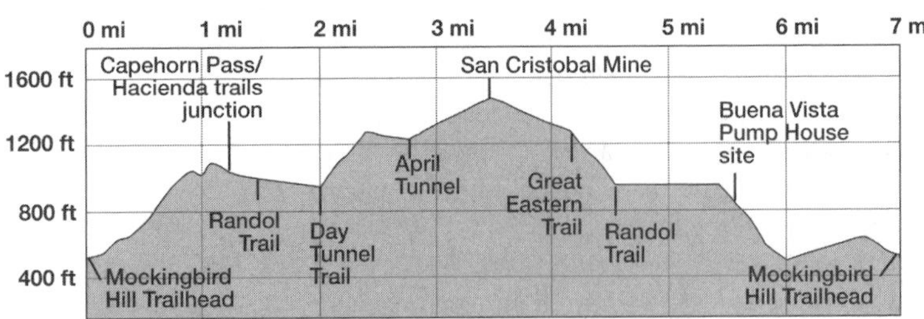

TRAIL 31 Almaden Quicksilver County Park Profile

On reaching the **Mine Hill Trail**, a dirt road,▶7 turn sharply right and climb across a forested hillside. Notice the deep red cinnabar ore in the slope above this road. At a junction▶8 with the **San Cristobal Trail**, turn left. This short trail climbs to the restored entrance of the **San Cristobal Mine.**▶9 The first 70 feet of tunnel are open to the public, providing the setting for you to imagine a miner's life in these hills. There is a shady picnic table adjacent to the mine entrance.

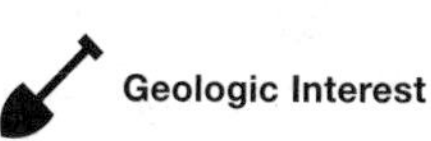

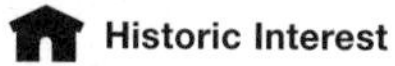

Now retrace your route to the junction of the Mine Hill and April trails.▶10 From here, follow the **Mine Hill Trail** as it curves right. Where the **Great Eastern Trail** joins on the left,▶11 use it and then the **Day Tunnel Trail** to retrace your route to the Randol Trail.▶12

Tunnels and mine shafts, including the April Tunnel, the St. George Shaft, and the Victoria Shaft, once provided entry to a dangerous, subterranean world. Mine tailings are scattered throughout the park.

Turning left on the **Randol Trail**, follow the dirt road on a level but curvy course that wanders past a large pile of mine tailings. At a junction with the Santa Isabel Trail, stay right and use the Randol Trail to descend past the granite foundations of the **Buena Vista Pump House.** A bit farther, turn right on the hiking-only **Buena Vista Trail**▶13 and descend through manzanita to an oak forest.

When you reach the **New Almaden Trail,**▶14 turn right. This trail, also for hiking only, drops to a creek, where you turn left and cross it on rocks. A moderate climb soon puts you briefly atop a ridge, but then the trail curves downhill again and lands you in a ravine with a seasonal creek. You cross several more seasonal creeks, and then the trail snakes its way uphill to the four-way junction with

OPTIONS

A Shorter Option

An enjoyable 4.4-mile loop omits the excursion to Mine Hill▶4 and continues along the Randol Trail.

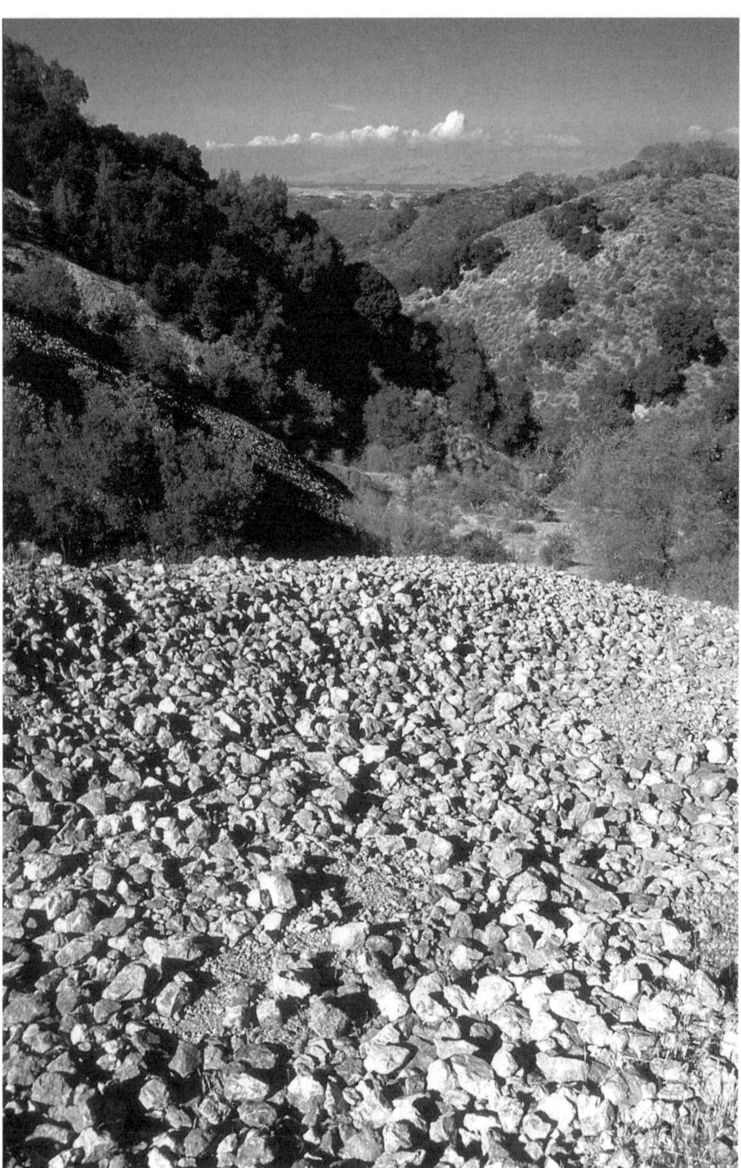

Tailings piles *spill down the hillside below the mines, contrasting with the verdant surroundings.*

the Hacienda Trail you passed near the start of this route. Continuing straight, you soon begin a series of S-bends that descend to the parking area.►15

MILESTONES

►1	0.0	From trailhead information board, go right on Hacienda Trail
►2	1.2	Right on Capehorn Pass Trail
►3	1.5	Right on Randol Trail, just before Mine Hill Trail junction
►4	2.0	Day Tunnel area, left on Day Tunnel Trail
►5	2.3	Right on Great Eastern Trail
►6	2.4	Right on April Trail at T-junction
►7	3.0	Right on Mine Hill Trail
►8	3.4	Left on San Cristobal Trail
►9	3.5	San Cristobal Mine
►10	4.0	Right to stay on Mine Hill Trail
►11	4.2	Straight on Great Eastern Trail; retrace to junction of Day Tunnel and Randol trails
►12	4.6	Left on Randol Trail
►13	5.5	Right on Buena Vista Trail
►14	5.8	Right on New Almaden Trail
►15	7.0	Back at parking area

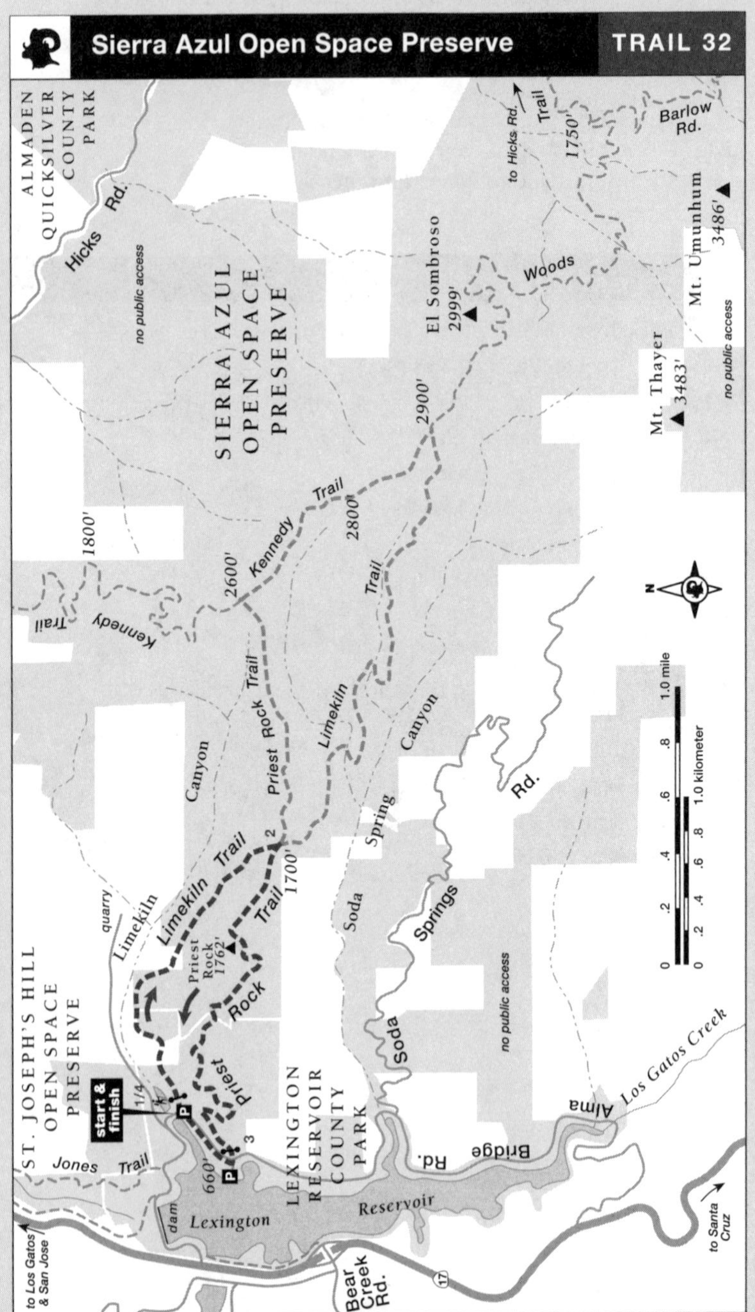
Sierra Azul Open Space Preserve
TRAIL 32
ALMADEN QUICKSILVER COUNTY PARK
SIERRA AZUL OPEN SPACE PRESERVE
ST. JOSEPH'S HILL OPEN SPACE PRESERVE
LEXINGTON RESERVOIR COUNTY PARK
Hicks Rd.
no public access
Kennedy Trail
Priest Rock Trail
Limekiln Trail
Woods
El Sombroso 2999'
Mt. Thayer 3483'
Mt. Umunhum 3486'
Barlow Rd.
to Hicks Rd.
1750'
1800'
2600'
2800'
2900'
1700'
660'
Priest Rock 1762'
Soda Springs Canyon
Soda Springs Rd.
Los Gatos Creek
Alma Bridge Rd.
Lexington Reservoir
dam
Jones Trail
quarry
start & finish
Bear Creek Rd.
to Los Gatos & San Jose
to Santa Cruz
1.0 mile
1.0 kilometer

Sierra Azul Open Space Preserve: Limekiln–Priest Rock Loop

This loop, which starts and ends in Lexington Reservoir County Park, visits the northwest corner of Midpeninsula Regional Open Space District's largest, most remote preserve. Much of the journey is over serpentine soil, which gives rise to a fascinating community of shrubs and wildflowers. Shrubs such as manzanita and currant may add splashes of unexpected color as early as December, and the bright red toyon berries attract numerous species of hungry songbirds. Often blazingly hot in summer, this route is perfect for a winter ramble if it's not muddy. Spring rains may reveal migrating newts.

TRAIL USE
Hike, Run, Bike, Dogs Allowed
LENGTH
5.2 miles, 2–3 hours
VERTICAL FEET
±1300'
DIFFICULTY
– 1 2 **3** 4 5 +
TRAIL TYPE
Loop
SURFACE TYPE
Dirt

FEATURES
Stream
Canyon
Autumn Colors
Wildflowers
Birds
Historic
Great Views
Secluded

FACILITIES
None

Best Time

Fall through spring, but trails may be muddy in wet weather.

Finding the Trail

From State Hwy. 17 northbound, exit at Alma Bridge Rd., south of Los Gatos. At 0.7 mile, you pass a parking area, right, for Lexington Reservoir. At 1.2 miles, stay right at a fork with the entrance road to Lexington Quarry. Roadside parking along Alma Bridge Rd is just ahead on the right, opposite gate SA22; there is additional parking 0.4 mile ahead opposite gate SA21. The trailhead is at gate SA22, on the southeast side of the road.

From Hwy. 17 southbound, take the Bear Creek Rd. exit south of Los Gatos. After 0.1 mile, you come to a stop sign at a four-way junction. Turn right,

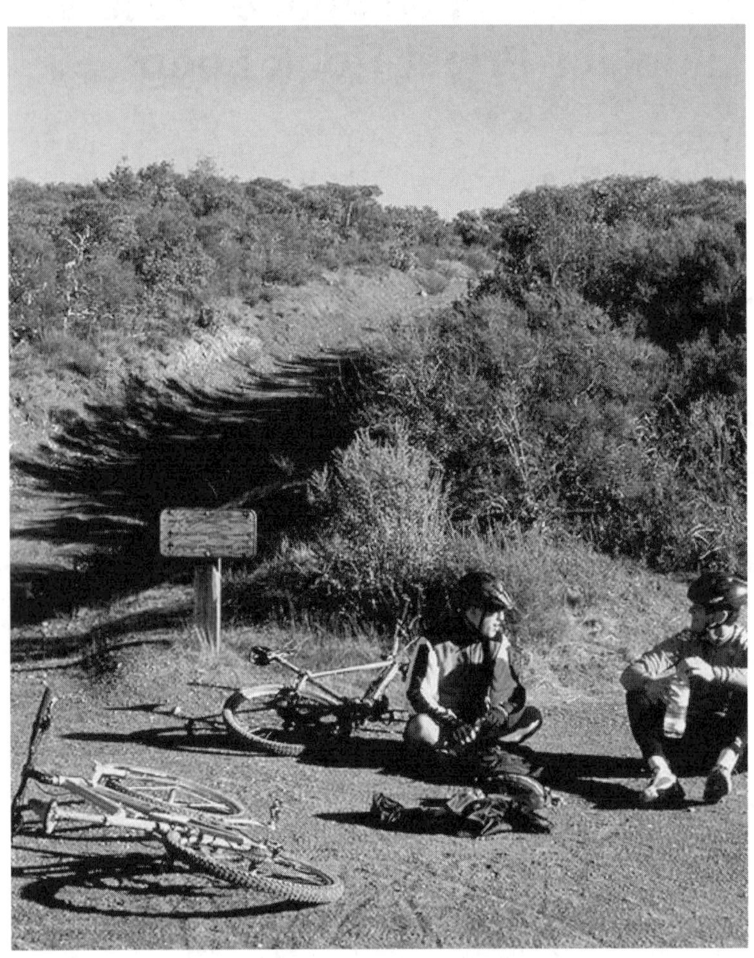

Cyclists *rest at the junction of the Limekiln and Priest Rock trails.*

cross over Hwy. 17, and turn left to get on Hwy. 17 northbound. Go 0.4 mile to Alma Bridge Rd., turn right, and follow the directions above.

Clumps of leather oak, a low shrub with curved and prickly leaves, indicate the presence of serpentine soil.

Trail Description

From the trailhead,▶1 pass around gate SA22 and begin climbing moderately northeast on the **Limekiln Trail,** a rough and rocky road. Eventually the grade eases to gentle, and you follow a winding course up a hillside that drops steeply left into **Limekiln Canyon,** named for furnaces used to reduce limestone to lime. Several kilns operated nearby from the late 1800s until the 1930s.

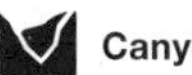

Now the road turns left and crosses a side canyon. This is a landslide-prone area, and the road may be wet, muddy, and uneven. Young manzanita bushes have sprouted in the displaced soil, helping to stabilize it. Beyond the slide area, the road swings right.

Now you descend into a cool and shady creekside forest. Soon you reach the boundary between Lexington Reservoir County Park and the **Sierra Azul Open Space Preserve.** Here the road begins a moderate-to-steep climb over very rocky ground. The massive Lexington Quarry, which is on the

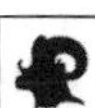

OPTIONS

More Sierra Azul Trails

The **Priest Rock Trail,** a rugged dirt road, climbs northeast from its junction with the Limekiln Trail▶2 nearly 1000 feet in 1.5 miles, to a junction with the Kennedy Trail. From there, you can make a 4.6-mile loop back to the Limekiln–Priest Rock junction▶2 by turning right onto the **Kennedy Trail** and right again onto the **Limekiln Trail.** Alternatively, you could follow the 6.2-mile **Woods Trail,** which descends east from this loop to a parking area at gate SA06 on Hicks Rd.

From the ridgetop, enjoy a fine view that stretches north from San Jose to the East Bay hills and Mt. Diablo.

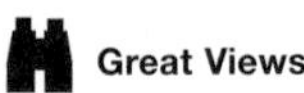

Great Views

north side of the canyon, is visible through openings in the dense bay forest.

You continue your uphill trek, eventually trading forest for thick stands of chaparral rooted in serpentine soil. Just beyond a fence and a gate is a four-way junction with the Priest Rock Trail, a dirt road that goes left and right along the ridgetop.►2 Here the Limekiln Trail continues straight, but you turn right on the **Priest Rock Trail**.

A gentle ascent ends with a short, steep pitch, and now you are on level ground. An unsigned dirt road joins sharply from the left, and then a short trail to a viewpoint departs right. Other spur roads branch left and right, but you stay on the main dirt road. Crossing under a set of power lines and a tower, the road bends sharply left. A fence is just to the right of the road, and **Priest Rock,** a modest outcrop, rises behind it, half hidden in the chaparral.

Now the road begins to snake its way downhill, and soon you reach gate SA23 and the preserve boundary. Your road continues into **Lexington Reservoir County Park,** and you descend on a grade that alternates between gentle, moderate, and steep. Leveling briefly, the road then climbs gently through a possibly wet area. Now overlooking Lexington Reservoir, you resume winding downhill to the bottom of the Priest Rock Trail. At gate SA21, turn sharply right to meet paved **Alma Bridge Road.**►3 Cross it carefully, turn right, and walk northeast along the road shoulder about 0.4 mile to the parking area.►4

MILESTONES

▶1	0.0	Take Limekiln Trail northeast
▶2	2.3	Right on Priest Rock Trail
▶3	4.8	Right on Alma Bridge Rd.
▶4	5.2	Back at parking area

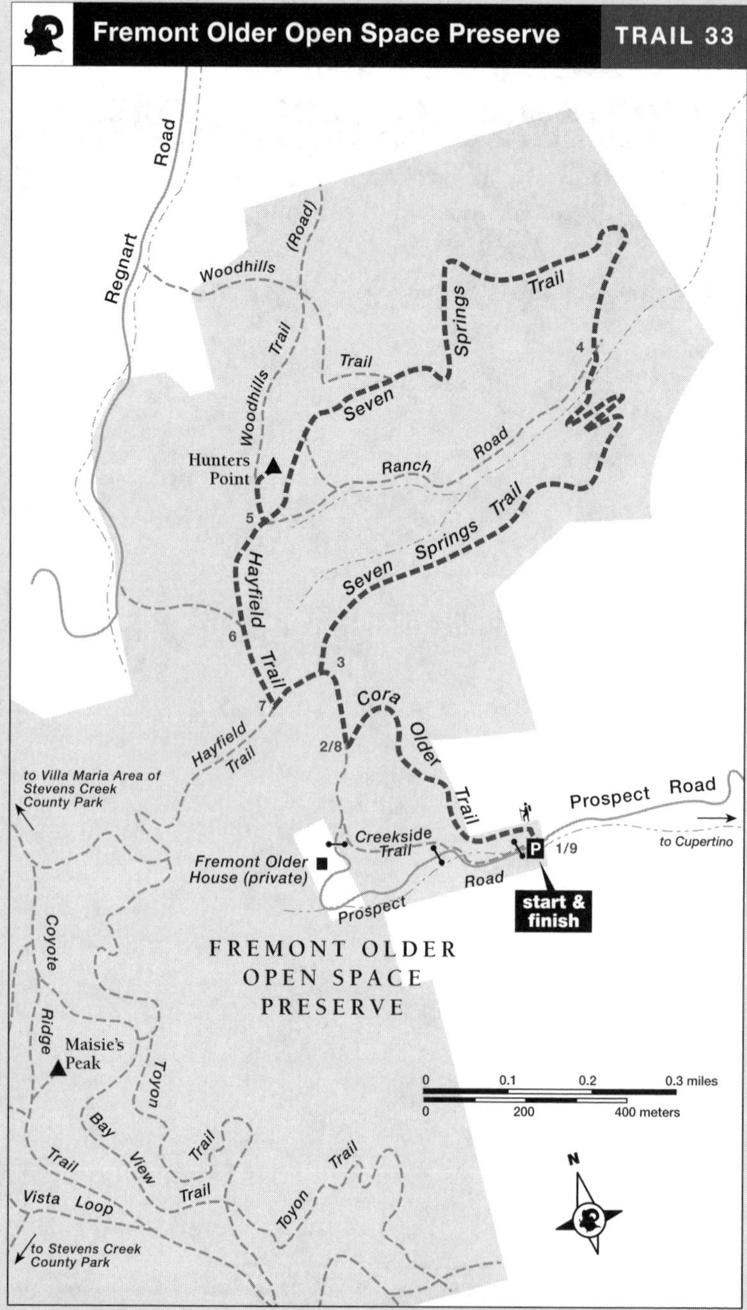
Fremont Older Open Space Preserve
TRAIL 33
Regnart Road
Woodhills
(Road)
Woodhills Trail
Trail
Seven Springs Trail
Hunters Point
Ranch Road
Seven Springs Trail
Hayfield Trail
Cora Older Trail
Hayfield Trail
Prospect Road
to Cupertino
to Villa Maria Area of Stevens Creek County Park
Creekside Trail
Fremont Older House (private)
Prospect Road
start & finish
1/9
2/8
3
4
5
6
7
FREMONT OLDER OPEN SPACE PRESERVE
Coyote Ridge
Maisie's Peak
Toyon
Bay View Trail
Trail
Trail
Vista Loop
Toyon Trail
to Stevens Creek County Park
0 0.1 0.2 0.3 miles
0 200 400 meters
N

Fremont Older Open Space Preserve

Varied terrain and superb views from Hunters Point make this semiloop route a favorite among South Bay hikers, bicyclists, and runners. In spring, the grasslands along the Cora Older and Hayfield trails come alive with wildflowers, and the secluded canyon traversed by the Seven Springs Trail offers shady respite on a warm day. Remnants of walnut and apricot orchards are reminders of Santa Clara Valley's heyday as an agricultural paradise.

TRAIL USE
Hike, Run, Bike, Child Friendly, Dogs Allowed

LENGTH
3.1 miles, 2–3 hours

VERTICAL FEET
±800'

DIFFICULTY
– 1 2 **3** 4 5 +

TRAIL TYPE
Loop

SURFACE TYPE
Dirt

FEATURES
Canyon
Summit
Wildflowers
Birds
Great Views

FACILITIES
Restrooms

Best Time

Fall through spring, but trails may be muddy in wet weather.

Finding the Trail

From State Hwy. 85 at the Cupertino–San Jose border, take the De Anza Blvd. exit, go south 0.5 mile to Prospect Rd., and turn right. After 0.4 mile you come to a stop sign, where you stay on Prospect Rd. by turning left and crossing a set of railroad tracks. When you reach the junction of Prospect Rd. and Rolling Hills Rd., follow Prospect Rd. as it bends sharply left. At 1.8 miles, you reach the preserve entrance and the parking area, left. (The parking area is adjacent to Saratoga Country Club—a sign here warns you to beware of flying golf balls and to park at your own risk.) The trailhead is on the north side of Prospect Rd., across from the parking area.

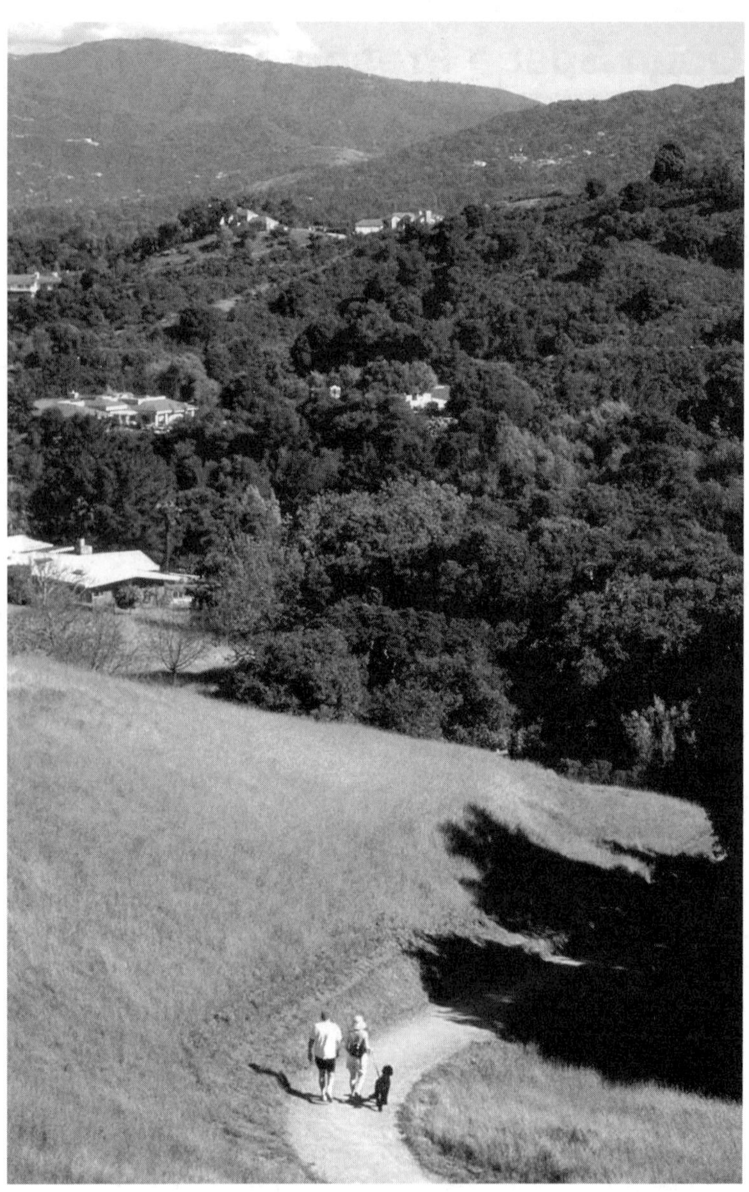

Looking south *from Fremont Older Open Space Preserve toward Black Mountain.*

Trail Description

From the trailhead,▶1 which has information boards and a map holder, follow the **Cora Older Trail** uphill. The single-track trail switchbacks left, then winds uphill and crosses several culverts draining seasonal creeks. Turning left and crossing an open hillside, you soon reach a T-junction.▶2 Here, you go right on a dirt road and after several hundred feet arrive at another junction.▶3 From this junction, the road curves left, but you angle right on the **Seven Springs Trail**, a single track.

With a ravine holding a seasonal creek on your left, you enter a cool and shady forest. Soon the ravine widens to a valley, whose north-facing slope holds the remnants of an orchard. Winding your way downhill, you pass stands of walnut trees and then meander through a brushy area. The trail turns left, crosses a culvert draining the seasonal creek, and then reaches a four-way junction.▶4 Here, Ranch Road joins from the left and descends right as a closed road.

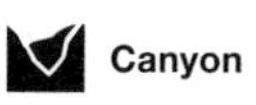

Your route, the Seven Springs Trail, continues straight and climbs toward the preserve boundary, then turns west to gain the ridgetop. On a level stretch you pass a junction with the single-track Woodhills Trail, right. Soon you pass a second junction, where an unnamed dirt road descends steeply left. Your trail traverses briefly across a hillside, then merges with **Ranch Road**, which ascends sharply from the left. Bear right a few steps to meet the **Hayfield Trail.**▶5 From this three-way junction, ascend right and soon come to a fork where the Woodhills Trail, a steep dirt road, goes left. Here you veer right and, in about 100 feet, find yourself atop **Hunters Point.** The view from Hunters Point takes in San Jose, the Santa Clara Valley, Mt. Hamilton, Mt. Umunhum, and most of the southern end of San Francisco Bay, the East Bay hills, and Mt. Diablo. On a clear day, you can even see Mt. Tamalpais and the San Francisco skyline.

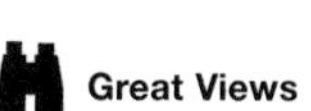

After enjoying a rest and the superb scenery, retrace your route to the junction with the Woodhills Trail, and then to the next junction, just west of where the Seven Springs Trail and Ranch Road merge.▶5 Now follow the **Hayfield Trail** as it angles right and descends on a moderate grade, passing in about 0.1 mile a dirt road signed REGNART ROAD, 0.2 MILE.▶6

Continue straight on a rolling course to a junction with a dirt road,▶7 signed PROSPECT ROAD PARKING, 0.8 MILE. Here turn left and, after several hundred feet, reach the junction with the Seven Springs Trail where you began this loop. Now turn right, go 0.1 mile, and then turn left on the **Cora Older Trail,**▶8 retracing your route to the parking area.▶9

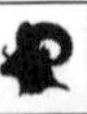

HISTORY

Fremont Older's Home

Fremont Older Preserve was named for a crusading San Francisco newspaper editor, who, with his wife, Cora, lived here for many years. After serving as a printer and editor in Redwood City, Older took over editorial duties at the San Francisco *Bulletin* in 1895. You can visit their home, "Woodhills," which was completed in 1914 and is on the National Register of Historic Places, during the annual house and garden tour, which usually takes place in the spring. Call the Midpeninsula Regional Open Space District office for details: (650) 691-1200.

MILESTONES

►1	0.0	Take Cora Older Trail
►2	0.4	Right on dirt road at T-junction
►3	0.5	Right on Seven Springs Trail
►4	1.2	Four-way junction; continue straight on Seven Springs Trail
►5	2.0	Right on Hayfield Trail, right at junction with Woodhills Trail, climb to Hunters Point; then retrace to previous junction
►6	2.4	Straight at junction with connector to Regnart Rd.
►7	2.5	Left on dirt road
►8	2.6	Retrace to parking area by going right on dirt road, then left on Cora Older Trail
►9	3.1	Back at parking area

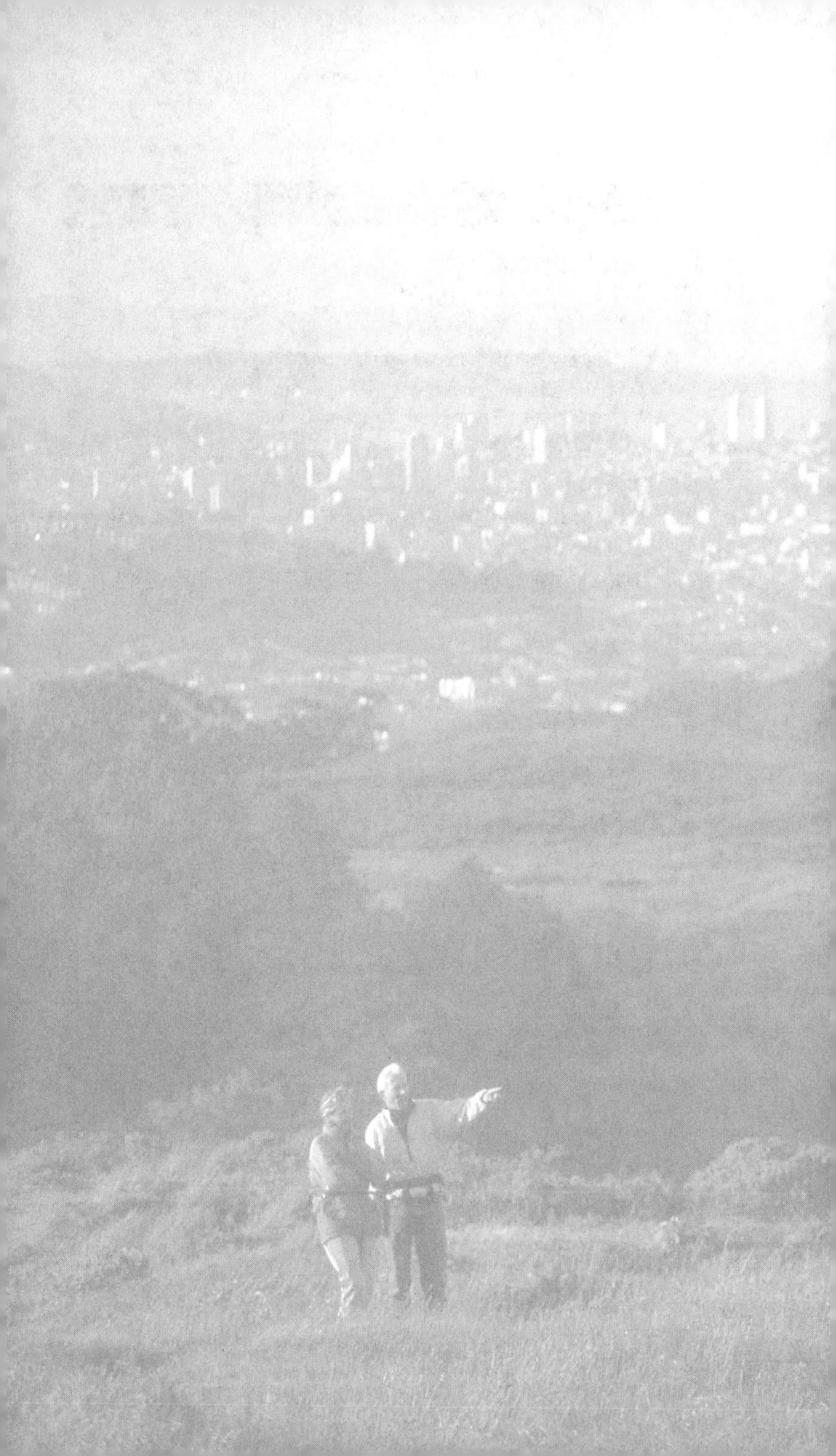

CHAPTER 4

Peninsula

34. Monte Bello Open Space Preserve
35. Long Ridge Open Space Preserve
36. Skyline Ridge Open Space Preserve
37. Russian Ridge Open Space Preserve
38. Windy Hill Open Space Preserve
39. El Corte de Madera Creek Open Space Preserve
40. Purisima Creek Redwoods Open Space Preserve
41. Kings Mountain
42. Montara Mountain
43. San Bruno Mountain State and County Park
44. Presidio of San Francisco

Peninsula

The Peninsula encompasses northwestern **Santa Clara County**, **San Mateo County**, and **San Francisco.** This great thumb of land between the Pacific Ocean and San Francisco Bay is centered on the Santa Cruz Mountains. On the west side of the range are forested canyons, stream-filled ravines, and grassy ridges extending west to the Pacific shore. On the east side are oak woodlands, mixed-evergreen forests, grasslands, and salt marshes. The mountains taper near the Golden Gate, allowing moist, cool air to stream inland from the Pacific, and the forests give way to wind-blown coastal scrub.

The history of the land begins with Native Americans, Spanish missionaries, and Mexican settlers. Later, under American rule, a string of settlements developed along the historic El Camino Real, with ranches and vineyards in the mountains. The logger's ax decimated the coast redwood forest, in a matter of decades, to build San Francisco and nearby cities. Railroads and then highways shaped the string of towns on the Peninsula into a major metropolitan corridor, and growth threatened to spread westward from the San Francisco Bay to the foothills and the coast.

By the late 20th century, the Peninsula had a scattering of state and county parks, but a comprehensive plan was needed to protect remaining open space. In 1972, voters approved creation of the Midpeninsula Regional Open Space District (MROSD), which now administers nearly 50,000 acres of open space. The Golden Gate National Recreation Area (GGNRA) expanded from San Francisco south into Pacifica in 1984 and to the Phleger Estate in 1996.

Thanks to public agencies and private nonprofits, the Peninsula's mosaic of federal, state, county, and local parks is one of the finest places to enjoy outdoor activities in the Bay Area. Many parks and open space preserves are contiguous, making possible extended hikes, runs, and bike rides.

No single hike could do justice to San Francisco, but we end our circuit of the Bay Area overlooking the Golden Gate, where the GGNRA has made great strides converting the Presidio army post for recreational use.

See Appendix 2 for agency contact information (page 314) and Appendix 6 for maps (page 321).

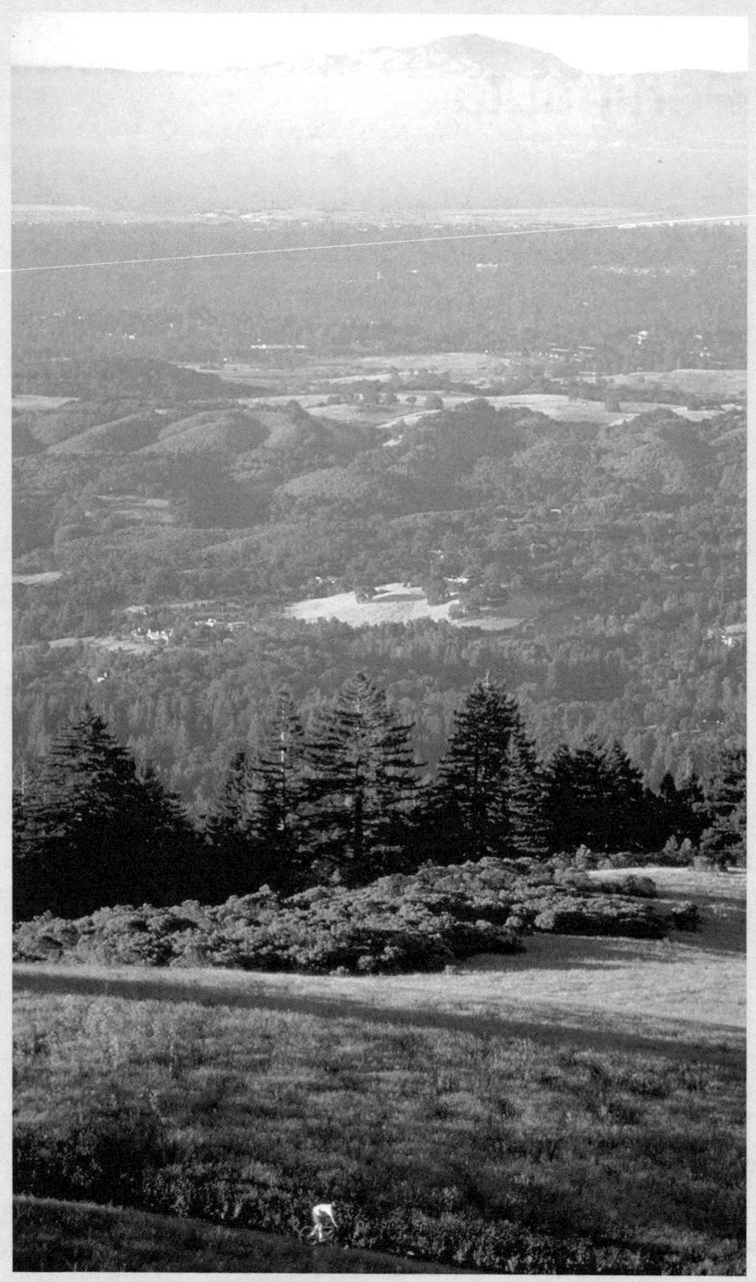

Windy Hill *(Trail 38) overlooks the Peninsula, San Francisco, and Mt. Diablo.*

Peninsula

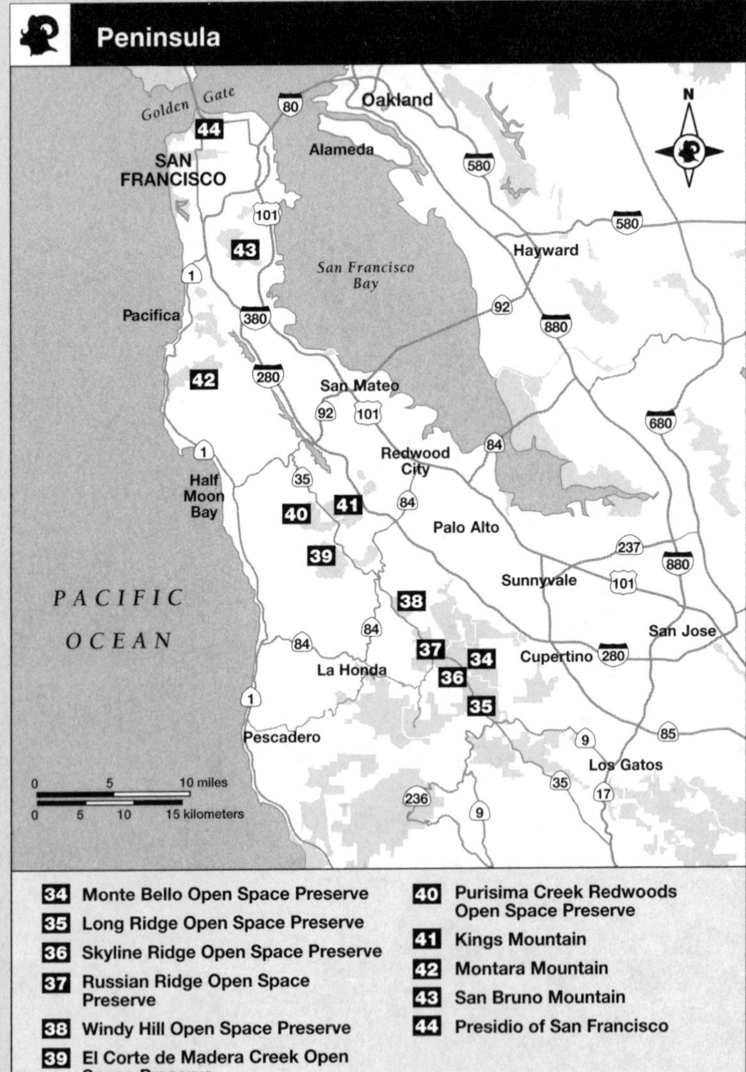
Peninsula
N
Golden Gate
80
Oakland
44
SAN FRANCISCO
Alameda
580
101
580
43
San Francisco Bay
Hayward
1
Pacifica
380
92
880
42
280
San Mateo
92
101
680
84
1
Redwood City
Half Moon Bay
35
40
41
84
Palo Alto
39
237
880
Sunnyvale
101
PACIFIC
OCEAN
38
84
84
37
34
Cupertino
280
San Jose
La Honda
36
1
35
Pescadero
9
85
Los Gatos
0 5 10 miles
0 5 10 15 kilometers
236
35
17
9
34 Monte Bello Open Space Preserve
35 Long Ridge Open Space Preserve
36 Skyline Ridge Open Space Preserve
37 Russian Ridge Open Space Preserve
38 Windy Hill Open Space Preserve
39 El Corte de Madera Creek Open Space Preserve
40 Purisima Creek Redwoods Open Space Preserve
41 Kings Mountain
42 Montara Mountain
43 San Bruno Mountain
44 Presidio of San Francisco

TRAIL FEATURE TABLE

Peninsula

TRAIL	Difficulty	Length	Type	USES & ACCESS	TERRAIN	FLORA & FAUNA	OTHER
34	4	6.0	Loop	Hiking, Running	River or Stream, Canyon, Mountain, Summit	Autumn Colors, Wildflowers, Birds	Geologic Interest, Great Views, Photo Opportunity, Camping
35	3	4.6	Loop	Hiking, Running, Biking	River or Stream, Canyon, Summit	Autumn Colors, Birds	Great Views, Secluded, Cool & Shady
36	3	4.2	Out & Back	Hiking, Running, Child Friendly	Lake or Shore, Mountain	Wildflowers, Birds	Great Views
37	3	4.6	Loop	Hiking, Running, Biking	Summit	Wildflowers, Birds, Wildlife	Great Views, Photo Opportunity
38	5	8.0	Loop	Hiking, Running	River or Stream, Canyon	Autumn Colors, Wildflowers, Birds	Great Views, Secluded, Cool & Shady
39	3	4.3	Loop	Hiking, Running, Biking	River or Stream, Canyon	Autumn Colors, Birds	Geologic Interest, Secluded, Cool & Shady
40	5	10.1	Loop	Hiking, Running	River or Stream, Canyon	Autumn Colors, Wildflowers, Birds	Historic, Great Views, Secluded, Cool & Shady
41	4	7.9	Loop	Hiking, Running, Fee	River or Stream, Canyon	Birds, Wildlife	Secluded, Cool & Shady
42	4	7.2	Out & Back	Hiking, Running, Fee	Mountain	Wildflowers	Geologic Interest, Great Views
43	3	3.1	Loop	Hiking, Running, Fee	Mountain	Wildflowers, Birds	Great Views, Photo Opportunity
44	3	4.1	Loop	Hiking, Running, Biking[1], Child Friendly, Dogs Allowed	Lake or Shore	Wildflowers, Birds	Historic, Great Views, Photo Opportunity

USES & ACCESS: Hiking; Running; Biking; Child Friendly; Dogs Allowed; $ Fee; Permit Required

TYPE: Loop; Out & Back; Point to Point

DIFFICULTY: - 1 2 3 4 5 + (less … more)

TERRAIN: River or Stream; Waterfall; Lake or Shore; Canyon; Mountain; Summit

FLORA & FAUNA: Autumn Colors; Wildflowers; Birds; Wildlife

OTHER: Historic; Geologic Interest; Great Views; Photo Opportunity; Secluded; Cool & Shady; Camping; Steep

[1] *Bicyclists use described alternate trails or trailheads*

Peninsula

TRAIL 34

Hike, Run
6.0 miles, Loop
Difficulty: 1 2 3 **4** 5

Monte Bello Open Space Preserve . . 249

This challenging but supremely rewarding loop climbs from the riparian corridor along Stevens Creek to the windswept grasslands of Monte Bello Ridge, capped by Black Mountain. The route includes a self-guiding nature trail and a trip across the San Andreas Fault.

TRAIL 35

Hike, Run, Bike
4.6 miles, Loop
Difficulty: 1 2 **3** 4 5

Long Ridge Open Space Preserve . . 257

Superb views are the reason to wander uphill from the shady confines of Peters Creek to the Wallace Stegner memorial bench high atop Long Ridge. On a clear day, the scene extends westward over the Pescadero Creek watershed, taking in thousands of acres of protected lands, which are truly a living monument to the open space movement.

TRAIL 36

Hike, Run, Child Friendly
4.2 miles, Out & Back
Difficulty: 1 2 **3** 4 5

Skyline Ridge Open Space Preserve 261

The Ridge Trail rises from the forested environs of Alpine Pond, to a breezy realm of grassland and chaparral, where views of Butano Ridge, Portola Redwoods State Park, and the Pacific coast await. The spring wildflowers here are superb.

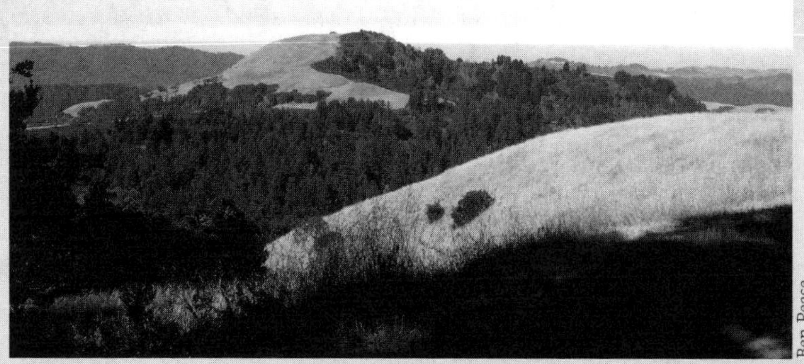

Ben Pease

View of *Mindego Hill at Russian Ridge Open Space Preserve (Trail 37)*

This remarkable ramble through what many consider the Peninsula's most scenic preserve samples a wide variety of habitats, from oak woodlands to the dazzling wildflower meadows atop Borel Hill. Have binoculars handy to pick out soaring hawks and falcons, as well as Bay Area landmarks.

TRAIL 37

Hike, Run, Bike
4.6 miles, Loop
Difficulty: 1 2 **3** 4 5

This adventurous semiloop explores one of the Midpeninsula Regional Open Space District's best-loved preserves. Dropping about 1000 feet, you follow cool and shady Hamms Gulch downhill through a lush forest, only to win back lost elevation via switchbacks. You then contour parallel to Skyline Boulevard for an easy last lap.

TRAIL 38

Hike, Run
8.0 miles, Loop
Difficulty: 1 2 3 4 **5**

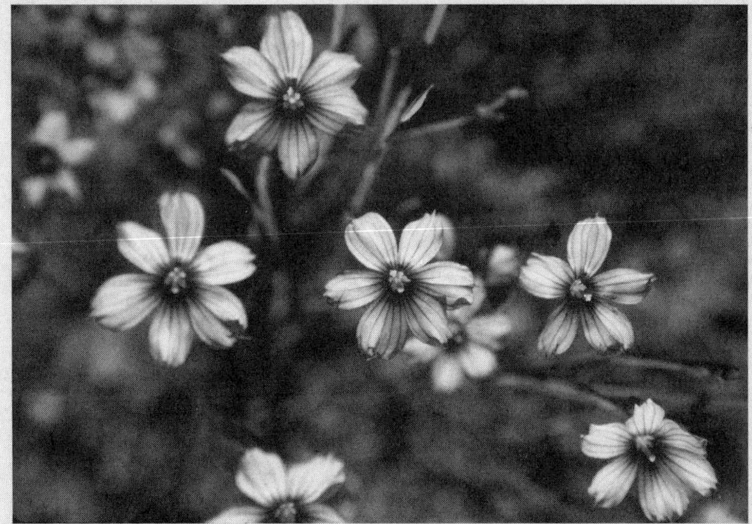

Blue-eyed grass *is a common spring wildflower in the grasslands throughout the Peninsula.*

TRAIL 43

Hike, Run
3.1 miles, Loop
Difficulty: 1 2 **3** 4 5

Despite its urban setting, San Bruno Mountain's rugged canyons and ridges host a remarkable array of rare and/or endangered species. When not fogbound, the trails afford views of San Francisco and beyond, and the spring wildflower displays are sensational.

TRAIL 44

Hike, Run, Bike, Child Friendly, Dogs Allowed
4.1 miles, Loop
Difficulty: 1 2 **3** 4 5

This loop through this former US Army post is both a historical walk and a hopeful look forward at efforts to reclaim developed lands for public enjoyment. Highlights include military buildings spanning three centuries and vantage points of the Golden Gate, San Francisco Bay, and beyond.

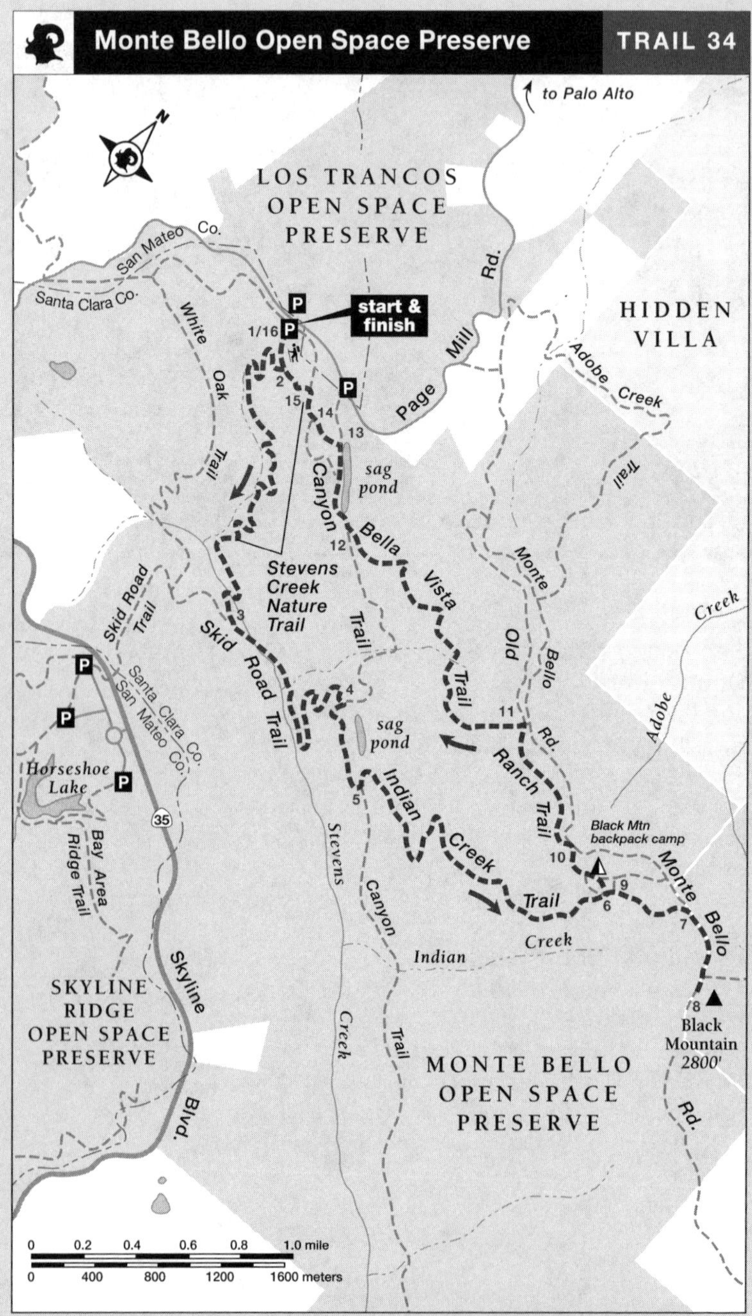
Monte Bello Open Space Preserve
TRAIL 34
to Palo Alto
LOS TRANCOS OPEN SPACE PRESERVE
HIDDEN VILLA
San Mateo Co.
Santa Clara Co.
start & finish
Page Mill Rd.
White Oak Trail
Adobe Creek Trail
Canyon Trail
sag pond
Bella Vista Trail
Stevens Creek Nature Trail
Skid Road Trail
Old Ranch Trail
Monte Bello Rd.
Santa Clara Co.
San Mateo Co.
Horseshoe Lake
Bay Area Ridge Trail
Indian Creek Trail
Black Mtn backpack camp
Stevens Creek
Canyon Trail
Indian Creek
Adobe Creek
Skyline Blvd.
35
SKYLINE RIDGE OPEN SPACE PRESERVE
MONTE BELLO OPEN SPACE PRESERVE
Black Mountain 2800'
0 0.2 0.4 0.6 0.8 1.0 mile
0 400 800 1200 1600 meters

Monte Bello Open Space Preserve

This challenging but supremely rewarding loop explores the riparian corridor of Stevens Creek, formed by the San Andreas Fault, and the windswept grasslands of Monte Bello Ridge, which forms the scenic backdrop for Sunnyvale, Cupertino, and Mountain View. The views from Black Mountain are superb, and the descent along the Old Ranch and Bella Vista trails offers some of the best hiking on the Peninsula.

TRAIL USE
Hike, Run

LENGTH
6.0 miles, 3–4 hours

VERTICAL FEET
±1400'

DIFFICULTY
– 1 2 3 **4** 5 +

TRAIL TYPE
Loop

SURFACE TYPE
Dirt

FEATURES
Stream
Canyon
Mountain
Summit
Autumn Colors
Wildflowers
Birds
Geologic Interest
Great Views
Photo Opportunity
Camping

FACILITIES
Restrooms

Best Time

Spring and fall; Stevens Creek may be impassable in wet weather.

Finding the Trail

From Interstate 280 in Los Altos Hills, take the Page Mill Rd./Arastradero Rd. exit and go south on Page Mill Rd. 7.2 miles to a parking area on your left.

From the junction of Skyline Blvd. and Page Mill Rd. southwest of Palo Alto, take Page Mill Rd. north 1.4 miles to a parking area on your right.

The hikers trailhead is on the south corner of the parking area, near information boards and a map holder. (A separate bicycle/equestrian trailhead is near the entrance to the parking area.)

Trail Description

From the trailhead,►1 follow the single-track **Stevens Creek Nature Trail** through open grassland.

Along the way are signs describing the flora, fauna, and geology of this wonderful preserve.

Canyon

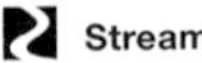

Near a rest bench is a junction,►2 where you turn sharply right and stay on the Stevens Creek Nature Trail, signed TO SKID ROAD TRAIL. Now descending via switchbacks, you soon enter a mixed evergreen forest. A canyon, right, holds a seasonal tributary of Stevens Creek. A sharp left-hand bend brings you to a set of wooden steps leading down to **Stevens Creek,** which formed along the **San Andreas Fault.** After crossing Stevens Creek on rocks (this may be impossible during wet weather), you climb an eroded bank to get back on the trail. A moderate climb that soon levels brings you to a junction with the **Skid Road Trail,** where you bear left.►3

Now a bridge takes you across Stevens Creek, and then the route temporarily narrows to single-track width. A moderate climb brings you to a bridge over a tributary that falls from Monte Bello Ridge. Curving right and climbing steeply, the trail takes you across a precipitous hillside and soon returns to dirt-road width.

Now ascending via S-bends, you reach a seasonal-closure gate that prevents access to the Skid Road Trail by bikes and horses during wet weather. In a clearing, you find a T-junction with the **Canyon Trail,** a dirt road.►4 Here you turn right.

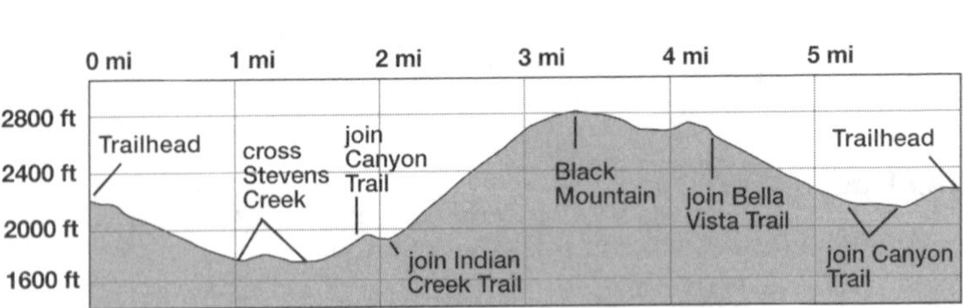

TRAIL 34 Monte Bello Open Space Preserve Profile

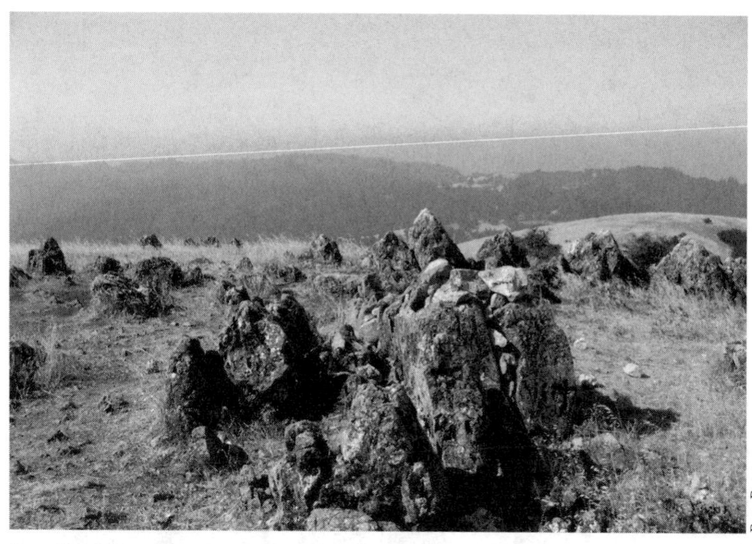

Ben Pease

Prominent limestone *outcroppings at Black Mountain*

The Canyon Trail angles left and almost immediately begins a steep climb that soon relents enough to provide an enjoyable ramble through wooded and open terrain. At a T-junction,►5 the Canyon Trail turns right, but you switch to the **Indian Creek Trail**, also a dirt road, by veering left. Now you begin a long, steady climb up the side of **Monte Bello Ridge**, which parallels the San

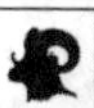

HISTORY

Skid Road

Skid Road was used by loggers driving teams of oxen dragging huge, cut Douglas-firs. To make the going easier, the road was inlaid with flat-topped logs called "skids," which were doused with water to reduce friction. In 19th-century western towns, the neighborhood frequented by loggers, which usually contained saloons, flophouses, and brothels, was often called Skid Road, or Skid Row.

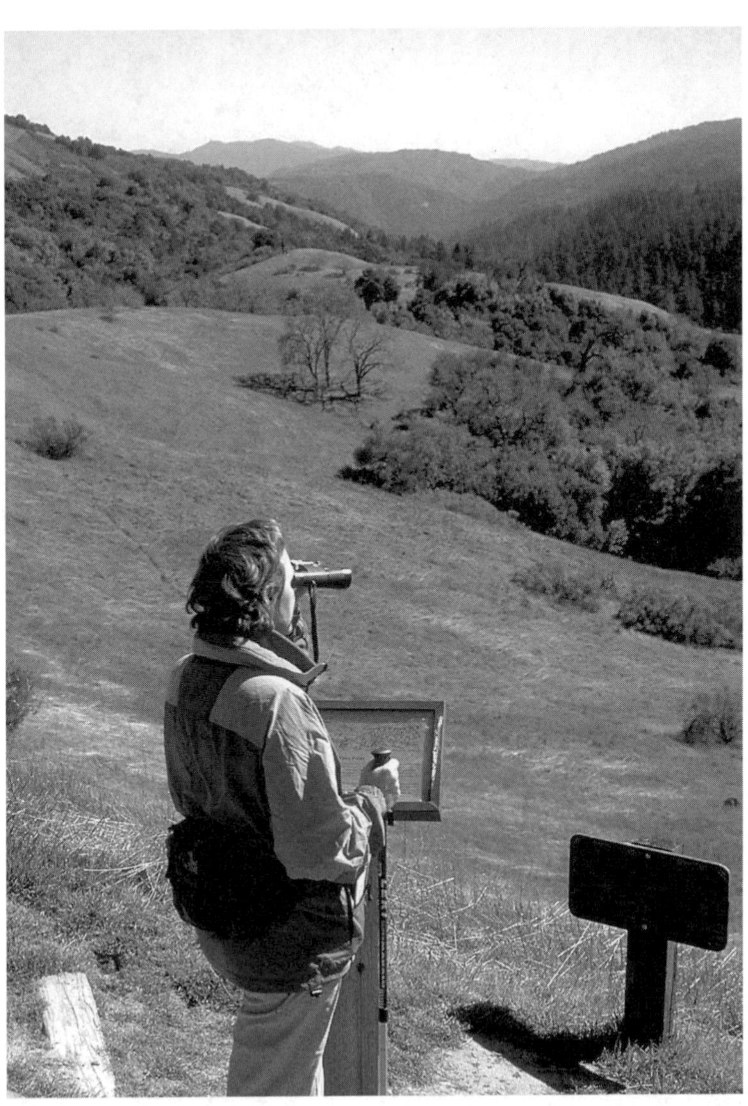

The view *across Stevens Creek headwaters follows the San Andreas Fault.*

Andreas Fault. A sea of coastal scrub studded with venerable valley oaks and young madrones soon yields to stands of chaparral, including chamise, toyon, and buckbrush.

The road eventually reaches two closely spaced junctions. At the first, a single-track trail leads left to Monte Bello Road. At the second, a dirt road veers left.▶6 To reach the **Black Mountain backpack camp** and a well-deserved rest spot, turn left on this dirt road. After about 100 feet, you come to a T-junction with a gravel road, where you turn left to reach the camp.

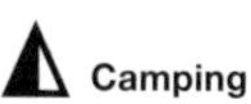

To press on to the summit of Black Mountain and save the backpack camp for later, stay on the Indian Creek Trail as it curves right and climbs past the turnoff to the backpack camp. The Indian Creek Trail ends at the next junction,▶7 where you join **Monte Bello Road** by bearing right. Continuing straight past the Black Mountain Trail, left, you soon stand atop **Black Mountain**, a broad, treeless vantage point studded with limestone outcrops.▶8 After soaking in the 360-degree views, retrace your route to the backpack-camp junction.▶9

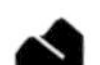

Mountain

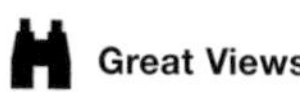

Here turn right and, after about 100 feet, meet the gravel road at the T-junction mentioned above. Turn left and walk through the backpack camp. Just past the camp, you pass the single-track connector to the Indian Creek Trail, left. Continuing straight, you follow the ridgetop to a four-way junction.▶10 Here, Monte Bello Road joins sharply from the right and continues by veering right. Your route, though, is the single-track **Old Ranch Trail**, which angles left.

At the next junction,▶11 you swing left onto the **Bella Vista Trail**, a single track that descends northwest across steep, grassy slopes and dips into shaded gulches.

From Black Mountain, on a clear day, you can see most of the San Francisco Bay Area, bounded by Mt. Tamalpais, Mt. Diablo, and Mt. Hamilton.

Finally reaching the **Canyon Trail,** a dirt road, you angle right.►12 After passing a seasonal wetland called a **sag pond,** where a rest bench awaits, you pass a junction with a hiking-only trail on the left. Continue straight for about 100 yards and then turn left on the **Stevens Creek Nature Trail,**►13 a multiuse single track that passes through an old orchard of mostly English walnut trees.

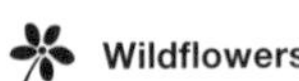

Soon the hiking-only trail joins, left,►14 and you bear right to make a rising traverse across an open slope. The nearby grasslands are decorated in spring and summer with wildflowers such as California poppy, checker mallow, owl's clover, bluedicks, and blue-eyed grass. At the next junction, equestrians and bicyclists go straight, contouring around the north side of a knoll to the parking area, but hikers turn left on a single-track trail overlooking the canyon holding Stevens Creek. Ahead, you close the loop at a familiar junction; veer right►15 and retrace your route to the parking area.►16

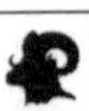

OPTIONS

More of Monte Bello

The 3-mile Stevens Creek Nature Trail is a great introductory hike by itself. From the end of the Skid Road Trail►4 turn left up the Canyon Trail. After 0.5 mile you come to the end of the Bella Vista Trail►12 and resume the described route.

Camping at **Black Mountain backpack camp** is by advance reservation only. The campground has picnic tables and a restroom but no water. Call the Midpeninsula Regional Open Space District office: (650) 691-1200.

MILESTONES

▶1	0.0	Take Stevens Creek Nature Trail
▶2	0.1	Right to stay on Stevens Creek Nature Trail at start of loop
▶3	1.2	Left on Skid Rd. Trail
▶4	1.8	Right on Canyon Trail
▶5	2.0	Left on Indian Creek Trail
▶6	3.0	Road to Black Mountain backpack camp on left
▶7	3.2	Right on Monte Bello Rd.
▶8	3.5	Summit of Black Mountain (2800')
▶9	4.0	Retrace to backpack-camp junction; right on dirt road, then left on gravel road through camp
▶10	4.1	Left on Old Ranch Trail
▶11	4.6	Left on Bella Vista Trail
▶12	5.4	Right on Canyon Trail
▶13	5.6	Left on Stevens Creek Nature Trail
▶14	5.8	Bear right where hiking-only trail joins from left
▶15	5.9	Right on Stevens Creek Nature Trail at end of loop
▶16	6.0	Back at parking area

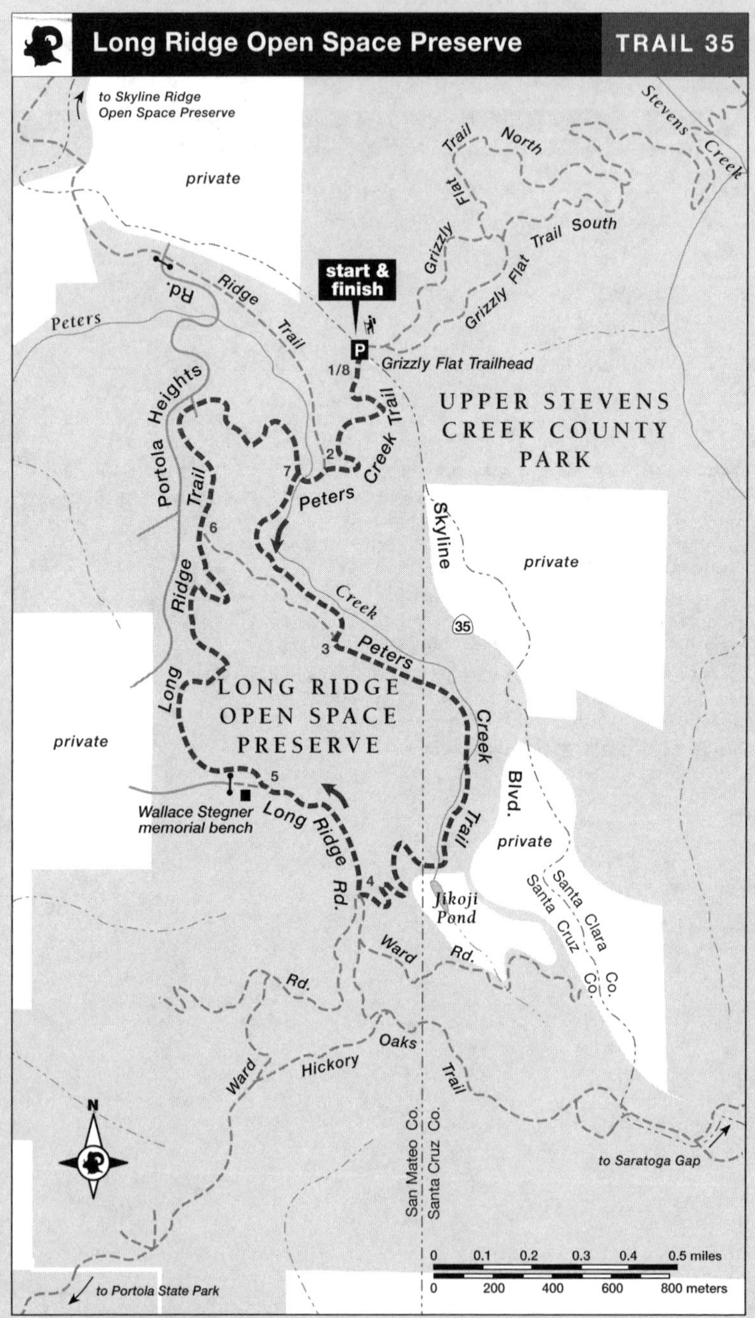
Long Ridge Open Space Preserve
TRAIL 35
to Skyline Ridge Open Space Preserve
private
Stevens Creek
North Trail
Grizzly Flat
Grizzly Flat Trail South
start & finish
Rd.
Ridge Trail
Peters
Grizzly Flat Trailhead
1/8
UPPER STEVENS CREEK COUNTY PARK
Portola Heights
Peters Creek Trail
2
7
Peters
Trail
6
Skyline
private
Ridge
Creek
35
3
Peters
LONG RIDGE OPEN SPACE PRESERVE
Long
Creek
private
Blvd.
5
Wallace Stegner memorial bench
Long Ridge Rd.
Trail
private
4
Jikoji Pond
Santa Clara Co.
Santa Cruz Co.
Ward Rd.
Rd.
Oaks
Hickory
Ward
Trail
N
San Mateo Co.
Santa Cruz Co.
to Saratoga Gap
0 0.1 0.2 0.3 0.4 0.5 miles
0 200 400 600 800 meters
to Portola State Park

Long Ridge Open Space Preserve

Superb views are the reason to wander uphill from the shady confines of Peters Creek to the dramatically situated Wallace Stegner memorial bench high atop Long Ridge. On a clear day, the scene extends westward over the Pescadero Creek watershed, taking in thousands of acres of protected lands, which are truly a living monument to the open space movement.

TRAIL USE
Hike, Run, Bike

LENGTH
4.6 miles, 2–3 hours

VERTICAL FEET
±850'

DIFFICULTY
– 1 2 **3** 4 5 +

TRAIL TYPE
Loop

SURFACE TYPE
Dirt

FEATURES
Stream
Canyon
Summit
Autumn Colors
Birds
Great Views
Secluded
Cool and Shady

FACILITIES
None

Best Time

All year, but trails may be muddy in wet weather. Peters Creek, Long Ridge, and Ridge trails are closed seasonally to bikes and horses.

Finding the Trail

From the junction of Skyline Blvd. and Page Mill Rd./Alpine Rd. south of Palo Alto, take Skyline Blvd. southeast 3.1 miles to a roadside parking area on the left. This parking area, sometimes called the Grizzly Flat Trailhead, serves both Long Ridge Open Space Preserve and Upper Stevens Creek County Park. The trailhead is on the southwest side of Skyline Blvd., across from the parking area.

Trail Description

From the trailhead▶**1** pass through a seasonal-closure gate that prevents access by bikes and horses during wet weather; ahead are information boards with dog-permit information and a map holder. From here, descend the **Peters Creek Trail** as it

A still-prolific apple orchard beside the Peters Creek Trail blooms beautifully in spring and in the fall is often heavily loaded with several varieties of apples.

wanders across a hillside that falls away to the right. Soon this single-track trail swings into a cool, dark forest of mostly Douglas-fir and California bay.

At a junction, a trail merges sharply from the right. This is the Ridge Trail, which heads north toward Skyline Ridge Open Space Preserve. The Ridge Trail and the Peters Creek Trail (from this point on) are both part of the Bay Area Ridge Trail. Dogs are prohibited beyond this point on the Peters Creek Trail. You continue straight on the Peters Creek Trail, and after several hundred feet cross the trail's namesake creek on a bridge. Stay straight at the next junction, where the Long Ridge Trail joins from the right.▶**2**

In a meadow, you pass a dirt road▶**3** which ascends right to the Long Ridge Trail. Follow the Peters Creek Trail, here a dirt road bordered by dense forest on the right and an open field with the willow-lined creek on the left. At an unsigned junction, a dirt road forks left and crosses a bridge over Peters Creek, but you angle right. Soon you cross to the east side of **Peters Creek**, enjoying a stroll beneath red alders, a moisture-loving tree often found beside creeks and rivers.

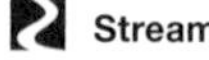

Where a gate blocks the road, turn right and cross an earthen dam. Built in the 1960s, this 200-foot-long dam turned part of Peters Creek into the cattail-fringed **Jikoji Pond** on your left. On the far side of the dam, you cross the pond's spillway on a wooden bridge. Now the trail zigzags uphill through forest and meadow to a seasonal-closure gate.

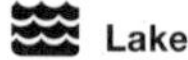

OPTIONS

Trail Options

Long Ridge Open Space Preserve borders Upper Stevens Creek County Park, Skyline Ridge Open Space Preserve, and Portola Redwoods State Park, making possible many extended loops and point-to-point routes.

Just beyond the gate is a four-way junction atop Long Ridge.►4 Here, Ward Road goes left and also straight, but you turn right on **Long Ridge Road.** This spectacularly situated road affords a fabulous view that extends westward across the Pescadero Creek drainage to the Pacific Ocean. A rolling course through mostly open terrain brings you in about 0.5 mile to the **Wallace Stegner memorial bench,**►5 which honors one of California's best-loved writers and open-space advocates.

Great Views

Since 1979, the pond at the headwaters of Peters Creek has been the property of a Buddhist group, now known as Jikoji, which runs a nearby meditation center.

Just past the bench, veer right from the road on the single-track **Long Ridge Trail.** Beyond a seasonal-closure gate, you enter dense forest and contour across a hillside that falls away to the right. Crossing a saddle, you descend to a junction in a clearing, where you cross a dirt road.►6

Go straight and continue on the Long Ridge Trail, which wraps around a wooded knoll studded with stands of black oak and manzanita. A moderate and then steep descent brings you to the junction with the **Peters Creek Trail** you passed earlier.►7 Here turn left and retrace your route to the parking area, remembering to stay right on the Peters Creek Trail where the Ridge Trail branches left.►8

MILESTONES

►1	0.0	Take Peters Creek Trail
►2	0.5	Long Ridge Trail on right
►3	0.9	Angle left to stay on Peters Creek Trail
►4	2.1	Right at four-way junction on Long Ridge Rd.
►5	2.6	Stegner memorial bench on left; veer right on Long Ridge Trail
►6	3.4	Straight across clearing to stay on Long Ridge Trail
►7	4.1	Retrace to parking area by going left and then right on Peters Creek Trail
►8	4.6	Back at parking area

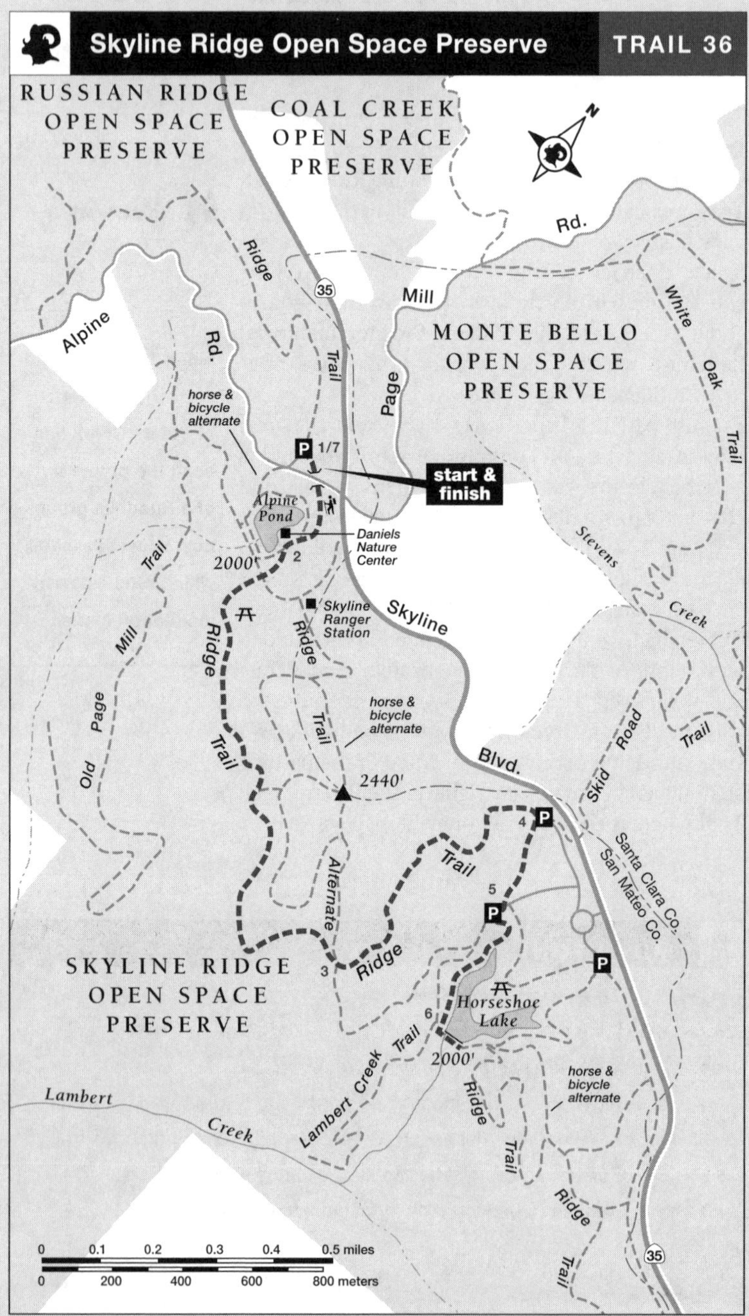
Skyline Ridge Open Space Preserve
TRAIL 36
RUSSIAN RIDGE OPEN SPACE PRESERVE
COAL CREEK OPEN SPACE PRESERVE
MONTE BELLO OPEN SPACE PRESERVE
SKYLINE RIDGE OPEN SPACE PRESERVE
N
Rd.
Mill
Page
Alpine
Rd.
Ridge
Trail
35
White Oak Trail
horse & bicycle alternate
1/7
start & finish
Alpine Pond
Daniels Nature Center
2000'
2
Trail
Mill
Old Page
Skyline Ranger Station
Ridge
Trail
Ridge
Trail
Skyline
Blvd.
Stevens Creek
horse & bicycle alternate
2440'
Skid Road
Trail
4
Trail
5
Santa Clara Co.
San Mateo Co.
Alternate
Ridge
3
Horseshoe Lake
6
2000'
Lambert Creek Trail
Lambert Creek
Ridge Trail
horse & bicycle alternate
Ridge Trail
0 0.1 0.2 0.3 0.4 0.5 miles
0 200 400 600 800 meters

Skyline Ridge Open Space Preserve

This out-and-back hike is a favorite among young and old alike. The trail rises from the forested environs of Alpine Pond to a breezy realm of grassland and chaparral—with views of Butano Ridge, Portola Redwoods State Park, and the Pacific coast—and then descends to Horseshoe Lake.

TRAIL USE
Hike, Run,
Child Friendly

LENGTH
4.2 miles, 2–3 hours

VERTICAL FEET
±250'

DIFFICULTY
– 1 2 **3** 4 5 +

TRAIL TYPE
Out & Back

SURFACE TYPE
Dirt

FEATURES
Lake
Canyon
Wildflowers
Birds
Great Views

FACILITIES
Nature Center
Restrooms

Best Time

All year, but trails may be muddy in wet weather.

Finding the Trail

From the junction of Skyline Blvd. and Page Mill Rd./Alpine Rd. south of Palo Alto, take Alpine Rd. west about 100 yards to a parking area on the right. This parking area serves both Skyline Ridge and Russian Ridge open space preserves. The trailhead is on the south side of the parking area.

If, as often happens on summer weekends, this parking area is filled, you can head 0.9 mile southeast on Skyline Blvd. to the Skyline Open Space Preserve entrance on the right. Then drive to the northernmost parking area▶**4** by bearing right at each of two forks. From here, you can hike the Ridge Trail by following the trail description below in reverse (3.4 miles out and back if you omit the Horseshoe Lake segment).

Trail Description

From the trailhead, walk down the wooden steps or the wheelchair-accessible path to an information

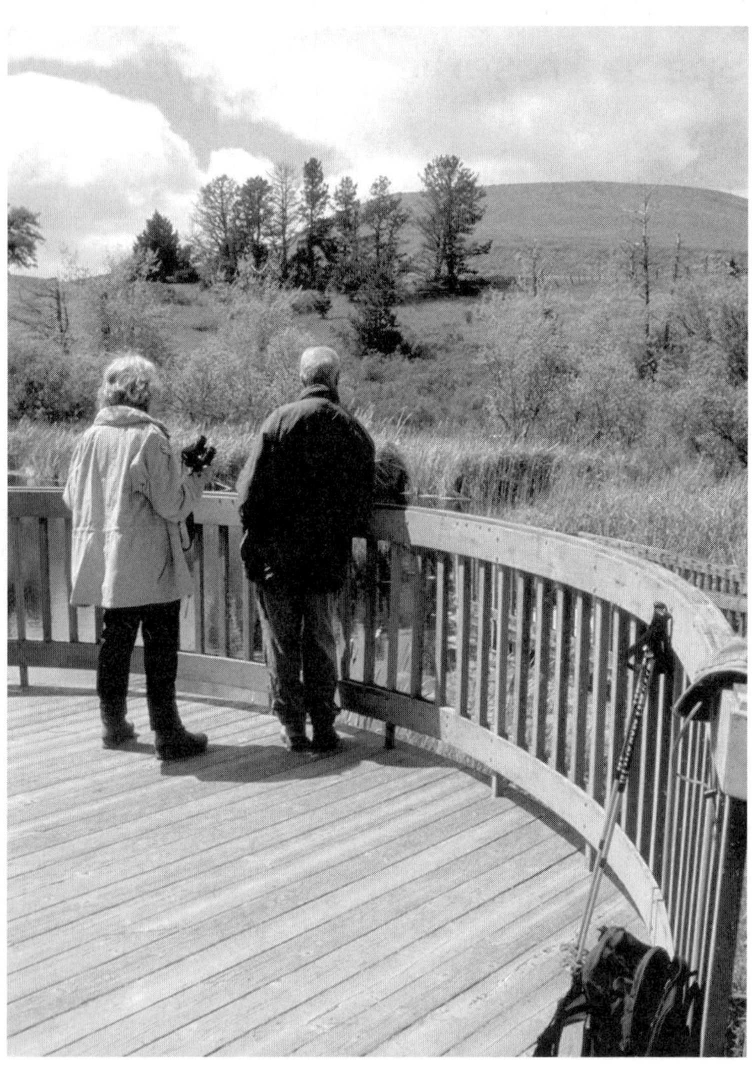

Daniels Nature Center *has an observation deck overlooking Alpine Pond.*

board.▶1 From here, your route, the **Ridge Trail**, goes through a tunnel under Alpine Road. Passing a gravel road that joins from the left, you soon arrive at cattail-lined **Alpine Pond** and the **Daniels Nature Center.**▶2

Just past the nature center, the Pond Loop Trail goes right, but you follow the Ridge Trail, a single track, by ascending left. When you reach the Ridge Trail Alternate, a paved road, you continue straight, and soon pass an unsigned trail and a fenced farm building, both uphill and left.

Emerging from forest, you make a rising traverse across an open hillside that drops west. From a tree-shaded rest bench, where the Pacific may be in view, climb steadily on a moderate grade into a zone of chaparral. Past a spur trail branching left, the Ridge Trail threads its way across a sandstone outcrop (edged by sturdy cable railings) from which you may gaze down the canyon of **Lambert Creek.**

The trail traverses through a wooded area that soon gives way to extensive stands of sage, manzanita, and silk tassel. As the trail descends sharply left, you begin to get sweeping views that extend southeast toward Mt. Umunhum. Monte Bello Ridge, topped by Black Mountain, is northeast.

At a four-way junction with the Ridge Trail Alternate, now a dirt road, continue straight,▶3 returning to forest. You wander steadily downhill across shady ravines and open meadows.

Much of the land that became Skyline Ridge Open Space Preserve was at one time owned by San Francisco mayor—and later California governor—James Rolph, Jr., known as "Sunny Jim."

Canyon

Great Views

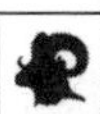
OPTIONS

Ridge Trail Alternate

The Ridge Trail is a hiking-only section of the **Bay Area Ridge Trail.** Bicyclists and equestrians must use another route, which starts across Alpine Rd. just south of the parking area. The **Ridge Trail Alternate** descends past Alpine Pond, then follows a several (mostly) dirt roads over the ridge and down to Horseshoe Lake. The two Ridge Trail alignments cross twice.

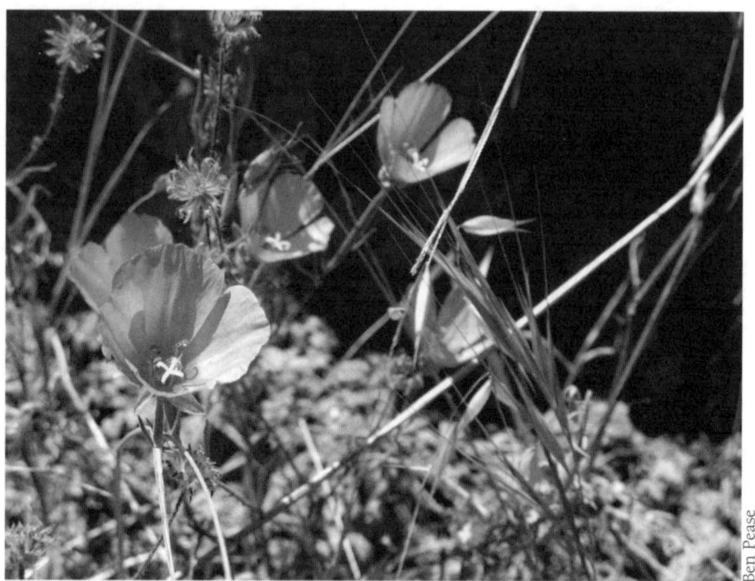

Clarkia *is a bright purple flower found in grasslands.*

Eventually, in a clearing, you arrive at the northernmost of Skyline Open Space Preserve's three parking areas,▶4 which has information boards and a toilet.

Bear sharply right on the Ridge Trail, now a multiuse path, through a grassy meadow. Soon you come to a gravel road and another parking area.▶5 Veer right, then angle left to the beginning of the parking area. Descending a set of wooden steps, you come to a T-junction at a bend in the **Horseshoe Lake Trail.** Angle right on the lower leg of this wheelchair-accessible trail and descend south. Soon the willows along the valley to your left give way to **Horseshoe Lake,** a cattail-fringed reservoir that may have rafts of ducks and American coots. At the next junction, keep left on a dirt road to reach the dam,▶6 from where you can gaze left up both arms of the lake and see how it got its name.

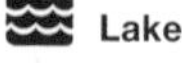
Lake

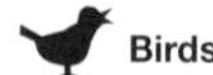
Birds

From here, retrace your route to the parking area.▶7

MILESTONES

- ▶1 0.0 Take Ridge Trail south under Alpine Rd.
- ▶2 0.2 Alpine Pond, Daniels Nature Center; stay left on Ridge Trail
- ▶3 1.2 Four-way junction with Ridge Trail Alternate road; go straight
- ▶4 1.7 Upper Horseshoe Lake trailhead, turn sharply right on Ridge Trail
- ▶5 1.9 Angle right on gravel road to parking area, then left to Horseshoe Lake Trail
- ▶6 2.1 Angle left on Ridge Trail to Horseshoe Lake dam
- ▶7 4.2 Back at parking area

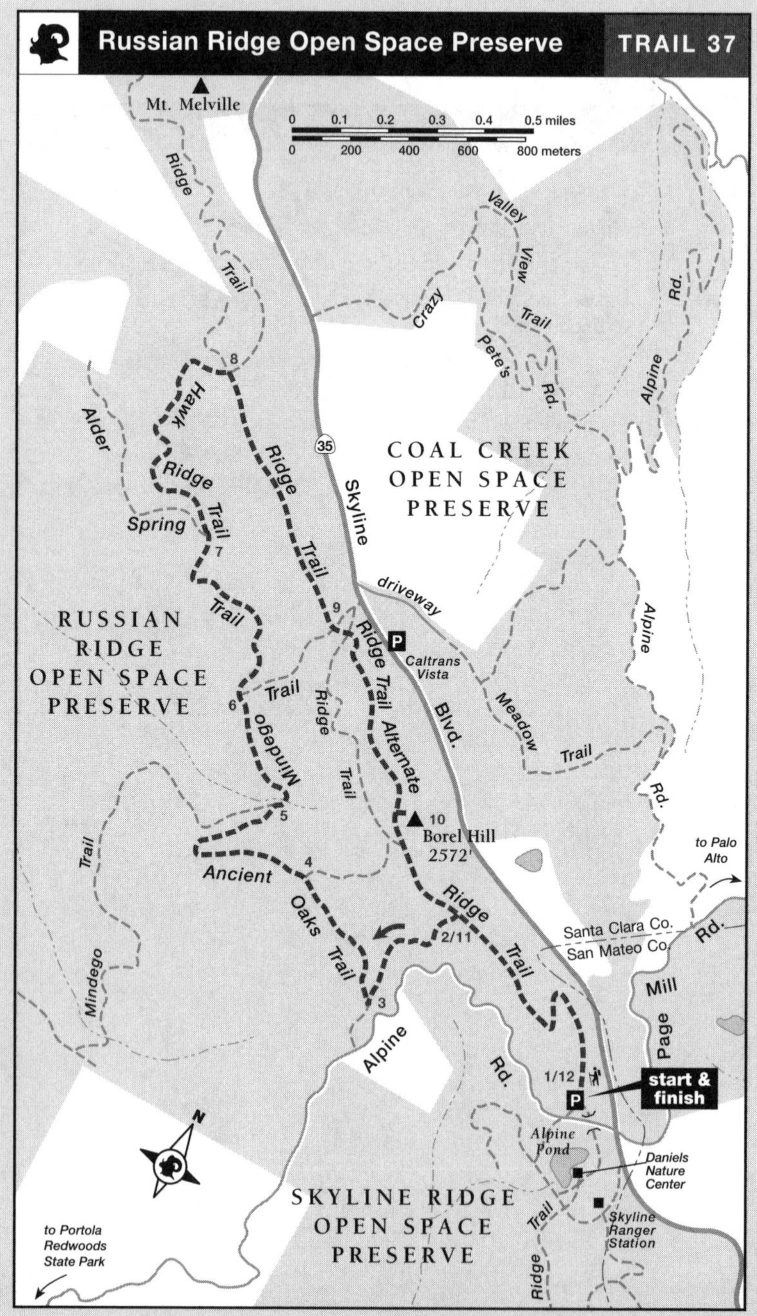

Russian Ridge Open Space Preserve
TRAIL 37
Mt. Melville
0.5 miles
800 meters
COAL CREEK
OPEN SPACE
PRESERVE
RUSSIAN
RIDGE
OPEN SPACE
PRESERVE
SKYLINE RIDGE
OPEN SPACE
PRESERVE
Ridge Trail
Hawk Ridge Trail
Alder Spring Trail
Mindego Trail
Ancient Oaks Trail
Ridge Trail Alternate
Skyline Blvd.
driveway
Caltrans Vista
Crazy Pete's Rd.
Valley View Trail
Alpine Rd.
Meadow Trail
Borel Hill
2572'
to Palo Alto
Santa Clara Co.
San Mateo Co.
Page Mill Rd.
start &
finish
Alpine Pond
Daniels Nature Center
Skyline Ranger Station
to Portola Redwoods State Park

Russian Ridge Open Space Preserve

This remarkable Peninsula ramble samples a wide variety of habitats, from oak forests perched on Pacific-facing slopes to dazzling wildflower meadows atop Borel Hill. Bring binoculars to pick out soaring hawks and falcons, along with various Bay Area landmarks.

TRAIL USE
Hike, Run, Bike

LENGTH
4.6 miles, 2–3 hours

VERTICAL FEET
±1050'

DIFFICULTY
– 1 2 **3** 4 5 +

TRAIL TYPE
Loop

SURFACE TYPE
Dirt

FEATURES
Summit
Wildflowers
Birds
Wildlife
Great Views
Photo Opportunity

FACILITIES
Restrooms

Best Time

All year, but spring wildflowers are the prime attraction; trails may be muddy in wet weather.

Finding the Trail

From the junction of Skyline Blvd. and Page Mill Rd./Alpine Rd. south of Palo Alto, take Alpine Rd. west about 100 yards to a parking area on the right. This parking area serves both Russian Ridge and Skyline Ridge open space preserves. On busy days parking may be unavailable. The trailhead is on the west side of the parking area.▶1

Additional parking for Russian Ridge is available at the Caltrans Vista Point parking area, 1.1 miles northwest on Skyline Blvd.

Trail Description

Your route, the single-track **Ridge Trail,** climbs northwest from the trailhead on a steady grade. This multiuse trail is part of the Bay Area Ridge Trail.

Aided by switchbacks, you gain the ridgeline and are rewarded by ever-improving views east across the San Andreas Fault to Monte Bello

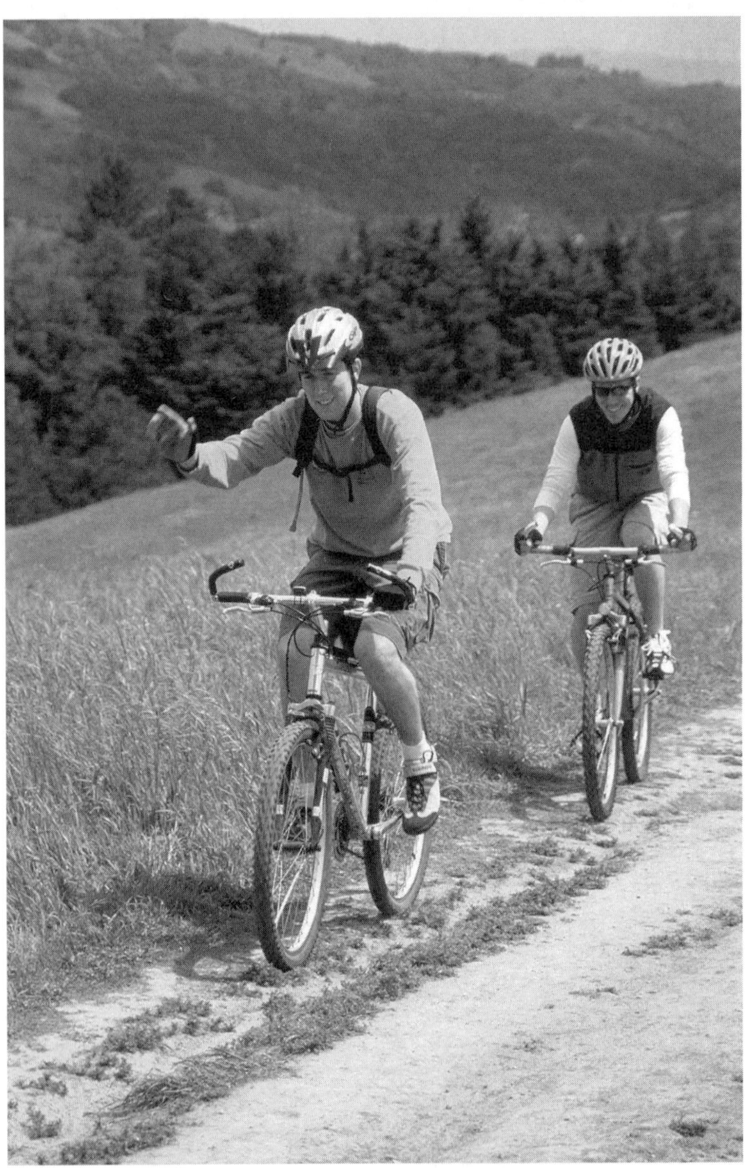

Bicyclists *ascend multiuse Ridge Trail toward Borel Hill. Black Mountain is on the horizon.*

Ridge and Black Mountain, and southeast to Mt. Umunhum and Loma Prieta.

After about 0.5 mile, you turn left at a junction▶2 with a dirt road connector to the Ancient Oaks Trail. Follow this road west, curving left above a wooded ravine. With Alpine Road immediately left, you meet a junction with the **Ancient Oaks Trail.**▶3

Lupine, poppies, mule ears, buttercups, blue-eyed grass, and checker mallow form a flowering foreground no matter which way you look.

Turning right on this single track, you enjoy a splendid view of the Pacific Ocean as you make a rising traverse across a grassy hillside. The trail levels briefly and then starts to descend. You pass a connector to the Ridge Trail, right▶4 in a grove of large coast live oaks. Continuing down the ridge, you skirt a steep hillside overlooking a canyon, then turn sharply right from grassland into shady bay forest.

Losing elevation, you come to a junction,▶5 where you turn right on the **Mindego Trail.** This dirt road wanders on a mostly level grade to a fork.▶6 Here the Mindego Trail ascends right, but you veer left on the **Alder Spring Trail**, a dirt road through open grassland. You descend gently between wooded and open areas, with views of Mindego Hill and, on a clear day, the Pacific Ocean.

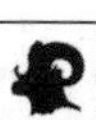

NOTE

Skyline Habitats

Russian Ridge is famous for its springtime displays of wildflowers. Lupine, clarkia, checker mallow, red maids, California buttercup, fiddleneck, owl's clover, Johnny jump-ups, mule ears, tidy-tips, and California poppies are among the most common grassland species found here. Westerly winds push coastal fog inland to Russian Ridge, where it helps keep plants moist during the dry season. Many of the large coast live oaks and California buckeyes are clad in dense layers of moss, and moisture dripping from trees may cause the ground underfoot to be wet and slippery. Shade-loving plants in the cool, forested canyons include trillium, fairy bells, mission bells, and hound's tongue.

Atop Borel Hill, the unrivaled vista extends northeast across San Francisco Bay to the East Bay hills, east to Mt. Hamilton, and west to the Pacific.

At a junction with the **Hawk Ridge Trail,▶7** angle right and uphill across a steep, grassy slope. The top-of-the-world feeling is enhanced as the narrow trail rises toward a gap in the crest of **Russian Ridge.**

At a four-way junction with the **Ridge Trail,** turn right on this dirt road.▶8 Ahead about 1 mile is Borel Hill, the geographic high point of this route. When you reach a four-way junction with the Mindego Trail,▶9 continue straight and begin a moderate climb. After about 75 feet, a single-track segment of the Ridge Trail veers right, to the west side of the ridge, but you stay on the nameless dirt road, which this guide calls the **Ridge Trail Alternate.** This eroded track snakes its way up the spine of the ridge. Though a little steeper than the trail, it has better views.

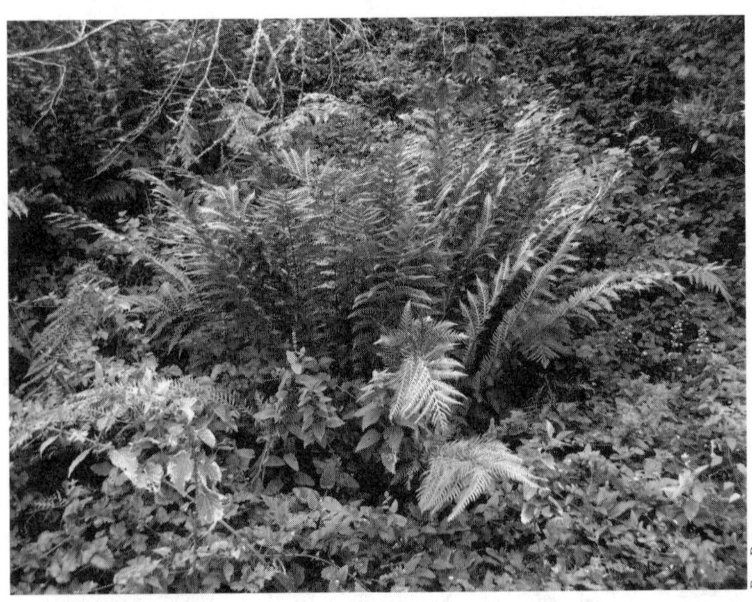

Ben Pease

Giant chain fern *on the Alder Spring Trail*

Near the summit of **Borel Hill** is truly a sea of wildflowers, a carpet of color. At a four-way junction,▶10 a trail goes right to a vantage point, but you turn left for the final push to the summit, where a sign shows you are 2572 feet above sea level. From this dramatic perch, most of the San Francisco Bay Area is revealed.

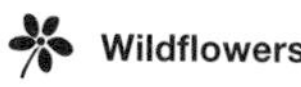

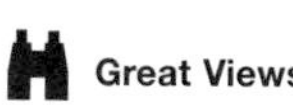

When you are ready to leave, put the elevation sign at your back and follow the trail in front of you. It soon joins the **Ridge Trail Alternate** at a T-junction. You turn left and, after about 100 feet, merge with the **Ridge Trail.** The next junction▶11 is with the connector to the Ancient Oaks Trail you used near the start of this trip. From here, retrace your route to the parking area.▶12

MILESTONES

▶1	0.0	Take Ridge Trail northwest
▶2	0.5	Left on connector road to Ancient Oaks Trail
▶3	0.8	Right on Ancient Oaks Trail
▶4	1.1	Pass a connector to the Ridge Trail
▶5	1.5	Right on Mindego Trail
▶6	1.8	Left on Alder Spring Trail
▶7	2.2	Straight on Hawk Ridge Trail
▶8	2.8	Right at four-way junction on Ridge Trail (dirt road)
▶9	3.4	Straight at four-way junction on Ridge Trail Alternate (dirt road)
▶10	3.9	Left to Borel Hill (2572'), then south to Ridge Trail Alternate and left at T-junction
▶11	4.1	Straight at junction with road to Ancient Oaks Trail, then retrace to parking area
▶12	4.6	Back at parking area

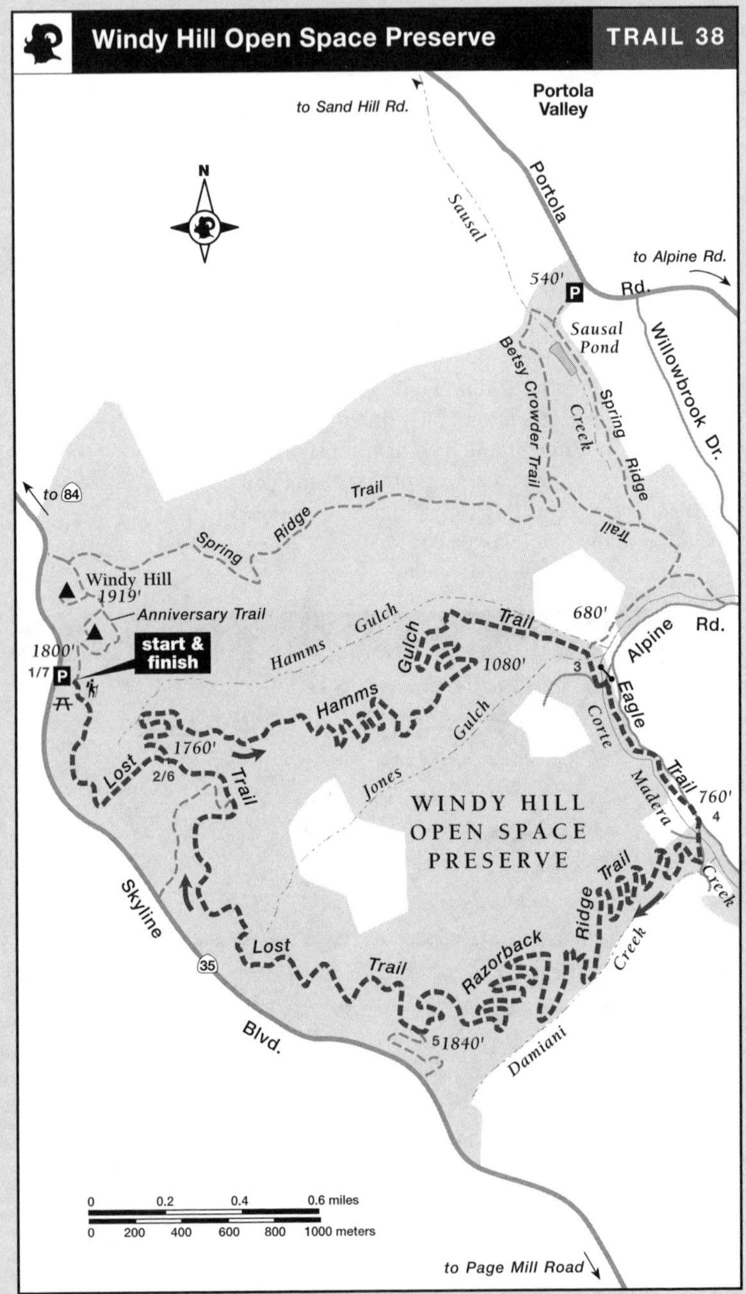
Windy Hill Open Space Preserve
TRAIL 38
Portola Valley
to Sand Hill Rd.
N
Sausal
Portola
Rd.
to Alpine Rd.
540'
P
Sausal Pond
Willowbrook Dr.
Betsy Crowder Trail
Creek
Spring Ridge Trail
to 84
Spring Ridge Trail
Windy Hill
1919'
Anniversary Trail
680'
Alpine Rd.
1800'
start & finish
Hamms Gulch Trail
1080'
1/7
3
Eagle
Hamms
Gulch
Corte Madera
Lost
1760'
2/6
Trail
Jones
Trail
760'
4
WINDY HILL OPEN SPACE PRESERVE
Ridge Trail
Creek
Skyline
Lost Trail
Razorback
Creek
35
Blvd.
5
1840'
Damiani
0 0.2 0.4 0.6 miles
0 200 400 600 800 1000 meters
to Page Mill Road

Windy Hill Open Space Preserve

This adventurous semiloop explores one of Midpeninsula Regional Open Space District's best-loved preserves. From Skyline Boulevard you follow cool and shady Hamms Gulch downhill through a lush forest of Douglas-fir, California buckeye, and bigleaf maple to the banks of lovely Corte Madera Creek before climbing back to Skyline Boulevard. Bring binoculars to catch glimpses of forest birds and scan the skies for raptors such as hawks and falcons. As its name implies, there is often wind at the upper reaches of this preserve, and also, in summer, fog.

TRAIL USE
Hike, Run

LENGTH
8.0 miles, 4–5 hours

VERTICAL FEET
±1650'

DIFFICULTY
– 1 2 3 4 **5** +

TRAIL TYPE
Loop

SURFACE TYPE
Dirt

FEATURES
Stream
Canyon
Autumn Colors
Wildflowers
Birds
Great Views
Secluded
Cool & Shady

FACILITIES
Restrooms
Picnic Tables

Best Time

This trail is best all year; often foggy and windy, especially near Skyline Boulevard.

Finding the Trail

From the junction of Skyline Blvd. and State Hwy. 84 in Sky Londa, take Skyline Blvd. southeast 2.3 miles to a parking area on the left. The trailhead is on the northeast corner of the parking area, near information boards and a map holder.

Trail Description

From the trailhead,▶1 go through a gap in a fence and turn right on the **Lost Trail,** part of the Bay Area Ridge Trail. After about 100 feet, pass through a seasonal-closure gate that prevents access by horses during wet weather. Now your single-track

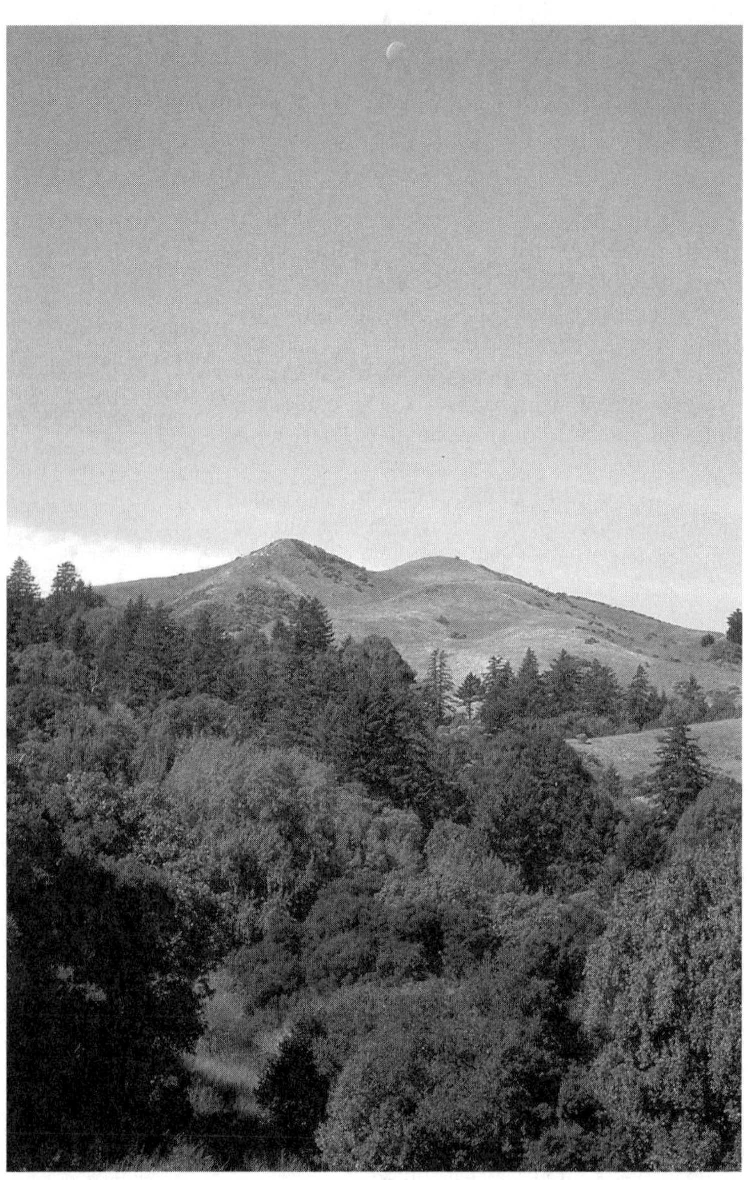

Windy Hill's twin grassy summits and wooded slopes *are prominent landmarks along the skyline on the central Peninsula.*

trail climbs on a gentle grade, with views that range from the Stanford University campus and Palo Alto to the East Bay hills and Mt. Diablo.

At a junction,►2 turn left on the single-track **Hamms Gulch Trail** and begin a long, delightful descent through a dense forest of towering Douglas-firs, fragrant California bays, and tanbark oaks. Passing a meadow, you ramble downhill past stands of madrone and California buckeye, enjoying a view of Windy Hill from a convenient bench. Near the bottom of the gulch are stands of coast redwood.

 **Great Views**

Enjoy the view along the ridgeline and from the summit! Aided by clear skies and binoculars, Oakland, San Francisco, and three of the Bay's bridges are visible.

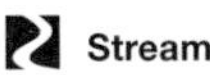

After nearly 2 miles along **Hamms Gulch,** you reach another seasonal-closure gate. Just beyond the gate, a connector to the Spring Ridge Trail branches left.►3 You veer right to stay on the Hamms Gulch Trail. After several hundred yards you cross a wooden bridge over a creek flowing from **Jones Gulch**, then arrive at a paved road. Turn left on this road to cross **Corte Madera Creek** on an old stone bridge.►4

Once across the creek, look right to find the start of the **Eagle Trail,** which is maintained by the town of Portola Valley and closed to bikes. Follow this single-track trail as it parallels the rocky bed of Corte Madera Creek, which is right. Soon the trail reaches **Alpine Road,** which you follow for about 100 yards, then regain the trail as it descends right.

Again returning to Alpine Road, follow it for about 100 feet, then turn right on a paved road that crosses Corte Madera Creek via a bridge. Beyond the

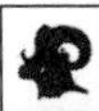

OPTIONS

Windy Hill

From the trailhead, the Anniversary Trail and a short spur trail climb to the summit of **Windy Hill,** for some of the best views on the Peninsula.

creek, a driveway branches right, but you continue straight on the narrow paved road. After climbing moderately for about 200 yards, you come to a trail post and turn right on the **Razorback Ridge Trail,** a single track.

Past a seasonal-closure gate, you climb steadily on a moderate grade, switchbacking across a narrow, forested ridge and making several forays toward the deep canyon of **Damiani Creek.** Near the top of the climb, a gap in the forest provides a view north to Windy Hill.

At a junction with the **Lost Trail,**►**5** angle right, pass a watering trough for horses, and then enjoy a mostly level grade. Now following a ridge downhill, you give up several hundred feet of hard-won elevation near the head of Jones Gulch before leveling again.

On a scrub-covered hillside, cross under a set of power lines and then reach a four-way junction with a dirt-and-gravel road. Continuing straight across the junction, climb gently to meet the Hamms Gulch Trail on the right.►**6** From here, retrace your route on the Lost Trail to the parking area.►**7**

MILESTONES

- ▶1 0.0 Take Lost Trail, right
- ▶2 0.4 Left on Hamms Gulch Trail
- ▶3 3.0 Right to stay on Hamms Gulch Trail; then left across bridge and right on Eagle Trail (which alternates with Alpine Rd.)
- ▶4 3.6 Right to cross Corte Madera Creek on bridge; climb paved road 200 yards, then right on Razorback Ridge Trail
- ▶5 5.9 Right on Lost Trail
- ▶6 7.6 Hamms Gulch Trail on right; stay left on Lost Trail and retrace to parking area
- ▶7 8.0 Back at parking area

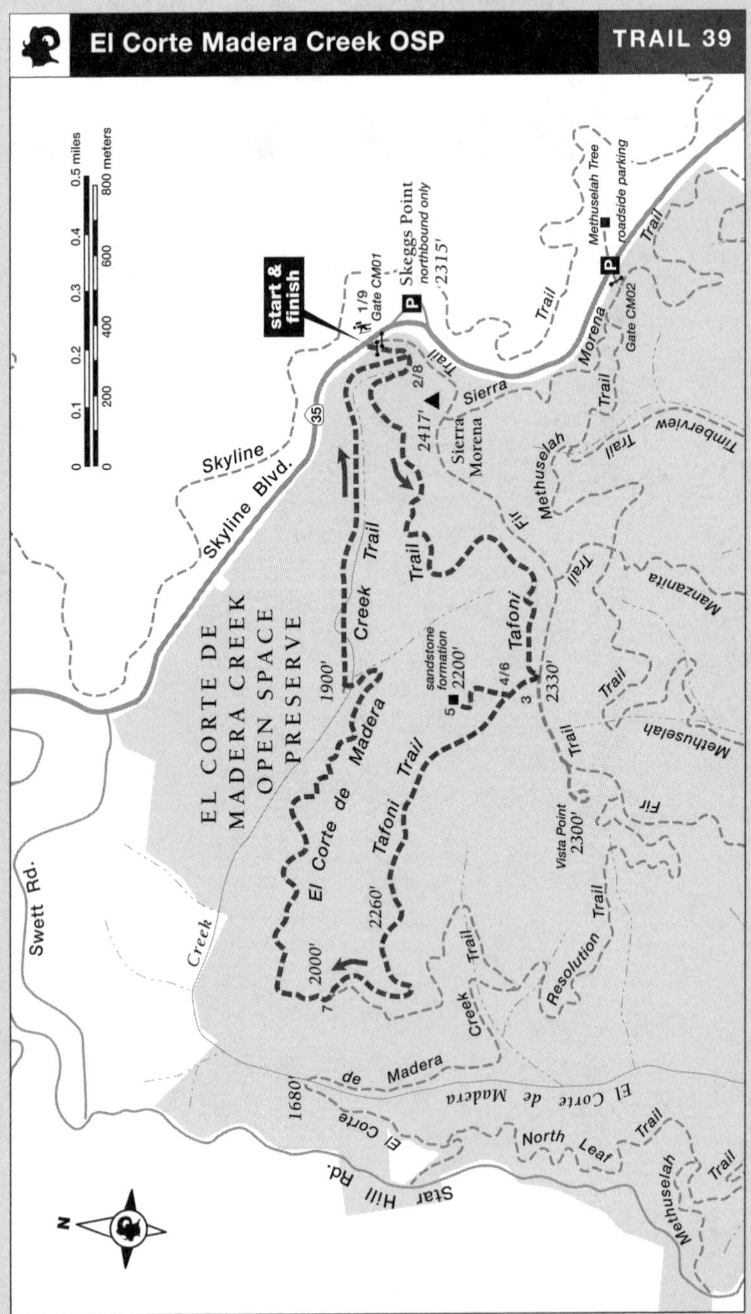
El Corte Madera Creek OSP
TRAIL 39
0 0.1 0.2 0.3 0.4 0.5 miles
0 200 400 600 800 meters
start & finish
1/9
Gate CM01
Skeggs Point
northbound only
2315'
Methuselah Tree
roadside parking
Gate CM02
Skyline
Skyline Blvd.
35
2/8
2417'
Sierra Morena
Sierra Morena Trail
Methuselah Trail
Timberview Trail
Fir Trail
Manzanita Trail
Creek Trail
Tafoni Trail
sandstone formation
2200'
4/6
5
3
2330'
1900'
EL CORTE DE MADERA CREEK OPEN SPACE PRESERVE
El Corte de Madera
2260'
2000'
7
Vista Point
2300'
Resolution Trail
Creek Trail
El Corte de Madera
1680'
North Leaf Trail
Methuselah Trail
El Corte
Star Hill Rd.
Swett Rd.
Creek
N

El Corte de Madera Creek Open Space Preserve

An unusual sandstone formation called tafoni is the main attraction of this invigorating loop at the north end of the preserve. Towering Douglas-firs and coast redwoods and a lush riparian corridor near the headwaters of El Corte de Madera Creek are some of the other highlights here.

TRAIL USE
Hike, Run, Bike
LENGTH
4.3 miles, 2–3 hours
VERTICAL FEET
±1300'
DIFFICULTY
– 1 2 **3** 4 5 +
TRAIL TYPE
Loop
SURFACE TYPE
Dirt

FEATURES
Stream
Canyon
Autumn Colors
Birds
Geologic Interest
Secluded
Cool & Shady

FACILITIES
Restrooms
Picnic Tables

Best Time

All year, but trails may be muddy in wet weather. The preserve is very popular with bicyclists, and the parking area fills early on weekends.

Finding the Trail

From the junction of Skyline Blvd. and State Hwy. 84 in Sky Londa, take Skyline Blvd. northwest 3.9 miles to the Caltrans parking area at Skeggs Point. The trailhead is at gate CM01, on the southwest side of Skyline Blvd. about 100 yards northwest of the parking area. Walk carefully along the east shoulder until opposite this gate, then cross when it is safe.

Trail Description

Two metal gates and a wood fence mark the trailhead.►1 An information board with a map holder is just past the right-hand gate. From here, follow the **Tafoni Trail**, a dirt road that soon curves right, bringing you to a junction, where you continue straight.►2 Towering Douglas-firs line the trail, and the hillside on your right falls steeply right into the canyon of **El Corte de Madera Creek.**

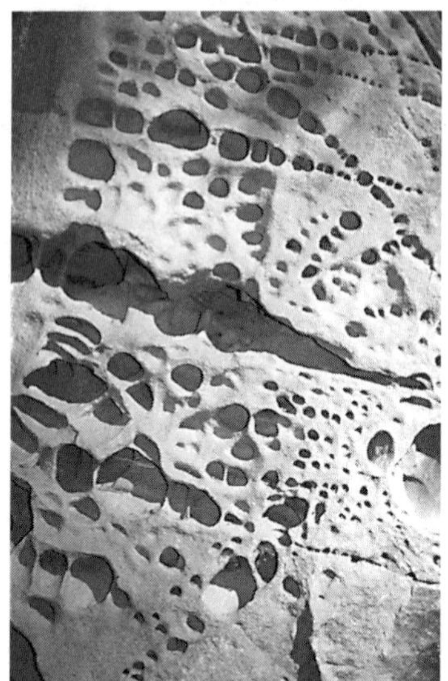

Tafoni *originated as undersea sand deposits.*

Turning right at a T-junction (left leg is closed), you enjoy a rolling course and then climb to a ridgetop, passing several old logging roads. Soon you come to a saddle and a four-way junction.►**3** Here, the Fir Trail goes left and straight, and your route, the Tafoni Trail, bears right.

The Tafoni Trail, a dirt road, descends gently along a ridge. At a junction signed SANDSTONE FORMATION, you turn right on a single-track trail►**4** that is closed to bikes and horses. Soon you come to an observation deck from where you can see the **eroded sandstone formations**, a form of rock that is called tafoni.►**5** The enormous outcrop is fragile, and the terrain around it is very steep: Please stay on the trail or the observation deck at all times.

When you have finished enjoying this unusual area, return to the **Tafoni Trail** and turn right.►**6** The road curves right and descends. Now on a ridgetop, you follow a rolling course which soon leads to a long, moderate descent. Far down the ridge, you turn right where the Tafoni Trail becomes a single track. Beside the trail are huge redwood stumps surrounded by family circles of second-growth trees, remnants of the area's logging past.

OPTIONS

Vista Point

For a quick trip to **Vista Point** that adds a half mile to your trip, from the junction of the Fir and Tafoni trails,►**3** go straight for 0.2 mile on the Fir Trail, then bear right on a spur road to Vista Point. Here the forest gives way to a sea of chaparral and broad views west toward the San Mateo coast and the Pacific Ocean. Retrace your route to the junction►**3** and turn left on the Tafoni Trail.

Now you merge with the **El Corte de Madera Creek Trail,**▶7 which joins sharply from the left. Continuing almost straight, you follow the single-track trail gently uphill through dense forest. El Corte de Madera Creek lies at the bottom of the steep drop to your left. You descend slightly as the canyon rises to meet you. Finally the trail bends sharply left and arrives at a bridge across El Corte de Madera Creek.

Across the bridge, you reach a T-junction with a dirt road; turn right to continue on the El Corte de Madera Creek Trail, which climbs steadily in a shady, steep-walled canyon. The road soon bends right and brings you to the junction with the **Tafoni Trail**, closing the loop.▶8 From here, turn left and retrace your route to the Skyline Boulevard trailhead.▶9 When walking back to the parking area, carefully cross Skyline Boulevard and walk on the east shoulder of the highway.

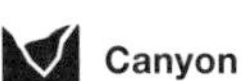

MILESTONES

▶1	0.0	Take Tafoni Trail southwest
▶2	0.1	El Corte de Madera Creek Trail on right; go straight
▶3	1.3	Stay on Tafoni Trail by veering right at four-way junction with Fir Trail
▶4	1.4	Trail to sandstone formation on right (no bikes)
▶5	1.5	Sandstone formation and observation deck; retrace to junction
▶6	1.6	At previous junction, turn right on Tafoni Trail
▶7	2.5	Straight on El Corte de Madera Creek Trail
▶8	4.2	Left on Tafoni Trail, retrace to trailhead
▶9	4.3	Back at trailhead

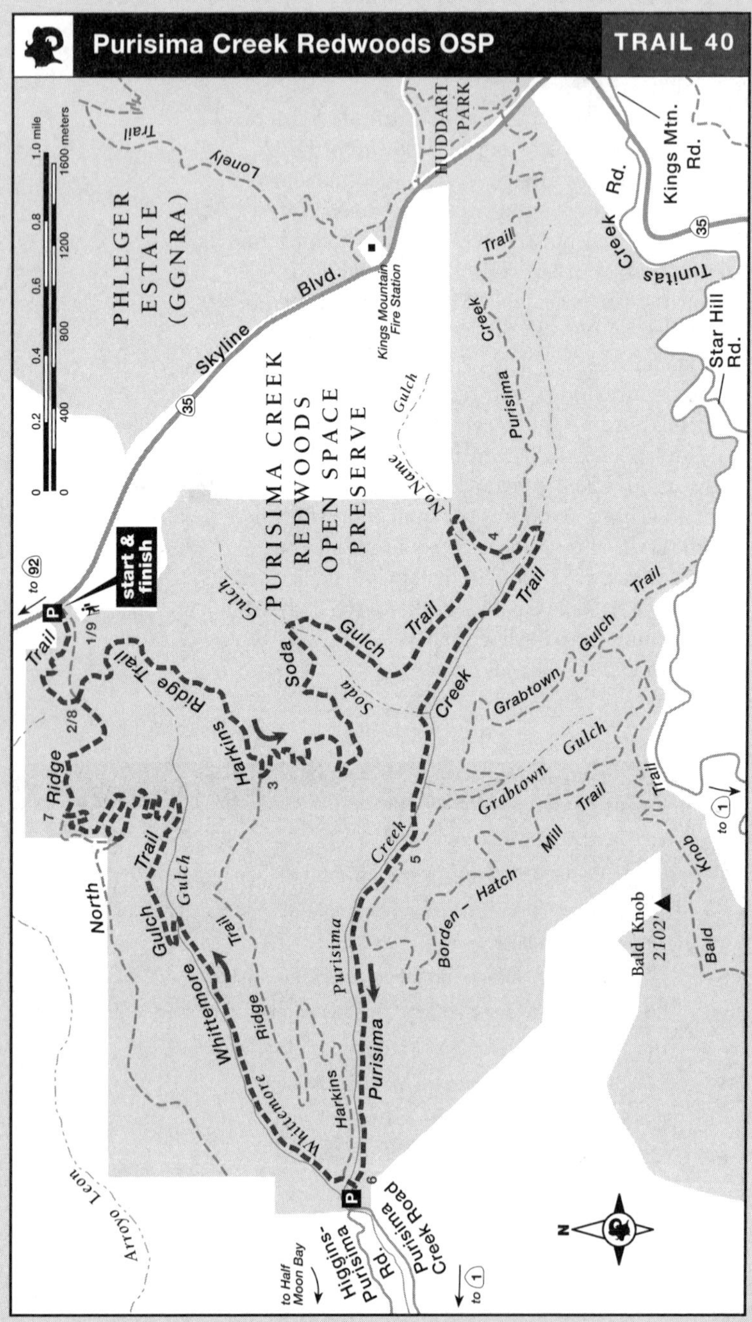

Purisima Creek Redwoods OSP
TRAIL 40
PHLEGER ESTATE (GGNRA)
PURISIMA CREEK REDWOODS OPEN SPACE PRESERVE
HUDDART PARK
Skyline Blvd.
Kings Mountain Fire Station
start & finish
to 92
Lonely Trail
Kings Mtn. Rd.
Tunitas Creek Rd.
Star Hill Rd.
Soda Gulch Trail
Purisima Creek Trail
Harkins Ridge Trail
North Ridge Trail
Whittemore Gulch Trail
Grabtown Gulch Trail
Borden - Hatch Mill Trail
Bald Knob Trail
Bald Knob 2102'
No Name Gulch
Arroyo Leon
Higgins-Purisima Rd.
Purisima Creek Road
to Half Moon Bay
to 1
1.0 mile
1600 meters

Purisima Creek Redwoods Open Space Preserve

One of the premier routes on the Peninsula, this challenging loop explores the north half of this expansive preserve. Dropping to Purisima Creek past the giant stumps of old-growth redwoods, you can imagine when these canyons echoed with the sounds of men and machinery harvesting a seemingly limitless resource. A vigorous climb through stands of Douglas-fir forest and coastal scrub make this one of the most botanically diverse routes in this guide.

TRAIL USE
Hike, Run

LENGTH
10.1 miles, 4–6 hours

VERTICAL FEET
±1600'

DIFFICULTY
– 1 2 3 4 **5** +

TRAIL TYPE
Loop

SURFACE TYPE
Dirt

FEATURES
Stream
Canyon
Autumn Colors
Wildflowers
Birds
Historic
Great Views
Secluded
Cool & Shady

FACILITIES
Restrooms
Phone

Best Time

All year, but trails may be muddy in wet weather.

Finding the Trail

From the junction of Skyline Blvd. and State Hwy. 92, take Skyline Blvd. southeast 4.5 miles to a parking area on the right. The trailhead is on the southwest corner of the parking area, near information boards and a map holder.

Trail Description

From the trailhead,►1 amble down a dirt road that goes left of the information boards and map holder. After 100 feet or so you reach a junction and bear right on the **North Ridge Trail**, a single track. This trail and several others on this route are part of the Bay Area Ridge Trail.

Switchback downhill to a four-way junction,►2 where you go on the multiuse **Harkins Ridge Trail.**

According to local historian Ken Fisher, San Mateo County's last grizzly bear was poisoned in Whittemore Gulch in 1879.

After winding through groves of coast redwood and California bay, you reach open ground on a scrubby hillside that drops to the right. Now you reach a T-junction with a closed road, left. Here, you turn right and descend a ridgetop dirt road. After a steep, eroded pitch, the road curves right, levels, and arrives at a junction.▶3

Turn left on the **Soda Gulch Trail,** a single track closed to bikes and horses that leads downhill across hillsides of coastal scrub into the realm of giant, although second-growth, redwoods. When you reach **Soda Gulch,** turn sharply right and cross a wood bridge over a tributary of Purisima Creek. After traversing an open hillside, cross a second tributary of Purisima Creek at the bottom of a steep canyon.

Canyon

Climb to a junction with the **Purisima Creek Trail**▶4 and then bear right. Follow this old dirt road as it curves left and descends to **Purisima Creek,** which flows under the road through a culvert. Soon a bridge takes you across Purisima Creek, which is now left. The creek from Soda Gulch joins from the right, and you cross it on the next bridge.

Stream

You descend on a moderate grade and cross Purisima Creek on a bridge, soon passing junctions with the Grabtown Gulch Trail and then the Borden–Hatch Mill Trail, both left.▶5 Now on a gentle grade, you descend along Purisima Creek beneath stately, second-growth redwoods.

Historic Interest

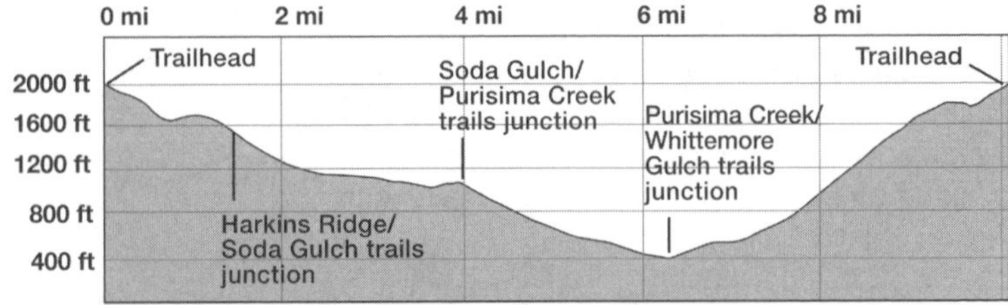

TRAIL 40 Purisima Creek Redwoods Open Space Preserve Profile

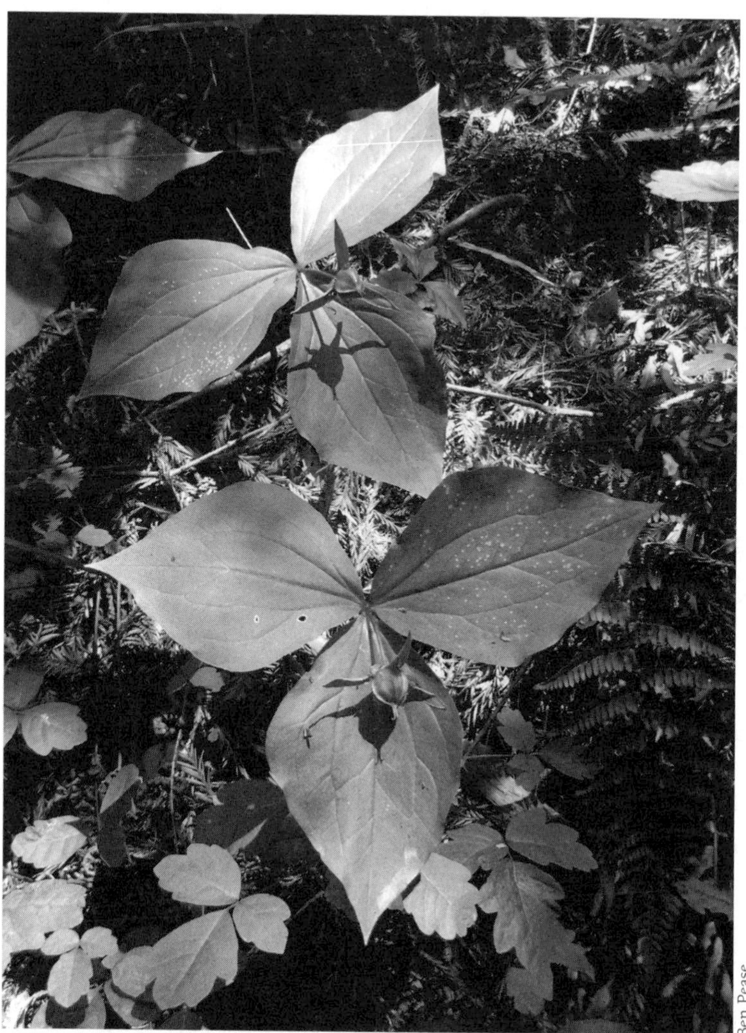

Ben Pease

Trillium *is an early bloomer in shady woodlands.*

Just before the Higgins Purisima parking area is a clearing with a junction, information boards, and a toilet.▶**6** Here turn right and cross Purisima Creek on a wood bridge. About 50 feet ahead, where the Harkins Ridge Trail goes right, turn left on the **Whittemore Gulch Trail.** The rocky dirt road soon narrows to a single track and passes a seasonal-closure gate that prevents access by bikes and horses during wet weather. (Use caution: This trail is popular with bicyclists.)

Canyon

The road curves right, narrows to a single track, and begins to climb **Whittemore Gulch,** which holds a tributary of Purisima Creek. Impressive rock cliffs, composed of marine sediments, provide a geological background to stands of coast redwood and red alder. You cross the creek on a small bridge and then climb easily along the forest edge, aided by switchbacks.

The elevation gain brings a brighter, more open feeling as you enter a zone of Douglas-fir and coastal scrub. After many twists and turns, you pass a short connector to the North Ridge Trail, beyond which is another seasonal-closure gate and then a T-junction with the **North Ridge Trail.**▶**7** Bear right on this dirt road and enjoy a mostly level walk along the ridge. At the four-way junction where you started this loop,▶**8** turn left on the hiking-only trail and retrace your route uphill to the parking area.▶**9**

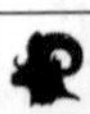

HISTORY

Borden–Hatch Sawmill

The **Borden–Hatch Sawmill** operated near Whittemore Gulch (1854), then at the foot of today's Borden–Hatch Mill Trail (1871) and Grabtown Gulch (1900). All three sites are now just clearings in the forest.

MILESTONES

▶1	0.0	Take dirt road southwest, then right on North Ridge Trail
▶2	0.5	Straight at four-way junction on Harkins Ridge Trail
▶3	1.4	Left on Soda Gulch Trail
▶4	4.0	Right on Purisima Creek Trail
▶5	5.3	Borden–Hatch Mill Trail on left; continue straight
▶6	6.3	Right across bridge, then left on Whittemore Gulch Trail
▶7	9.1	Right at T-junction on North Ridge Trail
▶8	9.6	Left at four-way junction, retrace to parking area
▶9	10.1	Back at parking area

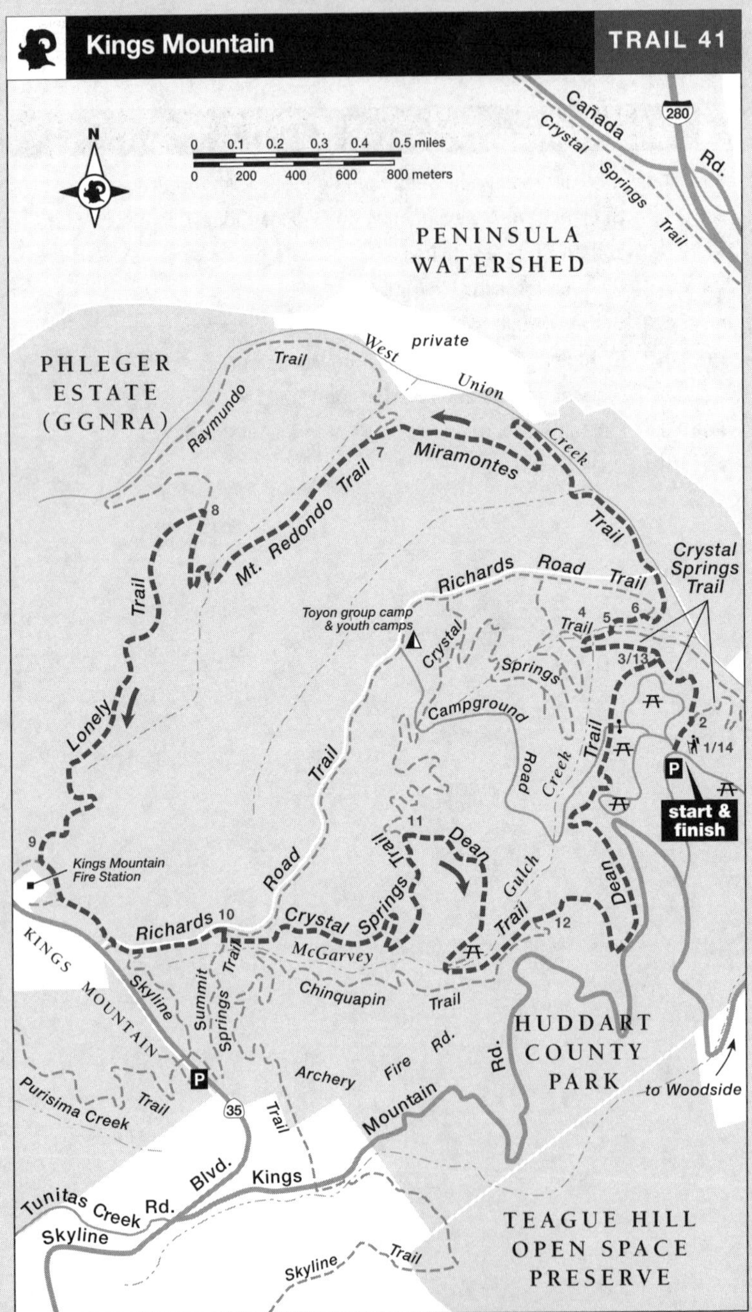
Kings Mountain
TRAIL 41
N
0 0.1 0.2 0.3 0.4 0.5 miles
0 200 400 600 800 meters
Cañada Rd.
280
Crystal Springs Trail
PENINSULA WATERSHED
PHLEGER ESTATE (GGNRA)
private
West Union Creek
Raymundo Trail
Miramontes Trail
Mt. Redondo Trail
Lonely Trail
Richards Road Trail
Crystal Springs Trail
Toyon group camp & youth camps
Crystal Springs Campground Road
Creek Trail
Dean Trail
Dean Gulch Trail
Crystal Springs Trail
McGarvey
Chinquapin Trail
Summit Springs Trail
Skyline
Kings Mountain Fire Station
KINGS MOUNTAIN
Purisima Creek Trail
Archery Fire Rd.
Kings Mountain Rd.
HUDDART COUNTY PARK
to Woodside
start & finish
Tunitas Creek Rd.
Skyline Blvd.
35
TEAGUE HILL OPEN SPACE PRESERVE
Skyline Trail
1/14
2
3/13
4
5
6
7
8
9
10
11
12

Kings Mountain

The contrast between Huddart County Park and its neighbor, Golden Gate National Recreation Area's Phleger Estate, could not be more extreme. Trading picnic areas and sports fields for serene groves of coast redwoods, you struggle up Kings Mountain on the aptly-named Lonely Trail, then saunter down to civilization on Huddart's well-graded equestrian trails.

TRAIL USE
Hike, Run
LENGTH
7.9 miles, 3–5 hours
VERTICAL FEET
±1500'
DIFFICULTY
– 1 2 3 **4** 5 +
TRAIL TYPE
Loop
SURFACE TYPE
Dirt

FEATURES
Fee
Stream
Canyon
Birds
Wildlife
Secluded
Cool & Shady

FACILITIES
Restrooms
Picnic Tables
Phone
Water

Best Time

All year, but trails may be muddy in wet weather.

Finding the Trail

From Interstate 280 in Woodside, take the Woodside Rd./Woodside/State Hwy. 84 exit and go southwest 1.6 miles to Kings Mountain Rd. Turn right, go 2.1 miles to the Huddart Park entrance, and turn right. At 0.2 mile there is an entrance kiosk and self-registration station. There are parking areas on both sides of the road just ahead. The trailhead▶1 is a few hundred feet north of the parking areas, on the east side of a paved road that is signed for Zwierlein, Werder, Madrone, and Miwok picnic areas.

Trail Description

The trailhead has information boards, a map holder, and water. You follow a single track that curves right and descends to a left-hand switchback amid stands of coast redwood, Douglas-fir, coast live oak, and tanbark oak. Soon the Bay Tree Trail departs sharply to the right, and you have a sports field, picnic area, and restrooms on your left. Now reach a junction with the **Crystal Springs Trail,**►**2** where you bear left and follow a rolling course. Soon you pass the Dean Trail, your return route, left.►**3**

Now the trail descends on a gentle grade, via more switchbacks, into a canyon holding a seasonal tributary of West Union Creek, shown on the park map as **McGarvey Gulch Creek.** At the canyon bottom, the Crystal Springs Trail turns left across the creek,►**4** but you go right on a connector. Soon you merge with the **Richards Road Trail** and turn sharply left.►**5**

Richards Road crosses McGarvey Gulch Creek via a culvert, then climbs to a junction►**6** where you veer right on the **Miramontes Trail.** The single-track trail gradually bends left and descends to **West Union Creek,** where you saunter through streamside groves of coast redwoods.

Stream

After following the shady stream, the Miramontes Trail climbs via switchbacks to a junction.►**7** You continue straight, now on the single-track **Mt. Redondo Trail,** which climbs steadily, and sometimes steeply, beside a deep canyon, right.

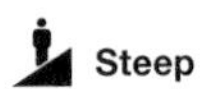

At the next junction, the Raymundo Trail goes straight and your route, the **Lonely Trail,** heads left.►**8** Ascending a ridge cloaked in toyon and tanbark oak, you begin to work your way across

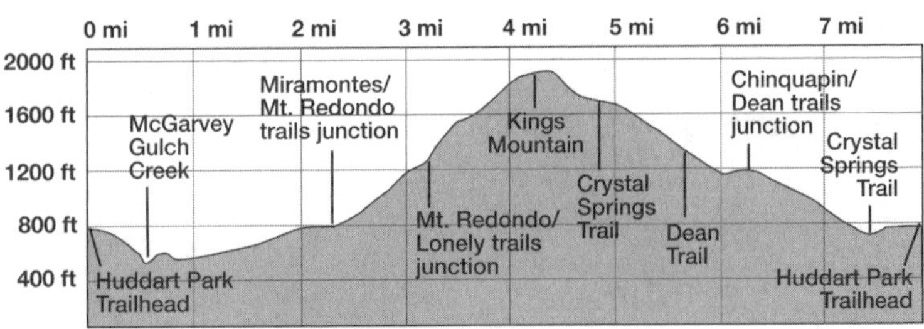

TRAIL 41 Kings Mountain Profile

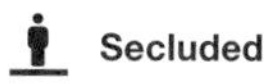

a canyon wall that drops steeply left. You are now high on the eastern flank of **Kings Mountain**, a long ridge extending from near State Highway 92 southeast to Bear Gulch Road.

After a brief respite, you resume a steady climb beside a deep ravine, left. The narrow trail perches on a steep hillside. Just below the Kings Mountain Fire Station, whose communication towers are just uphill, the Lonely Trail ends at an unsigned junction.►9 Bear left and follow a rolling course parallel to Skyline Boulevard, one of California's premier scenic roads. Stay left where another trail joins from the right.

At the boundary of **Huddart County Park**, angle left on the **Richards Road Trail**, a dirt road. After passing the Skyline Trail, right, turn right on the **Summit Springs Trail.**►10 After about 100 feet, find the **Crystal Springs Trail**, left, and a rest bench. From here, follow the Crystal Springs Trail past a seasonal-closure gate that prevents access by horses during wet weather. The wide path descends gently along a ridge and then through forest. At a junction with the **Dean Trail**,►11 turn sharply right and continue descending.

Just before reaching a bridge, you pass a spur to **McGarvey Flat**, a lovely spot with a picnic table and several rest benches hewn from logs. Continuing across McGarvey Gulch Creek, a gentle climb on an old road brings you to a junction with

HISTORY

More Phleger Trails

Explore the lower Phleger Estate property on this 6.9-mile semi-loop: From the top of the **Mt. Redondo Trail**►8 stay right on the **Raymundo Trail** and then descend along redwood-lined West Union Creek to the junction of the Mt. Redondo and Miramontes trails.►7 Return on the **Miramontes, Richards Rd.,** and **Crystal Springs trails** to Huddart Park.

the Chinquapin Trail, right.▶**12** Here veer left to stay on the Dean Trail, going straight through two crossings of Archery Fire Road ahead.

At the edge of a paved road near the Miwok picnic area, the Dean Trail turns sharply left and then begins a series of switchbacks, descending past the Madrone picnic area. Follow the Dean Trail, here a wide path, as it makes a curving descent past more picnic areas. At a T-junction with the **Crystal Springs Trail,**▶**13** turn right and retrace your route to the parking area.▶**14**

MILESTONES

▶1	0.0	Take single-track trail northeast; Bay Tree Trail on right
▶2	0.2	Left on Crystal Springs Trail
▶3	0.4	Dean Trail on left; straight to stay on Crystal Springs Trail
▶4	0.7	Right on connector to Richards Rd. Trail
▶5	0.8	Merge with Richards Rd. Trail, then left across creek
▶6	0.9	Right on Miramontes Trail
▶7	2.3	Straight on Mt. Redondo Trail
▶8	3.1	Left on Lonely Trail
▶9	4.1	Lonely Trail ends; bear left at unsigned junction below Kings Mountain Fire Station
▶10	4.9	Right on Summit Springs Trail, then left on Crystal Springs Trail
▶11	5.7	Sharply right on Dean Trail
▶12	6.3	Left at junction with Chinquapin Trail to stay on Dean Trail
▶13	7.5	Right at T-junction on Crystal Springs Trail, retrace to parking area
▶14	7.9	Back at parking area

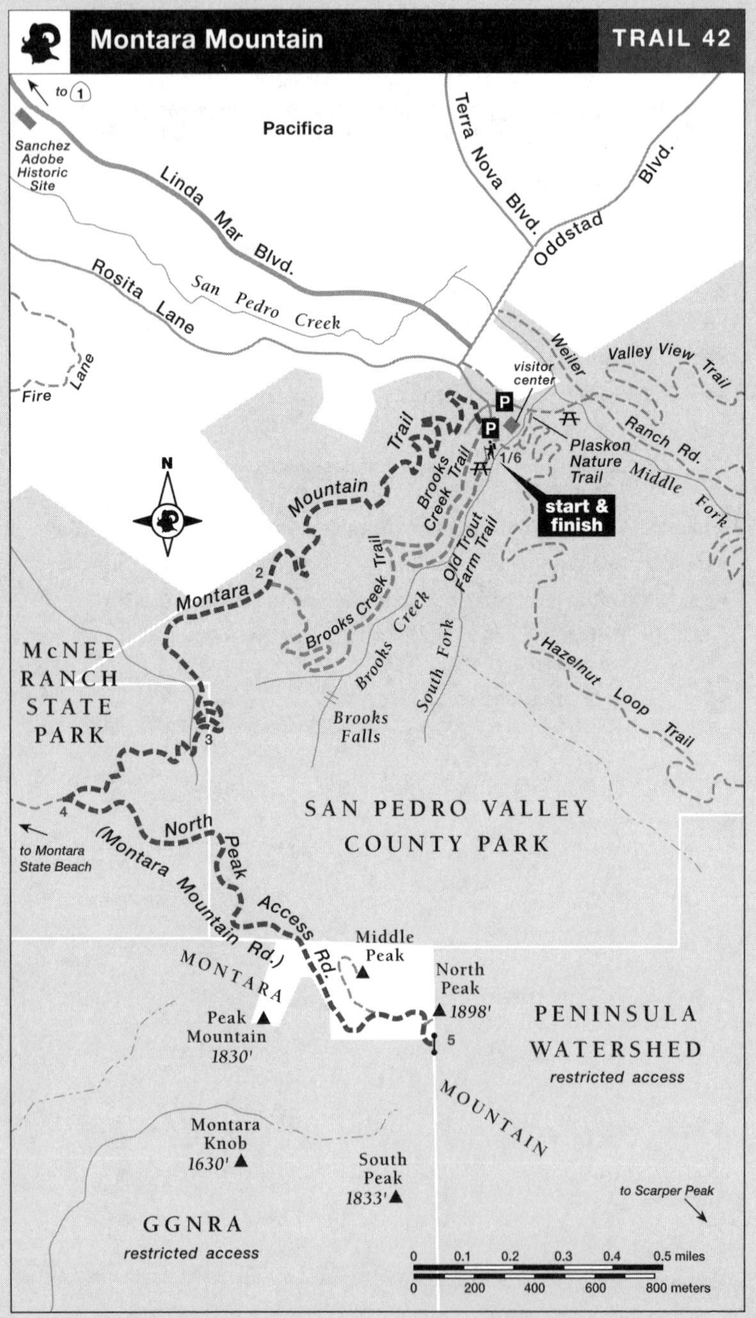
Montara Mountain
TRAIL 42
to 1
Pacifica
Sanchez Adobe Historic Site
Linda Mar Blvd.
Terra Nova Blvd.
Oddstad Blvd.
Rosita Lane
San Pedro Creek
Fire Lane
Weiler Ranch Rd.
Valley View Trail
visitor center
Plaskon Nature Trail
Middle Fork
1/6
start & finish
Mountain Trail
Brooks Creek Trail
Old Trout Farm Trail
Montara
2
N
Brooks Creek
South Fork
Hazelnut Loop Trail
McNEE RANCH STATE PARK
Brooks Falls
3
4
to Montara State Beach
North Peak Access Rd.
(Montara Mountain Rd.)
SAN PEDRO VALLEY COUNTY PARK
MONTARA
Middle Peak
North Peak 1898'
5
Peak Mountain 1830'
PENINSULA WATERSHED
restricted access
MOUNTAIN
Montara Knob 1630'
South Peak 1833'
to Scarper Peak
GGNRA
restricted access
0 0.1 0.2 0.3 0.4 0.5 miles
0 200 400 600 800 meters

Montara Mountain

Starting from San Pedro Valley County Park, you climb from eucalyptus forest through chaparral and coastal scrub, eventually finding yourself atop Montara Mountain, actually a long ridge with several summits. Although parts of the trail are rocky underfoot, the climbing is not difficult. Views of the Santa Cruz Mountains, the East Bay hills, and San Francisco landmarks reward your efforts.

TRAIL USE
Hike, Run

LENGTH
7.2 miles, 3–4 hours

VERTICAL FEET
±1650'

DIFFICULTY
– 1 2 3 **4** 5 +

TRAIL TYPE
Out & Back

SURFACE TYPE
Dirt

FEATURES
Fee
Mountain
Wildflowers
Geologic Interest
Great Views

FACILITIES
Restrooms
Picnic Tables
Phone
Water
Visitor Center (weekends and holidays)

Best Time

All year; expect dense fog in summer.

Trail Approach

From the junction of State Hwy. 1 and Linda Mar Blvd. in Pacifica, go southeast 1.9 miles on Linda Mar Blvd. to Oddstad Blvd. Turn right and then immediately left into San Pedro Valley County Park. Turn right past the entrance kiosk to a paved parking area. (If this lot is full, there is a second lot on the other side of the visitor center.) The trailhead is on the north side of the parking area, just north of the restrooms.

Trail Description

From the trailhead, walk west on a paved path to a junction. Here the Brooks Creek and Old Trout Farm trails go left, but you veer right on the **Montara Mountain Trail.**▶1 The single track crosses a paved driveway and heads gently uphill through a eucalyptus forest, steadily gaining elevation.

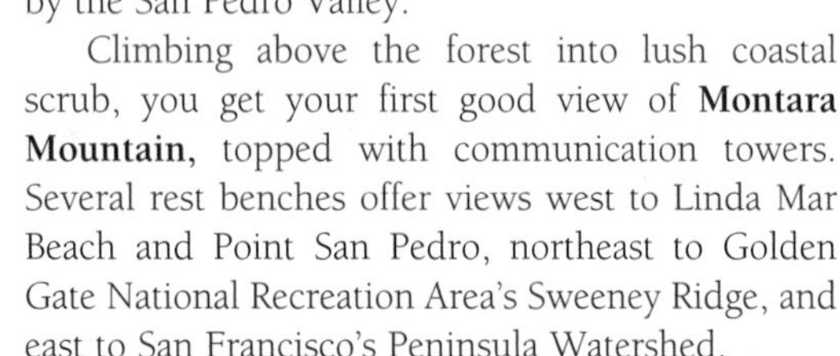

Soon you have a view of the Pacific Ocean, framed by the San Pedro Valley.

Climbing above the forest into lush coastal scrub, you get your first good view of **Montara Mountain,** topped with communication towers. Several rest benches offer views west to Linda Mar Beach and Point San Pedro, northeast to Golden Gate National Recreation Area's Sweeney Ridge, and east to San Francisco's Peninsula Watershed.

Great Views

Where the Brooks Creek Trail goes left, continue straight on the Montara Mountain Trail.►2 Rounding a brushy knoll with a view of Point San Pedro, the trail balances along a narrow ridge to attack the granite face of Montara Mountain. Rough, eroded switchbacks ascend on a moderate grade across rocky spurs and through ravines, all clad in a miniature forest of chinquapin and manzanita.

Montara Mountain is actually a long ridge crowned by several summits, including North Peak (1898'), South Peak (1833'), and distant Scarper Peak (1944').

Nearing the ridgeline, you enter **McNee Ranch State Park**►3 and meet the **North Peak Access Road** (also known as Montara Mountain Road).►4 Turn left on this wide gravel road and ascend a rolling ridgetop. Be alert for bicyclists and occasional utility vehicles. The locally rare granite outcrops and dense, windswept manzanita lend a high-elevation feel.

Continue past several communication facilities to a gate at the **Peninsula Watershed boundary.**►5 Montara Mountain's North Peak is just north of this

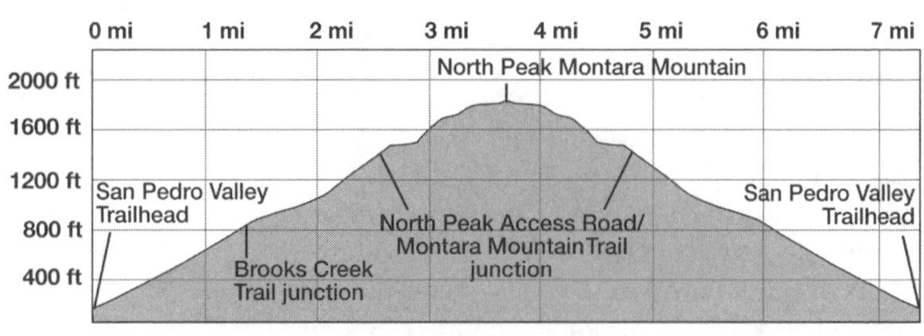

TRAIL 42 Montara Mountain Profile

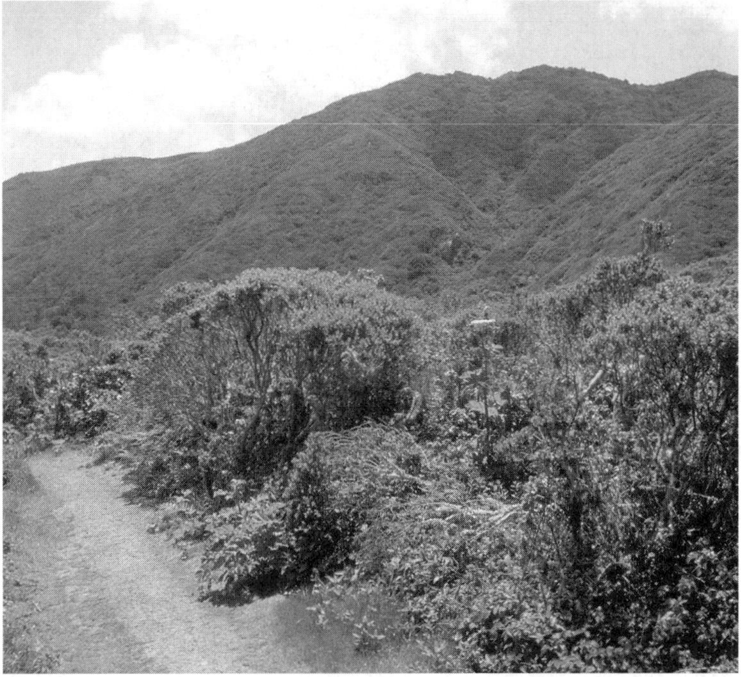

Montara Mountain's chaparral-clad slopes *form a scenic background to Pacifica.*

gate, on private property. Southeast, you have an uninterrupted vista of the Santa Cruz Mountains all the way to Mt. Umunhum. You may also spy Mt. Hamilton, with its white observatory domes, in the far distance. From nearby vantage points,

 **Great Views**

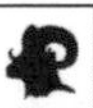

OPTION

Brooks Falls Overlook

A scenic variation on your descent is to turn right on the **Brooks Creek Trail.**►2 From this trail you can see Brooks Falls, which drops about 175 feet in three tiers from the north side of Montara Mountain in the rainy season. At the next junction take either the **Brooks Creek** or **Old Trout Farm trails** to San Pedro Valley.

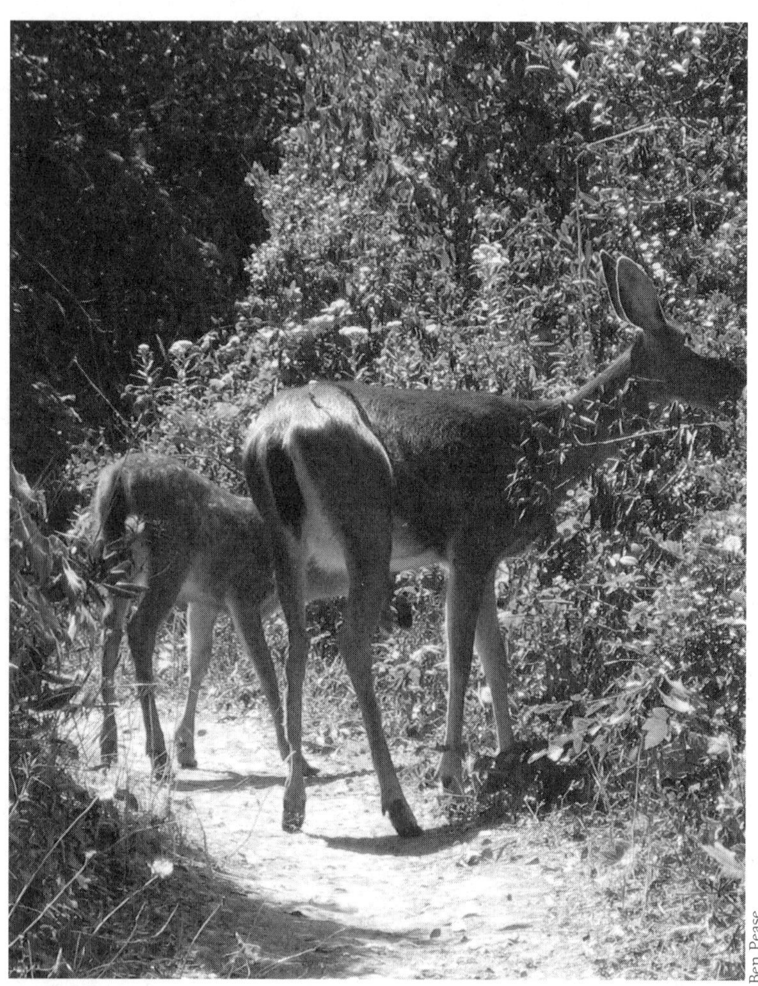

Deer *browse for huckleberries along the Montara Mountain Trail.*

you can look east to the Berkeley hills, capped by Vollmer Peak and Round Top. To the north, you can pick out features of San Francisco such as the Sunset District, Twin Peaks, and Golden Gate Park.

From here, retrace your route to the parking area.►**6**

MILESTONES

▶1	0.0	Take paved path west, then left on dirt path and right on Montara Mountain Trail
▶2	1.4	Brooks Creek Trail on left; continue straight
▶3	2.1	McNee Ranch State Park boundary
▶4	2.5	Left on North Peak Access Rd.
▶5	3.6	Road's end, retrace to parking area
▶6	7.2	Back at parking area

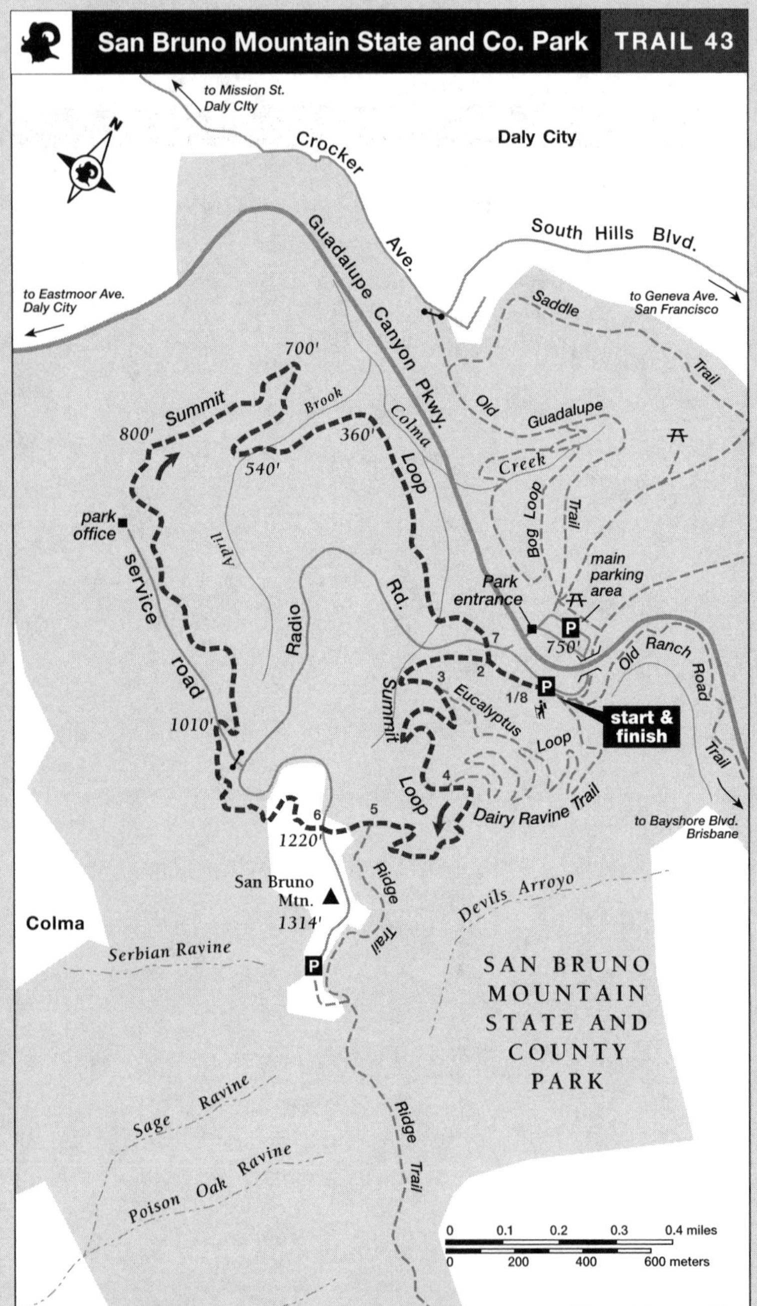
San Bruno Mountain State and Co. Park
TRAIL 43
to Mission St.
Daly City
Daly City
Crocker Ave.
N
Guadalupe Canyon Pkwy.
South Hills Blvd.
to Eastmoor Ave.
Daly City
to Geneva Ave.
San Francisco
Saddle Trail
700'
800'
Summit
Brook
360'
540'
Colma
Loop
Old Guadalupe
Creek
Bog Loop
Trail
park office
service road
April
Radio Rd.
Park entrance
main parking area
750'
Old Ranch Road
Trail
7
2
3
1/8
Summit
Eucalyptus
Loop
start & finish
1010'
4
Loop
Dairy Ravine Trail
6
5
1220'
to Bayshore Blvd.
Brisbane
Ridge Trail
San Bruno Mtn.
1314'
Devils Arroyo
Colma
Serbian Ravine
SAN BRUNO MOUNTAIN STATE AND COUNTY PARK
Sage Ravine
Poison Oak Ravine
Ridge Trail
0
0.1
0.2
0.3
0.4 miles
0
200
400
600 meters

San Bruno Mountain State and County Park

Despite its urban setting, San Bruno Mountain's rugged canyons and ridges host a remarkable array of rare and/or endangered species. Among these are several species of butterflies and more than a dozen plants, including three manzanitas. When not fog-bound, the trails here afford views of San Francisco and beyond, and the spring wildflower displays are sensational (something is in bloom nearly all year).

TRAIL USE
Hike, Run

LENGTH
3.1 miles, 2–3 hours

VERTICAL FEET
±700'

DIFFICULTY
– 1 2 **3** 4 5 +

TRAIL TYPE
Loop

SURFACE TYPE
Dirt

FEATURES
Fee
Mountain
Wildflowers
Birds
Great Views
Photo Opportunity

FACILITIES
Restrooms
Picnic Tables
Water
Phone

Best Time

All year; often foggy and windy; trails may be muddy in wet weather.

Finding the Trail

From US Hwy. 101 northbound in San Francisco, take the Third St. exit (not well signed). Go 0.5 mile to Paul Ave., turn left, go 0.1 mile to San Bruno Ave., and turn left again. At 0.9 mile San Bruno Ave. joins Bayshore Blvd. Continue straight another 1.5 miles to Guadalupe Canyon Pkwy. and turn right. Go 2.2 miles to the park entrance on the right. Just past the entry kiosk, turn right (passing the main parking area), pass under the bridge, and go 0.2 mile to a paved parking area on the south side of Guadalupe Canyon Pkwy. The trailhead is on the south side of the parking area.

From US Hwy. 101 southbound in San Francisco, take the Cow Palace/Third St. exit, staying right toward the Cow Palace. At 0.3 mile you reach Bayshore Blvd. and go straight. Go another 1.8 miles to Guadalupe Canyon Pkwy., turn right, and follow the directions above.

Eucalyptus trees are not native to California, and they encroach on native habitat. Logging here in the 1990s removed many to restore migration corridors for endangered butterflies.

Facilities

None at the trailhead; restrooms, picnic tables, phone, and water are at the main parking area, near the park entrance.

Trail Description

Past an information board and a map holder►1 turn right on the **Summit Loop Trail** (shown as Summit Trail on the park map). This single track soon comes to a junction where the Summit Loop Trail divides.►2 Here you stay left and climb through coastal scrub, then briefly enter a stand of eucalyptus.

After a switchback on the left, you pass the Eucalyptus Loop Trail, also on the left,►3 and bear right to stay on the Summit Loop Trail. As you gain elevation through grassland decorated with spring wildflowers, the views of San Francisco, San Francisco Bay, and the East Bay hills become more and more dramatic. Where the Dairy Ravine Trail angles left,►4 stay right on the Summit Loop Trail.

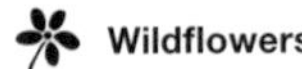

Gaining a ridgetop, you pass the Ridge Trail on the left.►5 Continue on the Summit Loop Trail to Radio Road, which climbs from the park entrance to just below the mountain's summit.►6 **San Bruno Mountain** itself is actually a long ridge, topped by communication towers, which angles northwest toward Daly City from Brisbane. This airy vantage point may help you appreciate the value—scenic, recreational, and spiritual—of preserving open space.

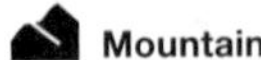

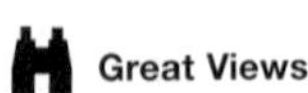

Your route resumes on the south side of Radio Road, just right of a metal gate across a paved driveway. The Summit Loop Trail zigzags its way downhill on a steep then moderate grade, past communication towers and satellite dishes, to a paved service road, which you cross. You traverse a north-facing slope, descend a ridgetop, then follow the trail as it bends sharply right and slices across a hillside.

At the bottom of the canyon, the trail bends left, then veers right to cross **April Brook.** Now heading downstream, your route soon curves right, then climbs on a moderate grade through tall coastal scrub. Several plank bridges help you across springs and seeps. As the trail levels, you cross paved Radio Road and then reach the junction where this loop began.►7 From here, turn left and retrace your route to the parking area.►8

Among the hundreds of wildflower species you may see are Douglas-iris, clarkia, goldfields, pearly everlasting, and mission bells, a chocolate-colored lily.

MILESTONES

►1	0.0	Go past information board, then right on Summit Loop Trail
►2	0.1	Left on Summit Loop Trail
►3	0.3	Eucalyptus Loop Trail on left; stay right
►4	0.7	Dairy Ravine Trail on left; go straight
►5	0.9	Pass Ridge Trail on left
►6	1.0	Cross paved Radio Rd. and continue southwest down Summit Loop Trail
►7	3.0	Cross paved Radio Rd., then left at junction, and retrace to parking area
►8	3.1	Back at parking area

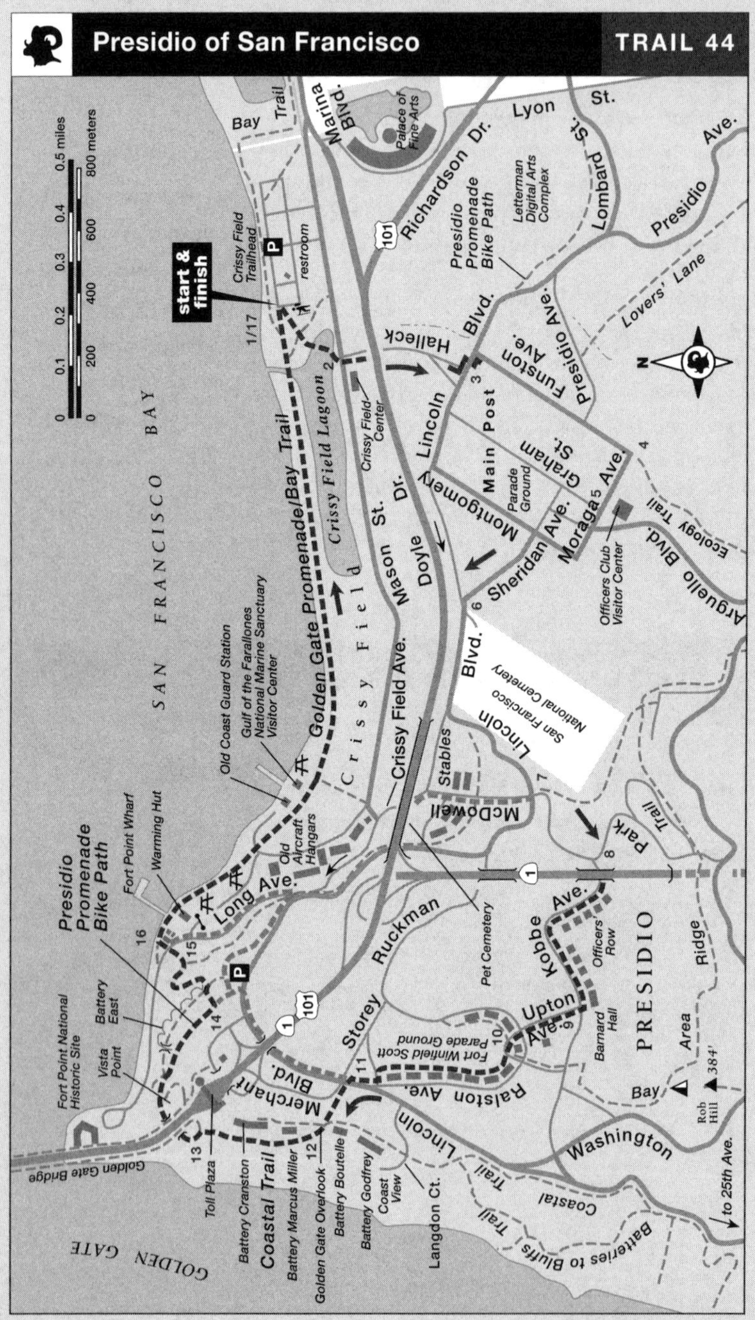
Presidio of San Francisco
TRAIL 44
SAN FRANCISCO BAY
GOLDEN GATE
PRESIDIO
start & finish
Crissy Field Trailhead
restroom
Golden Gate Promenade/Bay Trail
Bay Trail
Crissy Field Lagoon
Crissy Field
Crissy Field Center
Crissy Field Ave.
Marina Blvd.
Palace of Fine Arts
Richardson Dr.
Lyon St.
Lombard St.
Presidio Ave.
Letterman Digital Arts Complex
Presidio Promenade Bike Path
Lovers' Lane
Halleck
Lincoln Blvd.
Funston Ave.
Presidio Ave.
Main Post
Graham St.
Parade Ground
Montgomery
Moraga Ave.
Sheridan Ave.
Mason St.
Doyle Dr.
Officers Club Visitor Center
Arguello Blvd.
Ecology Trail
San Francisco National Cemetery
Stables
McDowell
Park Trail
Old Coast Guard Station
Gulf of the Farallones National Marine Sanctuary Visitor Center
Old Aircraft Hangars
Long Ave.
Fort Point Wharf
Warming Hut
Presidio Promenade Bike Path
Fort Point National Historic Site
Battery East
Vista Point
Pet Cemetery
Ruckman
Kobbe Ave.
Officers' Row
Upton Ave.
Barnard Hall
Storey
Fort Winfield Scott Parade Ground
Ralston Ave.
Merchant Blvd.
Lincoln
Washington
Bay Area Ridge Trail
Rob Hill 384'
to 25th Ave.
Coastal Trail
Batteries to Bluffs Trail
Golden Gate Bridge
Toll Plaza
Battery Cranston
Battery Marcus Miller
Golden Gate Overlook
Battery Boutelle
Battery Godfrey
Coast View
Langdon Ct.
0 0.1 0.2 0.3 0.4 0.5 miles
0 200 400 600 800 meters
N

Presidio of San Francisco

This guide's only urban route is both an enjoyable walk back in time and a hopeful look forward at efforts to reclaim developed lands for public enjoyment. The US Army transferred the Presidio to the National Park Service in 1994, ending more than 200 years of military history dating back to the Spanish era. On this route you pass military buildings from the 19th and 20th centuries, vantage points with views of San Francisco Bay, a famous orange bridge, and a popular waterfront path.

TRAIL USE
Hike, Run, Bike, Child Friendly, Dogs Allowed

LENGTH
4.1 miles, 2–3 hours

VERTICAL FEET
±300'

DIFFICULTY
– 1 2 **3** 4 5 +

TRAIL TYPE
Loop

SURFACE TYPE
Dirt, Paved

FEATURES
Shore
Wildflowers
Birds
Historic
Great Views
Photo Opportunity

FACILITIES
Restrooms
Phone
Picnic Tables
Water
Concessions

Best Time

All year; expect fog in summer.

Finding the Trail

From the west end of Marina Blvd., get in the right lane and stay straight, heading west on Mason St. through the Presidio's Marina Gate. After two blocks, turn north into the Crissy Field parking area. The trailhead is on the west end of the parking area, due west of the restrooms.

From southbound US Hwy. 101 heading east on Doyle Dr., get in the left lane and take the Marina Blvd. exit. After one block, turn right on Baker St., left on Jefferson St., left on Broderick St., and left on Marina Blvd., now heading west. In the right lane, stay straight on Mason St. into the Presidio as Marina Blvd. veers left toward the Golden Gate Bridge. Then follow the directions above.

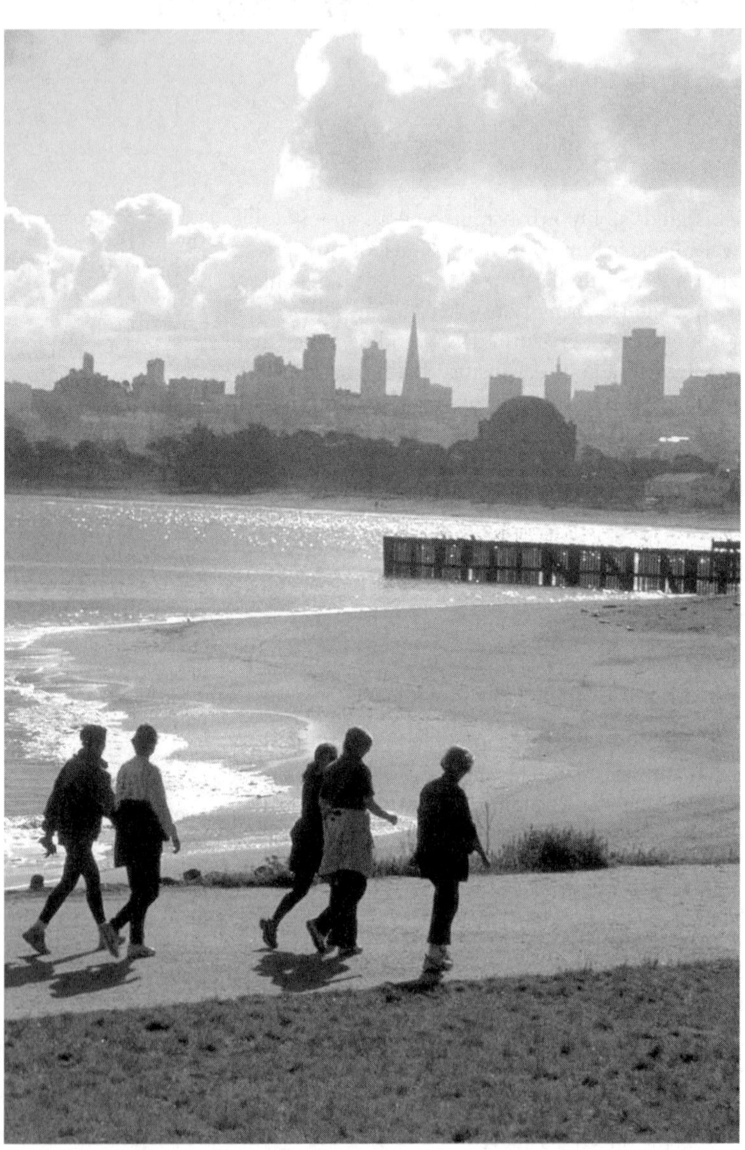

The Golden Gate Promenade/Bay Trail *follows the north shore of the Presidio, connecting the Golden Gate Bridge with Marina Green and Fort Mason.*

Trail Description

From the trailhead,►1 start southwest across a lawn on a gravel path. Soon you cross a curving footbridge over the east end of **Crissy Field Lagoon,** an artificial tidal lagoon that attempts to recreate the original marshes here. The effort has been successful, at least from an avian standpoint, and you may spot wading birds, shorebirds, ducks, gulls, and other species.

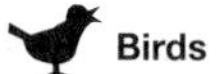

On the far side of the bridge, cross Mason Street►2 and go straight on **Halleck Street** with Crissy Field Center on your right. After passing under US Highway 101, traverse the wooden porch of Building 201 and climb past the old Sixth Army Headquarters.

Before the Golden Gate Bridge was built, Crissy Field was a landing strip for US Army airplanes.

At the end of Halleck Street,►3 turn left across it, turn right across Lincoln Boulevard, and then go left 100 feet to **Funston Avenue,** where you turn right. Climb gently past the old Post Hospital and a row of Victorian cottages, then meet **Moraga Avenue.**►4 Cross to the south side of Moraga Avenue and turn right. Amble past Pershing Hall, a small chapel, and the Officers Club, a corner of which incorporates adobe walls from the original Spanish military post.

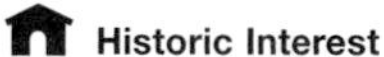

Beyond the Officers Club,►5 cross Moraga Avenue and go north one block on **Graham Street.** Cross to the north side of **Sheridan Avenue** and turn left. After about 100 feet along the edge of a lawn, regain the sidewalk. The Parade Ground, right, is flanked by the brick Montgomery Barracks on the west. From here the view north to San Francisco Bay is splendid. (The Presidio Trust intends to remove the nearby paved parking lot and make the Parade Ground more parklike.)

In a few blocks, Sheridan Avenue merges with **Lincoln Boulevard.** Continue west on the north side of Lincoln Boulevard.►6 With noisy Highway 101 on your right, the orderly rows of white

At Halleck and Lincoln,►3 go east along the stone wall a few steps to overlook a restored section of Tennessee Hollow Creek. The US Army filled this valley from the 1950s to 2006.

gravestones march up the hillside of San Francisco National Military Cemetery, left. Passing Crissy Field Avenue, stay left on Lincoln Boulevard. An old road (a future link in the Presidio Promenade) descends right toward the slate-roofed Cavalry Stables, built in 1914, visible in the wooded valley below.

Soon you come to an intersection with McDowell Avenue, right, and Park Boulevard, left.►7 Carefully cross Lincoln Boulevard (cross-traffic does not stop). Follow **Park Boulevard** about 50 yards, then angle left on a red gravel path that rises steadily through a forest of Monterey cypress and eucalyptus, planted in the 1880s. Meeting Park Boulevard again and crossing it, go right on **Kobbe Avenue**►8 past Officers Row, beautiful homes built in 1912. Just beyond Barnard Hall, an imposing brick guest house with white columns, turn right on **Upton Avenue,**►9 following a sidewalk on its left side. After one block, cross Ralston Avenue and enter **Fort Winfield Scott.**►10

Turn left in front of the tile-roofed barracks, keeping the parade ground on your right. This sidewalk, shared by the **Juan Bautista de Anza National Historic Trail** and the Bay Area Ridge Trail, has views from the Golden Gate Bridge to Angel Island and Mt. Diablo. Just past Building 1208, turn left to the intersection of Ralston and Lincoln avenues, then turn right on the shoulder of **Lincoln Avenue** to a four-way intersection with Storey and Merchant roads.►11 Here, cross Lincoln Boulevard and go west on the sidewalk of **Merchant Road.** As the road curves right, stay straight on the **Anza and Ridge trails** to a junction with the **Coastal Trail,**►12 on which you turn right. All three trails now share a single route north to the Golden Gate Bridge.

The gravel path bends west between Batteries Boutelle and Marcus Miller, two of several gun emplacements built to defend the Golden Gate from the 1890s until the 1940s. (There may be a short, clearly-signed detour here.) Now the footpath

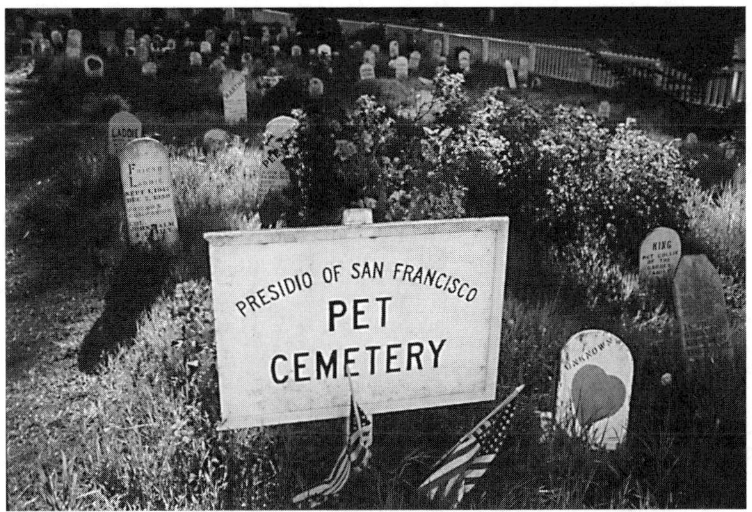

The Presidio Pet Cemetery *is located beneath the Doyle Dr./US Hwy. 101 bridge.*

ambles northward along the windswept bluff, with dramatic views left toward North Baker Beach and Point Bonita, and ahead to the Golden Gate Bridge.

Soon you come to a paved path,►**13** the bike route to the west sidewalk of the Golden Gate Bridge on afternoons and weekends. Go left beneath US Highway 101. (Be alert for cyclists and strolling tourists from here on!) Here a busy bike path ascends right toward Vista Point, but you stay left on the lower bike path, which is part of the **Bay Trail** and the **Presidio Promenade.** On a clear day you may enjoy a panoramic view from Point Bonita to the East Bay hills. Pass a brick path leading right to Vista Point and the toll plaza. The level bike path overlooks Battery East, a Civil War–era brick gun emplacement, left.

Near Lincoln Boulevard, turn left down a gravel path signed for Fort Point.►**14** Veer slightly right across a wide junction, cross the lip of Battery East, and descend gently via S-curves through coastal

The Presidio Visitor Center will eventually relocate from the Officers Club to Building 102, one of the Montgomery Barracks.

 **Great Views**

Fort Scott is named for Winfield Scott, who served in the army from before the War of 1812 until the Civil War. He is best known as a commander during the US–Mexican War.

scrub. Turn left down a long flight of wooden steps▶15 through a verdant gulch. Carefully cross Marine Drive, the busy road to Fort Point. At the seawall, pause a moment to gaze west toward Fort Point, then turn right on the **Golden Gate Promenade,** a paved path that is part of the San Francisco Bay Trail.▶16 Opposite an old fishing pier, you pass restrooms, water, and the Warming Hut, which has a cafe and bookstore, right.

Continuing east on the wide, gravel path, you pass a large picnic area and Long Avenue, then bend left along the edge of **Crissy Field,** the site of a historic Army airfield. An old Coast Guard station, left, includes a visitor center for Gulf of the Farallones National Marine Sanctuary. Soon the lawn ends and you follow the edge of Crissy Field Lagoon, enjoying views of Angel Island and Alcatraz. After crossing the lagoon outlet on a wide bridge, bear right to reach the parking area.▶17

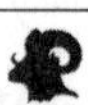

OPTIONS

Regional Trails from the Golden Gate

From the Golden Gate Bridge, the **Coastal Trail** goes south and then west to Baker Beach, Lands End, and the Cliff House. The **Ridge Trail** goes south into the city. Eastward, the **Golden Gate Promenade/Bay Trail** extends past Fort Mason to Aquatic Park. Northward, the **Bay, Ridge,** and **Coastal trails** follow the bridge's east sidewalk to Marin County.

MILESTONES

►1	0.0	Southwest on gravel path to footbridge over east end of Crissy Field Lagoon.
►2	0.2	Cross Mason St., straight on Halleck St.
►3	0.4	Left across Halleck St., right across Lincoln Blvd., left on Lincoln Blvd. 100 feet, right on Funston Ave.
►4	0.7	Cross Moraga Ave. and turn right to Officers Club
►5	0.8	Cross Moraga Ave., right on Graham St. one block, then left on Sheridan Ave.
►6	1.1	Merge with Lincoln Blvd. and follow it west; stay left on Lincoln Blvd. past Crissy Field Ave.
►7	1.8	Cross Lincoln Blvd., left on Park Blvd. for 50 yards, then angle left on red gravel path
►8	2.0	Cross Park Blvd., go right on Kobbe Ave. past Officers Row
►9	2.3	Right on Upton Ave.
►10	2.4	Cross Ralston Ave., enter Fort Scott, go left beside parade ground
►11	2.6	Just past building 1208, go left to intersection of Ralston and Lincoln avenues, then turn right on Lincoln Blvd.
►12	2.6	Cross Lincoln Blvd., go straight on Merchant Rd., then straight on Anza and Ridge trails to Coastal Trail; turn right.
►13	2.9	Left on paved bike path under Golden Gate Bridge, then left on lower bike path
►14	3.1	Left on gravel path signed for Fort Point
►15	3.2	After S-curves turn left down wooden steps
►16	3.3	Right on Golden Gate Promenade past Warming Hut and old Coast Guard Station
►17	4.1	Back at Crissy Field east parking area

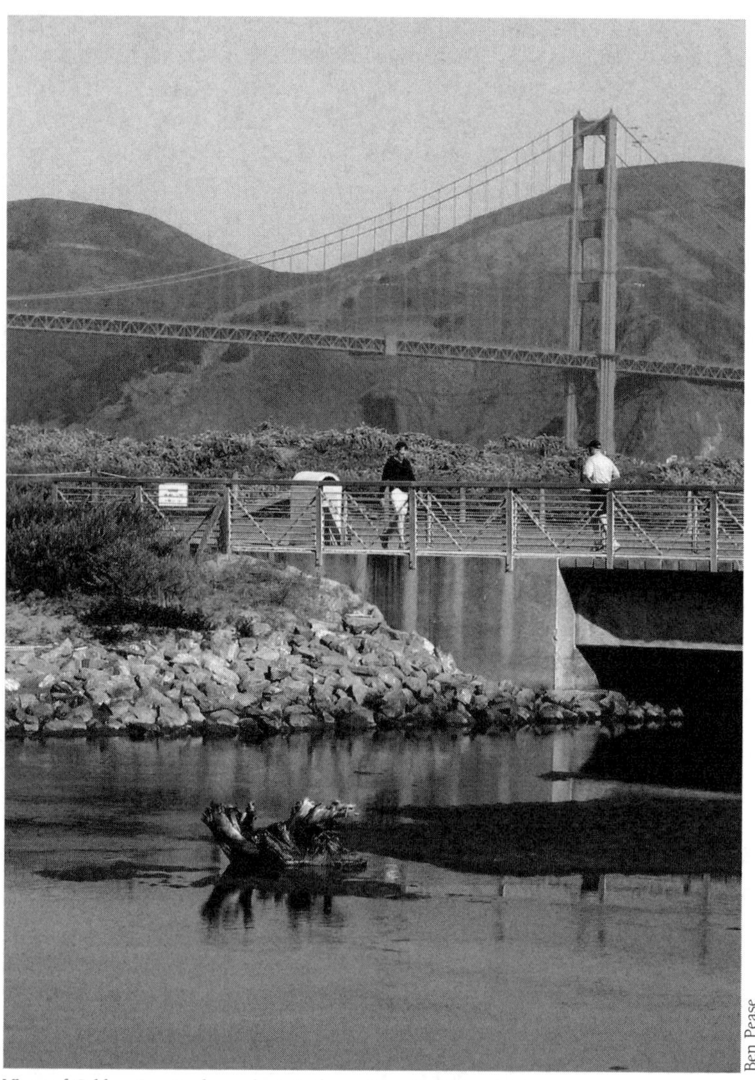

Ben Pease

View *of Golden Gate Bridge and Marin from Crissy Field (Trail 44)*

Appendix 1

Top-Rated Trails

North Bay

4. Mount Tamalpais: Middle Peak
7. Point Reyes National Seashore: Sky Trail
9. Mt. Burdell Open Space Preserve

East Bay

20. Black Diamond Mines Regional Preserve: Stewartville Loop
21. Mount Diablo State Park: Grand Loop
25. Pleasanton Ridge Regional Park

South Bay

30. Henry W. Coe State Park
31. Almaden Quicksilver County Park

Peninsula

37. Russian Ridge Open Space Preserve
40. Purisima Creek Redwoods Open Space Preserve
43. San Bruno Mountain State and County Park

Appendix 2

Governing Agencies

Chapter 1: North Bay

National Park Service (NPS)

Golden Gate National Recreation Area (GGNRA
www.nps.gov/goga
(415) 561-4700

Point Reyes National Seashore
www.nps.gov/pore
(415) 464-5100

California State Parks (CSP)
http://parks.ca.gov
(800) 777-0369

Marin County Open Space District (MCOSD)
www.marinopenspace.org
(415) 499-6387

Marin Municipal Water District (MMWD)
www.marinwater.org/controller?action=menuclick&id=242

Sky Oaks Ranger Station
(415) 945-1181

Skyline Park Citizens Association (Napa)
www.skylinepark.org
(707) 252-0481

Sonoma County Parks and Recreation
www.parks.sonoma.net

Chapter 2: East Bay

California State Parks (CSP)
http://parks.ca.gov
(800) 777-0369

Mt. Diablo Interpretive Association
www.mdia.org
(925) 927-7222

Mt. Diablo State Park
Information: (925) 837-2525
Reservations: (800) 444-7275

East Bay Regional Park District (EBRPD)
www.ebparks.org
Information: (510) 562-7275
Reservations:
Contra Costa County (925) 676-0192
Hayward Area (510) 538-6470
Livermore Area (925) 373-0144
Oakland Area (510) 636-1684

Chapter 3: South Bay

California State Parks (CSP)
http://parks.ca.gov
(800) 777-0369

Henry W. Coe State Park
www.coepark.org
Information: (408) 779-2728
Reservations for campsites:
(800) 444-7275
Reservations for backcountry access are first come, first served:
www.coepark.org/sites-backpacking.html#fl

Midpeninsula Regional Open Space District (MROSD)
www.openspace.org
(650) 691-1200

Santa Clara County Parks
www.parkhere.org and
www.gooutsideandplay.org
Information: (408) 355-2200
Reservations: (408) 355-2201

Chapter 4: Peninsula

Golden Gate National Recreation Area (GGNRA)
www.nps.gov/goga
(415) 561-4700

Midpeninsula Regional Open Space District (MROSD)
www.openspace.org
(650) 691-1200

San Mateo County Parks
www.eparks.net
Information: (650) 363-4020
Reservations: (650) 363-4021

Appendix 3

Outfitters

North Bay

REI
213 Corte Madera Town Center
Corte Madera
(415) 927-1938

2715 Santa Rosa Ave.
Santa Rosa
(707) 540-9025

Sonoma Outfitters
145 Third St.
Santa Rosa
(800) 290-1920

East Bay

Marmot Mountain Works
3049 Adeline St.
Berkeley
(510) 849-0735

REI
1338 San Pablo Ave.
Berkeley
(510) 527-4140

1975 Diamond Blvd., Ste. B100
(The Willows Shopping Center)
Concord
(925) 825-9400

43962 Fremont Blvd.
Fremont
(510) 651-0305

Sunrise Mountaineering
2455 Railroad Ave.
Livermore
(925) 447-8330

South Bay

REI
400 El Paseo de Saratoga
San Jose
(408) 871-8765

San Francisco and the Peninsula

Lombardi Sports
1600 Jackson St.
San Francisco
(415) 771-0600

The North Face
217 Alma St.
Palo Alto
(650) 327-1563

180 Post St.
San Francisco
(415) 433-3223

REI
840 Brannan St.
San Francisco
(415) 934-1938

1119 Industrial Rd., Ste. A
San Carlos
(650) 508-2330

2450 Charleston Rd.
Mountain View
(650) 969-1938

Appendix 4

Internet Resources

Note: See Appendix 2: Governing Agencies and Appendix 3: Outfitters for more listings.

Bay Area Hiker
www.bahiker.com

Bay Area Open Space Council
www.openspacecouncil.org

Bay Area Ridge Trail Council
www.ridgetrail.org

***Bay Nature* magazine**
www.baynature.com

California Native Plant Society
www.cnps.org

Committee for Green Foothills
www.greenfoothills.org

Greenbelt Alliance
www.greenbelt.org

Marin Trails
www.marintrails.com

Metropolitan Transportation Commission (public transit)
http://511.org

Mt. Diablo Interpretive Association
www.mdia.org

Mt. Tamalpais Interpretive Association
www.mttam.net

National Audubon Society
www.audubon.org

National Geographic Maps/TOPO!
http://maps.nationalgeographic.com/topo

Peninsula Open Space Trust
www.openspacetrust.org

Pine Ridge Association
http://coepark.org

Point Reyes Bird Observatory
www.prbo.org

San Mateo County Parks Foundation
www.supportparks.org

Save Mt. Diablo
www.savemountdiablo.org

Sempervirens Fund
www.sempervirens.org

Sierra Club
www.sierraclub.org

Sonoma County Trails Council
http://sonomacountytrails.org

Tamalpais Conservation Club
www.tamalpais.org

Trail Center
www.trailcenter.org

Trails.com, Hikes with Dogs in Northern California
http://www.trails.com/activity.aspx?area=15271

National Weather Service
www.nws.noaa.gov

Weather.com
www.weather.com

Whole Access
www.wholeaccess.org

Wilderness Press
www.wildernesspress.com

Appendix 5

Useful Books

Bay Area Trail Guides

Heid, Matt. *Camping and Backpacking in the San Francisco Bay Area.* Berkeley: Wilderness Press, 2003.

Lage, Jessica. *Point Reyes.* Berkeley: Wilderness Press, 2004.

——. *Trail Runner's Guide: San Francisco Bay Area.* Berkeley: Wilderness Press, 2003.

Lorentzen, Robert. *The Hikers' Hip Pocket Guide to Sonoma County.* 2nd ed. Mendocino: Bored Feet Publications, 2008

Margolin, Malcolm. *The East Bay Out.* Revised ed. Berkeley: Heyday Books, 1988.

Martin, Don, and Kay Martin. *Hiking Marin.* San Anselmo: Martin Press, 1995.

——. *Mt. Tam.* San Anselmo: Martin Press, 1994.

——. *Point Reyes National Seashore.* 2nd ed. San Anselmo: Martin Press, 1997.

Rusmore, Jean. *The Bay Area Ridge Trail.* 3rd ed. Berkeley: Wilderness Press, 2008.

—— et al. *Peninsula Trails.* 4th ed. Berkeley: Wilderness Press, 2005.

—— et al. *South Bay Trails.* 3rd ed. Berkeley: Wilderness Press, 2001.

Spitz, Barry. *Open Spaces.* San Rafael: Marin County Open Space District, 2000.

——. *Tamalpais Trails.* 4th ed. San Anselmo: Potrero Meadow Publishing Co., 1998.

Stanton, Ken. *Great Day Hikes in and around Napa Valley.* Mendocino: Bored Feet Publications, 1997.

Wayburn, Peggy. *Adventuring in the San Francisco Bay Area.* Revised ed. San Francisco: Sierra Club Books, 1995.

Weintraub, David. *Afoot & Afield San Francisco Bay Area.* Berkeley: Wilderness Press, 2004.

——. *East Bay Trails.* Berkeley: Wilderness Press, 1998.

——. *North Bay Trails.* Berkeley: Wilderness Press, 1999.

——. *Peninsula Tales & Trails.* Portland, Ore.: Graphic Arts Books, 2004.

Bay Area History Books

Lavender, David. *California*. Lincoln: University of Nebraska Press, 1972.

Richards, Rand. *Historic San Francisco*. San Francisco: Heritage House Publishers, 1999.

Natural History Books

Alt, David, and Donald W. Hyndman. *Roadside Geology of Northern and Central California*. Missoula, Mont.: Mountain Press Publishing Company, 2000.

Barbour, Michael, et al. *Coast Redwood*. Los Olivos: Cachuma Press, 2001.

Burt, William H., and Richard P. Grossenheider. *A Field Guide to the Mammals, North America, North of Mexico*. 3rd ed. Boston: Houghton Mifflin Company, 1980.

Clark, Jeanne L. *California Wildlife Viewing Guide*. Helena, Mont.: Falcon Press, 1992.

Coffeen, Mary. *Central Coast Wildflowers*. San Luis Obispo: EZ Nature Books, 1996.

Faber, Phyllis M., and Robert F. Holland. *Common Riparian Plants of California*. Mill Valley, Calif.: Pickleweed Press, 1988.

Faber, Phyllis M. *Common Wetland Plants of Coastal California*. 2nd ed. Mill Valley, Calif.: Pickleweed Press, 1996.

Kozloff, Eugene N., and Linda H. Beidleman. *Plants of the San Francisco Bay Region*. Revised ed. Berkeley: University of California Press, 2003.

Lanner, Ronald M. *Conifers of California*. Los Olivos: Cachuma Press, 1999.

Little, Elbert L. *National Audubon Society Field Guide to North American Trees, Western Region*. New York: Alfred A. Knopf, 1994.

Lyons, Kathleen, and Mary Beth Cooney-Lazaneo. *Plants of the Coast Redwood Region*. Boulder Creek: Looking Press, 1988.

National Geographic Society. *Field Guide to the Birds of North America*. 4th ed. Washington, D.C.: National Geographic Society, 1999.

Niehaus, Theodore F., and Charles L. Ripper. *A Field Guide to Pacific States Wildflowers*. Boston: Houghton Mifflin Company, 1976.

Pavlik, Bruce M., et al. *Oaks of California*. Los Olivos: Cachuma Press, 1991.

Peterson, Roger T. *A Field Guide to Western Birds*. 3rd ed. Boston: Houghton Mifflin Company, 1990.

Schoenherr, Allan A. *A Natural History of California*. Berkeley: University of California Press, 1992.

Sibley, David Allen. *The Sibley Guide to Birds*. New York: Alfred A. Knopf, Inc., 2000.

Stebbins, Robert C. *A Field Guide to Western Reptiles and Amphibians*. 2nd ed. Boston: Houghton Mifflin Company, 1985.

Stuart, John D., and John O. Sawyer. *Trees and Shrubs of California*. Berkeley: University of California Press, 2001.

Appendix 6

Maps

Finding the Trails

The California State Automobile Association (CSAA) gives its members free road maps–our favorites are *San Francisco Bay* and *Monterey Bay* in CSAA's California Regional series. Thomas Guide's *Metropolitan Bay Area Street Guide and Directory* is a helpful driving atlas. Online map services such as Google Maps and MapQuest can also help you find the best routes to the parks.

Privately Published and Agency Maps

Park maps and brochures of all the trails in this guide would fill a large shoebox. Style, quality, and accuracy vary. A fair number of maps are drawn with full trail detail and elevation contours. Others are simple sketch maps, and for a few parks, no map is available. Agencies are increasingly augmenting printed maps with digital maps on their Web sites. Sources for maps are listed below, by chapter.

At parks with staffed entrance kiosks or visitor centers, ask there for maps. Visitor centers may also have maps for nearby parks. Other trailheads have map holders where you can pick up park brochures and maps. Also check the Web site of the agency administering the park or open space to see if downloadable maps are available.

North Bay Trail Maps

Privately Published Maps

The *Rambler's Guide to Mt. Tamalpais and the Marin Headlands* by Olmsted & Bros. Map Co. has long been the best overall map for the Marin Headlands, Muir Woods National Monument, Mt. Tamalpais, and Pine Mountain areas (Trails 1–5). Wilderness Press's map of *Point Reyes National Seashore and West Marin Parklands* extends east from Point Reyes to show Pine Mountain and Samuel P. Taylor State Park (Trails 5–7). Pease Press's map *Trails of Northeast Marin County* shows the area from China Camp State Park to Mt.

Burdell (Trails 8 and 9). A new series of maps by Tom Harrison Maps covers most of Marin in excellent detail, from the Golden Gate to Point Reyes and Mt. Burdell (Trails 1–9). 360Geographics publishes several excellent trail maps showing China Camp, Annadel, Jack London, and Sugarloaf state parks (Trails 8 and 11–13).

Agency Maps

The basic Golden Gate National Recreation Area (GGNRA) brochure includes a simple trail map of the Marin Headlands (Trail 1). The brochure for Muir Woods National Monument includes only a sketch trail map of the main coast redwood grove, but the park store sells an excellent map of Muir Woods National Monument published by Golden Gate National Parks Conservancy (Trail 2).

State park maps for the North Bay are problematic—typically they have been available only at entrance kiosks or visitor centers, which may be open only on weekends. Brochures and maps currently available on the Web site include Mt. Tamalpais, China Camp, and Annadel state parks (Trails 3, 4, 8, and 11). The old two-color map for Samuel P. Taylor State Park (Trail 6) should be taken with a grain of salt. There is no state park map for Robert Louis Stevenson State Park (Trail 2) and the entrance station at Sugarloaf Ridge State Park (Trail 13) provides only a simple sketch map.

Marin Municipal Water District has print and online trail maps that include the Pine Mountain area (Trail 5). You can get a map of Mt. Burdell Open Space Preserve (Trail 9) at Marin County Open Space District's Web site and by mail. A simple but accurate map of Skyline Wilderness Park is available at the entrance kiosk and from the Skyline Park Citizens Association Web site.

East Bay Trail Maps

Privately Published Maps

Olmsted's *Rambler's Guides to the Northern East Bay* and *Central East Bay* give a great overview of the Oakland Hills, showing Wildcat Ridge, Tilden, Sibley, Redwood, and Briones Regional Parks (Trails 15–19).

Save Mt. Diablo's excellent new map of *Mt. Diablo, Los Vaqueros, and Surrounding Parks* extends from Mt. Diablo State Park east to Black Diamond Mines and Morgan Territory regional preserves (Trails 20–22). Mt. Diablo Interpretive Association publishes a smaller map focused solely on Mt. Diablo State Park (Trail 21).

Agency Maps

East Bay Regional Park District has excellent trail maps at trailheads, by mail, and from its Web site. A basic trail map of Mt. Diablo State Park is available at the state park Web site and (when staffed) at ranger stations.

South Bay Trail Maps

Privately Published Maps

The Pine Ridge Association publishes the excellent *Trail and Camping Map of Henry W. Coe State Park* (Trail 30), which can be purchased at the park's visitor center. The visitor center also has free handouts describing hikes of varying lengths.

Agency Maps

Santa Clara County Parks has printed maps at its trailheads and PDF maps on its Web site; these are also available by mail (Trails 28, 29, and 31). Midpeninsula Regional Open Space District maps are available at its trailheads, by mail, and as PDFs from its Web site (Trails 32 and 33).

Peninsula Trail Maps

Privately Published Maps

The most detailed maps of the parks and preserves from Monte Bello Ridge north to Kings Mountain are the Trail Center's *Trail Map of the Southern Peninsula* (Trails 34–38, distributed by Wilderness Press) and Wilderness Press's *Central San Francisco Peninsula Trails* (Trails 39–41, with data provided by the Trail Center). Pease Press's *Trails of the Coastside* map includes Montara Mountain and San Bruno Mountain (Trails 42 and 43).

Agency Maps

Midpeninsula Regional Open Space District maps are available at its trailheads, by mail, and from its Web site (Trails 34–40). Maps for San Mateo County Parks are also available at entrance stations, by mail, and from its Web site (Trails 41, 42, and 43). Maps for GGNRA's Phleger Estate (Trail 41) and the Presidio (Trail 44) are available at the Presidio's visitor centers and from the GGNRA Web site.

USGS Topographic Maps

The US Geological Survey's topographic quadrangles are great, general-purpose maps showing roads, streams, tree cover, and elevation contours. The 7.5 minute, 1:24,000 scale series are best for hiking. They usually show major trails and dirt roads, but trails and public land boundaries can be incomplete or outdated. You may find that the privately-published trail maps and the agency maps listed above are more useful on the trail (many of them are based on USGS maps).

Although few outdoor retailers now carry printed USGS maps, you can purchase maps for the entire western US at the USGS's Western Regional Office in Menlo Park, now jointly operated by the California Geological Survey (open weekdays, 10 A.M.–4 P.M.). Several online retailers including Map Link also sell printed USGS maps by mail.

Using TOPO!, a computer program from National Geographic Maps, you can view and print USGS maps from a CD-ROM on your computer. Using a slightly awkward interface, you can also draw routes, insert labels, measure distance, plot elevation gain and loss, and locate landmarks. If you have a GPS unit you can load waypoints from a TOPO! map into your GPS (so you can find them in the field), and also take waypoints stored in your GPS during a hike and plot them in TOPO!

Another alternative is to view and print USGS maps over the Internet, either via members-only services such as Trails.com, or for free at Acme Mapper (as seamless maps) and the Internet Archive (as scanned quadrangles). See below for complete Web addresses.

Useful Map Web Sites

The following Web sites will help you find the maps mentioned in this appendix, as well as several others that you might find useful:

- **360Geographics:** www.360geographics.com/360maps
- **Acme Mapper:** http://mapper.acme.com
- **Internet Archive:** www.archive.org/details/maps_usgs
- **Map Link Map Distributors:** www.maplink.com
- **Pease Press:** www.peasepress.com
- **Tom Harrison Maps:** www.tomharrisonmaps.com
- **TOPO! Software:** http://maps.nationalgeographic.com/topo
- **Trails.com:** www.trails.com
- **USGS Western Region/California Geological Survey Map and Publication Sales:** http://online.wr.usgs.gov and www.conservation.ca.gov/cgs

Index

Authors

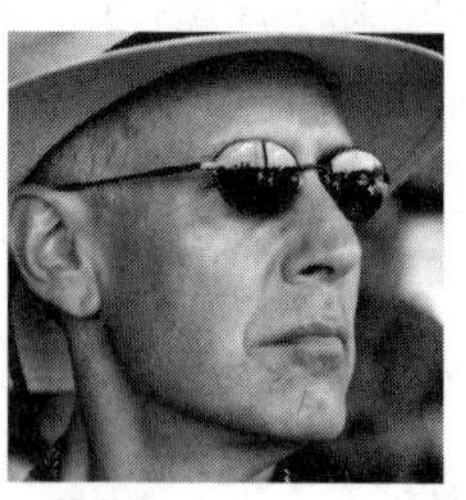

David Weintraub

David Weintraub is an educator, writer, editor, and photographer based in South Carolina and Cape Cod. A former long-time San Francisco resident, he has authored a number of books for Wilderness Press, including *East Bay Trails, North Bay Trails, Monterey Bay Trails*, and *Adventure Kayaking: Cape Cod and Martha's Vineyard.*

In 2004, Wilderness Press published David's *Afoot & Afield San Francisco Bay Area*, a comprehensive guide to hiking routes in the North Bay, East Bay, and South Bay and on the Peninsula.

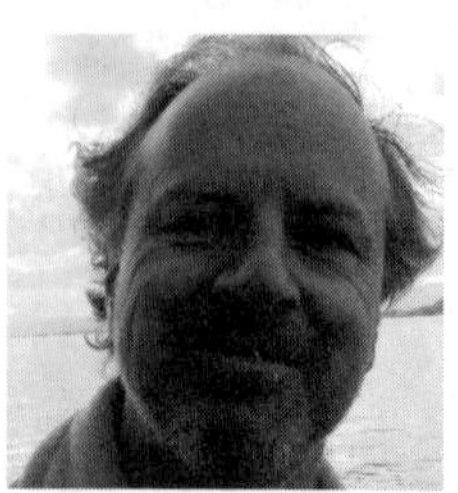

Ben Pease

Ben Pease is a cartographer and trail advocate based in San Francisco. He has explored Bay Area parks and trails for more than 30 years. Ben has created countless maps for Wilderness Press books, and he publishes a series of Pease Press trail maps, which champion lesser-known Bay Area parks.

Series Creator

Joe Walowski

Joe Walowski conceived of the Top Trails series in 2003, and was series editor of the first three titles: *Top Trails Los Angeles, Top Trails San Francisco Bay Area*, and *Top Trails Lake Tahoe*. He currently lives in Seattle.